AREA OF SPEECH PATHOLOGY-AUDIOLOGY
DEPARTMENT OF SPEECH AND DRAMATIC ART
UNIVERSITY OF MISSOURI-COLUMBIA
COLUMBIA, MISSOURI 65201

SO-EBA-339

CLEFT PALATE: A MULTIDISCIPLINE APPROACH

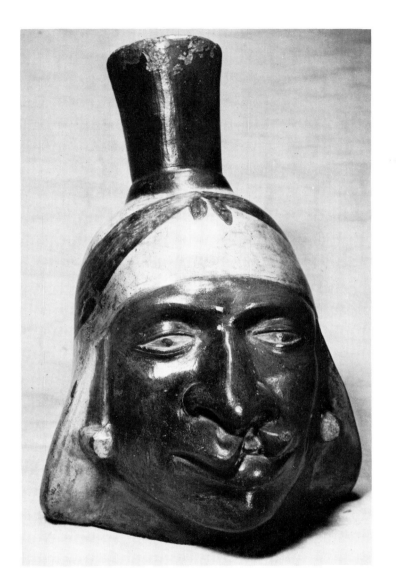

RELIC OF INCAS OF THE ANDES
Ceramic huaco
depicting unilateral complete cleft of the primary palate.
(Courtesy Ernesto Ferreyros, Lima, Peru.)

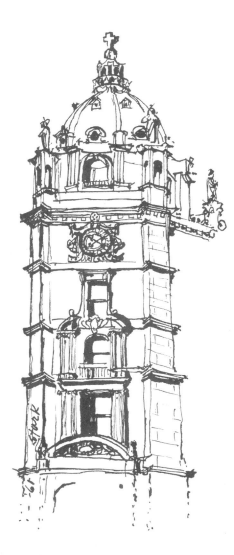

With Chapters by
Members of the
St. Luke's
Cleft Palate Clinic,
St. Luke's Hospital Center,
New York City

With 302 Illustrations

CLEFT PALATE

A MULTIDISCIPLINE APPROACH

By 19 Authors

Edited by   RICHARD B. STARK, M.D., F.A.C.S.

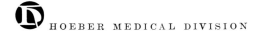

HOEBER MEDICAL DIVISION

HARPER & ROW, PUBLISHERS · NEW YORK, EVANSTON, AND LONDON

To
ROBERT ABBE
(*1851–1928*)
Inquisitive and inventive
St. Luke's surgeon,
founder of radium therapy in America,
creative artist,
humanist, and gentleman
this book is dedicated

CLEFT PALATE: A MULTIDISCIPLINE APPROACH

Copyright © 1968 by HOEBER MEDICAL DIVISION
HARPER & ROW, PUBLISHERS, INCORPORATED
Printed in the United States of America

All rights reserved · For information address
HOEBER MEDICAL DIVISION · HARPER & ROW, PUBLISHERS
49 East 33rd Street, New York, N.Y. 10016

Library of Congress catalog card number: 67-29727

CONTENTS

LIST OF AUTHORS

WILLIAM H. CANFIELD, ED.D.
  Consultant, Hearing and Speech Department, St. Luke's Hospital
  Center, New York City; Associate Professor of Speech Pathology and
  Audiology, Adelphi University, Garden City, New York

ANTHONY S. CARUSO, D.D.S.
  Attending Dental Surgeon, St. Luke's Hospital Center; Instructor in
  Prosthesis, Post-Graduate Division, New York University School of
  Dentistry, New York City

CLAYTON R. DEHAAN, M.D.
  Associate Attending Surgeon, St. Luke's Hospital Center; Instructor in
  Surgery, College of Physicians and Surgeons, Columbia University,
  New York City

ENNIO GALLOZZI, M.D.
  Associate Attending Anesthesiologist, St. Luke's Hospital Center,
  New York City

MARGIE DE FOREST HAIGHT, A.A.
  Research Associate in Plastic Surgery, St. Luke's Hospital Center, New
  York City

DESMOND A. KERNAHAN, M.B., F.R.C.S.(C.)
  Associate Professor and Chief, Department of Plastic Surgery, University of Manitoba, Winnipeg, Manitoba, Canada

NORMAN N. OSTROV, M.D.
  Attending Otolaryngologist, New York Polyclinic Hospital; Attending
  Otolaryngologist, St. Luke's Hospital Center, New York City

ANN M. RICHARDS, R.N.
  Formerly Charge Nurse, Pediatric Nursery, St. Luke's Hospital
  Center, New York City

MARGARET ROUILLION, M.S.W.
  Director, Social Service Department, St. Luke's Hospital Center, New
  York City

DAVID E. SAUNDERS, M.D.
  Attending Surgeon, Wilmington Medical Center; Consultant, Alfred
  I. duPont Crippled Children Institute, Wilmington, Delaware

EDWARD G. STANLEY-BROWN, M.D.
> Associate Attending Surgeon in Charge of Pediatric Surgery, St. Luke's Hospital Center; Assistant Clinical Professor of Surgery, College of Physicians and Surgeons, Columbia University, New York City

RICHARD B. STARK, M.D., F.A.C.S.
> Attending Surgeon in charge of Plastic Surgery, and Director, Cleft Palate Clinic, St. Luke's Hospital Center; Associate Clinical Professor of Surgery, College of Physicians and Surgeons, Columbia University, New York City

STUART SHELTON STEVENSON, M.D.
> Director of Pediatrics, St. Luke's Hospital Center; Clinical Professor of Pediatrics, College of Physicians and Surgeons, Columbia University, New York City

EDWARD STROH, JR., D.D.S., F.A.C.D.
> Director of Dentistry, St. Luke's Hospital Center; Director of Oral Surgery, Metropolitan Hospital Center, New York City

E. CLINTON VOLLMER, D.D.S.
> Instructor in Dentistry, Department of Orthodontics, Columbia University, College of Dental and Oral Surgery; Assistant Attending Dental Surgeon, Department of Orthodontics, St. Luke's Hospital Center, New York City

HIROSHI WASHIO, M.D.
> Associate Plastic Surgeon, Tokyo Metropolitan Police Hospital, Tokyo, Japan

R. C. A. WEATHERLEY-WHITE, M.D.
> Instructor in Surgery, University of Colorado School of Medicine, Denver

STANLEY WHITFIELD, M.D.
> Attending Surgeon and Director of the Department of Otolaryngology, St. Luke's Hospital Center; Assistant Otolaryngologist, Presbyterian Hospital; Associate Clinical Professor of Otolaryngology, College of Physicians and Surgeons, Columbia University, New York City

JANE DORSEY ZIMMERMAN, PH.D.
> Professor Emeritus of Speech, Teachers College, Columbia University, New York City; Adjunct Professor of Speech, Adelphi University, Garden City, New York; Director, Speech and Hearing Department, St. Barnabas Hospital, Bronx, New York; Consultant, Speech and Hearing Department, St. Luke's Hospital Center, New York City

PREFACE

Approximately 1 child in 1,000 is born with a cleft of the lip, of the palate, or of both structures. His disfigurement not only has a profound emotional effect on his family, but seriously compromises his own physical and psychological well-being. For example, since the cleft impares sucking, the infant cannot be fed in the usual way. On swallowing, the child often expels food through his nostrils. The chilling and drying effect of the air flow through the cleft causes a seemingly continuous sore throat, and if the infection ascends to the middle ear, otitis media and possibly mastoiditis may permanently impair hearing. Teeth may erupt in an abnormal arrangement and malocclusion may be severe. Speech is often unintelligible, provoking cruel taunts and mimicry from playmates. The psychological effect of an obvious facial cleft may be devastating.

Surgical procedures for the repair of facial clefts have long been available, but only in the last two decades have special cleft palate clinics been established offering multidisciplinary services which coordinate specific treatment with the child's needs at various stages of his growth and development. The St. Luke's Cleft Palate Clinic was formed in 1956. It offers the services of plastic surgeon, pediatrician, dentist, oral surgeon, orthodontist, prosthodontist, social worker, speech pathologist, anesthesiologist, otolaryngologist, audiologist, psychologist, psychiatrist, nurse and researcher in a coordinated individualized treatment program designed to achieve the best possible results in the shortest possible time with the least possible trauma to the child.

This book presents a multidisciplinary approach to the management of facial clefts. Its authors are staff members of the services which make up the St. Luke's Cleft

Palate Clinic. Its purpose is to detail newer surgical and ancillary procedures used in the treatment of the cleft palate child; to narrate older procedures that might profitably undergo a renaissance; to stress the value of a coordinated treatment plan involving many people and disciplines; to illustrate the operation of one cleft palate clinic; to indicate the worth of objective speech evaluation; to plead for a standard classification of facial cleft anomalies; and to encourage continued research into factors producing congenital defects.

No book is a solo effort, least of all this one. I am indebted to all the writers who have cooperated so fully in this venture. But there are many others who have labored to make our Cleft Palate Clinic a reality and who must be thanked publicly: Louis S. Blancato, M.D., Edgar L. Buehler, D.D.S., Paul Burgess, M.A., John M. Cotton, M.D., James C. Kirkbright, M.D., Constance Lamb, M.S., Mary Marcellus, M.A., Diane Meyers, M.A., Sylvia Rivera, M.A., Frances Schacter, Ph.D., Thomas C. Sumners, M.D., and Stanley Frileck, M.D.

The illustrations, the result of the artistry of Leonard Dank, speak for themselves. For the photography, I am indebted to Mr. George Tannis and Mr. Thomas Wood. Miss Elma Wadsworth has been of invaluable editorial help. Miss Margary Woodworth has cheerfully typed and retyped the material too many times to mention. She has been helped by Mrs. Helen Jacoby and Miss Mary Mason. Sam Broque has checked the bibliography. A grant from the National Institutes of Health has helped in part to support this project financially.

RICHARD B. STARK, M.D.

New York City

CHAPTER 1

History of
Cleft Lip
Surgery

HIROSHI WASHIO

Although Velpeau alluded to Celsus' treatment of harelip, Franco (?1505–1579) and Paré (1510–1590) were the first to describe in detail the principles and techniques involved in surgical treatment of cleft lip. Thereafter, Paré's twisted sutures (Fig. 1-1) became popular. Paré wrote:

> This kind of suture is used in the wounds of the lips, as also in hare-lips, for so we commonly call lips which are cleft from the first conformation in the wombe by the error of the forming faculty.
>
> But such a suture will help nothing to agglutination, if there lye or remain any skin between the lips of the wound; wherefore you shall cut away whatsoever thereof shall be there, otherwise you must expect no union. Other kinds of sutures are of no great use in wounds of these parts, for out of necessity of eating and speaking, they are in perpetual motion; wherefore a third would cut the flesh; for which reason you shall take up much flesh with such needle mentioned in this last described kind of suture.

Franco (1556) stated that two or three of the through-and-through needles could be used if expedient.

Tagliacozzi (1597) described the repair of the congenitally cleft lip:

> It is Art's task to excoriate the parts, and keep them close together, that they may unite in their Blood, to sew them when united, to keep them sewed, and to reduce them to a right temper and health. Let the Artist therefore take up that part of the Lip, which must be excoriated, in his Left Hand, and then take off the Skin equally with a very short Knife, till the Blood comes, to the very Angle of the

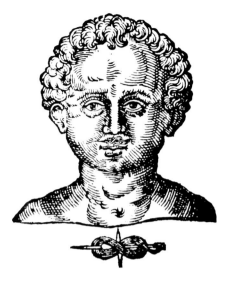

FIG. 1-1 *Paré's (1634) repair of "hare-lip." He pared the margins of the cleft, inserted a needle through-and-through the lip substance, then held it immobile by twisting the suture into a figure-of-eight.*

Hiatus, and then he must smooth the Wound. This Operation may also be performed very quickly and safely with a pair of Scissars. The same must be done on the other side. Then he must draw the parts together with his Hand, and stitch them. We must observe this, not to take our stitches superficially, but thorow all. The Artist must therefore pass his Needle streight through the Lip from the outside inwards, and on the other side he must pass the Needle from the inside outwards. He must tie the threads and fasten the ends, and then cut them off. He must take his stitches not too near the edges of the Wound, but at a good distance, lest the hold should break.

Velpeau (1838), who marks the end of the first period in cleft lip repair, summarized the following principles: "To effect cure these indications are to be fulfilled: Its borders are to be abraded, its two sides approximated and the two lips of the division maintained in perfect contact until they have become agglutinated." Many other great surgeons of that period sought better methods of attaining these basic principles.

The second period, which began with Malgaigne and Mirault (1844) and ended with Blair and Brown (1930), was characterized by remarkable strides in all branches of surgery. In cleft lip surgery, for example, the new concept of developing flaps led to a variety of designs. Other advances were the inception of anesthesia, improved antisepsis and asepsis, the technique of interrupted sutures, and better suture material and instruments.

This period ushered in all the classic incisions for lip repair. Even more important, individual surgeons began to realize that good results depended upon refinements of technique rather than a single and particular type of repair.

Blair and Brown wrote in 1930:

> If he learns to use any one of the standard methods, the surgeon who essays the correction of nose and lip defects will expend his energy to greater profit than if he attempts to exercise eclecticism, or, more dangerous yet, to contrive new methods. It is true that operative skill rather than breadth of acquaintance will bring greater satisfaction to the patient thus afflicted.

In the third period of cleft lip surgery, which extends to the present day, LeMesurier became an outstanding pioneer who shed new light on the classic Hagedorn methods (1884, 1892) with dramatic results in 1949. The desire for a repair that would give fullness to the upper lip and achieve a cupid's bow as well as nostril symmetry, was soon reflected in new techniques by Steffensen, Tennison, and Millard, whose work marked the beginning of a golden era in cleft lip surgery.

REPAIR OF UNILATERAL CLEFT LIP

The First Period

Many surgeons of the eighteenth century delayed repair of unilateral cleft lip until the child reached the age of 4 or 5 years on grounds that a young infant's crying and agitation led to violent movements conducive to convulsions; that the child would be terrorized by the mere sight of a surgeon; that emaciation from several days on a rigid diet would result in flabby cheeks and therefore relaxation of the sutures; and that fragility and lack of resistance of the tissues would disrupt the sutures on even slight traction.

Of contrary opinion were Busch, Roonhuysen, La Drau, and Heister, who claimed that crying and movement could be controlled. Interrupting the infant's sleep for several days preoperatively and administering an opium preparation shortly before surgery were calming measures that would result in sleep immediately after the procedure. They considered an infant easier to restrain than a child of 4 or 5 years; felt that his incisions healed faster and better; and that early correction of the deformity fostered good physical and mental development. Heister, in 1739, wrote:

> It has been an opinion of the ancients that it is not safe to perform the operation for a harelip upon infants before they are two years of

age or even four or five, the contrary of which is taught by experience, from whence we are furnished with instances of infants happily cured of a harelip, when they have not been above five or six months old, if they are well in other respects, and the operation rightly performed.

Despite the lack of anesthesia, the design of surgery was based upon many ingenious and progressive ideas. It was already well established that removal of tissue along the cleft margin was essential to successful repair. Excision of tissue with a hot iron, caustics, or blister plaster—common in the seventeenth century—gradually gave way to the more exact method of excision with sharp instruments. According to Velpeau, Celsus had used this method in the first century. Thick-bladed scissors with a large handle were preferred during the eighteenth and early nineteenth centuries. It was felt that the tissue could be excised instantly without prolonging pain, leaving a straight, smooth wound.

In the eighteenth century, the bistoury or knife was used sporadically. Velpeau credits Severin and Aerel with early use of this instrument, while Louis was another strong proponent. Indeed, the bistoury made possible the flap techniques of closure introduced in the nineteenth century. The bistoury was believed to reduce pain and produce a neater wound margin with little tendency to suppurate. Incision by scissors, relying more on compression than sawing, caused contusion of the tissues; the wound was beveled and thus unfavorable for primary union. An exponent of the scissors. Velpeau erroneously stated that these objections were without foundation.

To approximate the wound margins and to hold them in close contact. Franco used only adhesive strips across the upper lip. The most common method in the eighteenth century was the figure-of-eight suture around a perforating needle, as described by Paré. Heister (1739), a strong advocate of this method, mentioned the earlier use of interrupted suture by "German quacks." Louis, who used adhesive plaster and a supportive bandage, said that good surgeons never used interrupted sutures. His theory was that the fissure was created by muscle traction of the cheeks, and that the cleft margins could be easily united by mobilizing the cheeks medially.

Velpeau suggested that more pins or finer needles would achieve better union of the wound. Needles were usually removed after 3 or 4 days, and the sutures and supportive bandage remained in place until the latter came off by itself. Franco suggested the innovation of freeing the lip from the alveolus to decrease wound tension.

It was generally agreed that good postoperative care included bed rest, restriction of talking, and a diet of broth, milk, emulsions, and water for 3 or 4 days, after which solid foods were gradually added.

The Second Period

In January 1844, Malgaigne described his new "deux lambeaux" technique of lip repair (Fig. 1-2). Roux informed him that Clemot, a surgeon of Rochefort, had developed a similar procedure but had never published it. Since then, it became known as the Clemot-Malgaigne method.

Malgaigne, whose contribution cannot be overemphasized, wrote in 1843: "I came to the conclusion that with all the surgical skill available, we could only transform the severe case of cleft lip to its mildest form. It is virtually impossible to remove the notch of the vermilion." The "inevitable notch" became his prime target. In the "deux lambeaux" procedure, an incision starting at the base of the nostril was carried downward along the cleft edge to within a few millimeters of the vermilion border. A horizontal incision was then made into the lip substance on either side which lengthened the lip as it opened into a V. The released soft tissue was pulled downward, and the raw margins approximated. The lip thus was lengthened on the cleft side.

Shortcomings included the production of a tubercle of the vermilion instead of a notch, which placed the longest point of the lip lateral to the midline, and interruption of the natural and continuous mucocutaneous junction. However, the two-flap method gave better results than straight-line closures had previously. Above all, Malgaigne introduced the concept of shifting and rotating tissues from a site of abundance to a site of paucity. The procedure won many followers in the next 50 years, although Malgaigne's originality was further questioned by Mason in 1877:

> It appears that this operation was, as M. Roux states, previously performed by Clemot, but Dr. Maurice Colles of Dublin, writing in

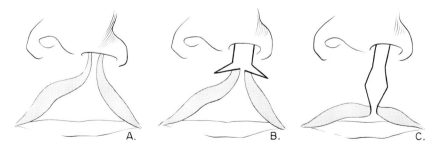

FIG. 1-2 *In 1844, Malgaigne described his two-flap technique to avoid the omnipresent postoperative notch. By means of horizontal incisions upon either side, the lip was lengthened, since the incisions opened as a V. This is the principle of the pantograph.*

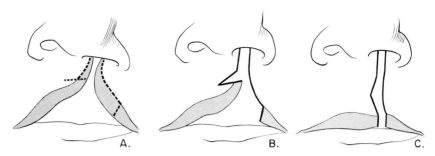

FIG. 1-3 *Mirault (1844) removed one of the two flaps described by Malgaigne, thus avoiding the formation of an unnatural eccentric vermilion tubercle. At the same time Mirault added tissue above the vermilion to afford pout to the profile.*

1868, claimed it as the device of an English surgeon. He says: "I learnt it twenty-one years ago from a fine old English surgeon, the late Samuel Smith of Leeds. He told me that he had devised it some twenty or thirty years previously (about 1820).

Because of his clear description, however, Malgaigne rightly deserves credit for the two-flap method. Several months after his report appeared in 1844, Mirault wrote to Malgaigne suggesting a minor modification of the method: removal of one of the two flaps with an oblique incision, affording an adequate raw surface to accommodate the other flap (Fig. 1-3). This represented an improvement in that less extensive advancement of the flaps prevented the unnatural formation of a unilateral vermilion tubercle, but its merit was not fully appreciated at that time. Mirault did not specify which side of the cleft should yield the flap. Lack of illustrations in his description of his own original method led to various interpretations of how it was performed.

The illustration of Mirault's operation which appeared in the first work of Blair and Brown in 1930, *Mirault Operations*, was taken from H. H. Smith's *A System of Operative Surgery*, published in 1852. Smith, in turn, had reproduced from a surgical text by Bernard and Huette (1846). However, in 1871 Mirault presented a modified method with his own drawing, featuring a rectangular flap in the vermilion.

The original Mirault operation was later modified by other surgeons, among them Colles of Dublin, who wrote in 1868: "I never throw away a particle of the parings. My incisions are made so as to make every fragment of them useful. On one side they are preserved to make the thick lip, and on the other side to increase its depth."

Furthermore, Colles rotated one small flap upward into the

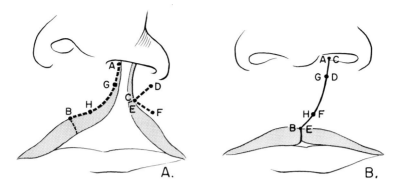

FIG. 1-4 *Colles (1868) of Dublin modified Mirault's procedure by adding tissue below the nostril as well as above the vermilion.*

floor of the nostril, while the other produced fullness above the muco-cutaneous junction, imparting a pouting profile (Fig. 1-4).

Jalaguier (1880) applied Mirault's method, forming the triangular flap from the medial or uncleft side (Fig. 1-5). In 1890 Edmund Owens described his modification, predicated upon rotating a large triangular flap and using vermilion from the medial side of the cleft to create the major portion of the vermilion of the upper lip (Fig. 1-6). Although Berry and Legg reported their modification of the Mirault operation in 1912, its greatest refinement came about later through the efforts of Blair and Brown.

The Malgaigne and Mirault procedures both were popular during the last half of the nineteenth century, and their respective merits were widely discussed by the profession.

In 1868 Prince wrote: "The proceeding of Malgaigne is better than leaving the flap of prolabium [vermilion] all on one side, and paring off the prolabium on the other to receive it, as in Mirault tech-

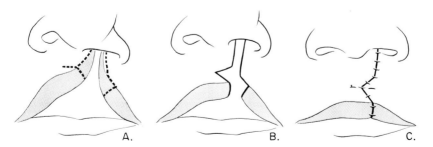

FIG. 1-5 *Jalaguier (1880) staggered the lateral incision on the cleft side, but added a triangular flap above the vermilion from the medial or uncleft side.*

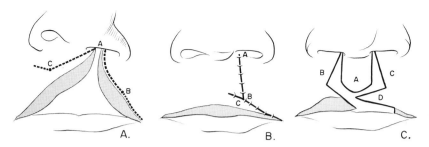

FIG. 1-6 *Owens (1890) used a large triangular flap from the medial side,*
A and B, thus affording virtually all the vermilion of the upper lip. The
same method adapted to bilateral cleft lip is shown in C.

nique." He advised the use of wire sutures (which should not be removed early) and, in some cases, a combination of sutures and pins.

Concerning wound closure, Heister had relegated interrupted
sutures to the realm of quacks. Thus the twisted suture method, employing a pin and figure-of-eight suture, proved popular up to the late
nineteenth century.

Before antisepsis and asepsis, pins and needles caused relatively
little suppuration of the wound. Interrupted sutures may have been
condemned because of their susceptibility to infection. Postoperative
splinting of the wound varied as well. The amount of tissue fixed between figure-of-eight sutures wrapped around the pin afforded more
stability to the incision than interrupted sutures, which therefore
required firmer external splinting.

With gradual improvement in splinting devices and reduction
in wound tension through surgical undermining of adjacent tissues
(Franco, 1561; Owen, 1890; Rose, 1891; Berry and Legg, 1912), the
twisted suture became replaced by interrupted sutures.

Certainly, the development of anesthesia (ether by Long in
1842, and cocaine by Koller in 1884) and Lister's concept of asepsis
(1867) contributed largely to the changes in surgical technique that
transpired late in the nineteenth century.

To obviate the shortcoming in Malgaigne's procedure—failure
of the longest portion of the lip to fall in the midline—König, in 1881,
devised a new technique (Fig. 1-7). Since there are two points in
unilateral cleft lip and three points in bilateral cleft lip where three
incisions meet in a T-shape, the high incidence of failure in wound
healing (33 per cent) with this method is not surprising.

It should be noted that in bilateral cleft lip, flaps lateral to the
clefts were added beneath the prolabium to increase its length,
whereas in the older methods the prolabium formed the entire central
portion of the lip (Paré, Heister, Desault). Only recently have sur-

geons recognized that adding tissue beneath the prolabium inevitably produces an overly long lip.

In 1884, Hagedorn suggested a unique operation (Fig. 1-8) which is historically important because it formed the basis of LeMesurier's operation and hence of most modern methods of cleft lip repair.

Rose (1891) attempted to avoid contraction with notching of the straight-line closure; he made the closure longer by opposing concave incisions on either side of the cleft. To shape the naris, he dissected the alar base from the maxilla.

Most of these complicated lip operations were possible only after the development of anesthesia. Both ether and chloroform were widely used late in the past century.

Although numerous cheiloplasties have been introduced since Malgaigne and Mirault published their work over 100 years ago, the Mirault repair has persisted. Surgeons have begun to realize that understanding the problems involved and developing technical skill, not any particular procedure, have produced these increasingly good results.

Berry and Legg (1912), in modifying the Mirault operation, recommended correction of the alar deformity of the cleft side and

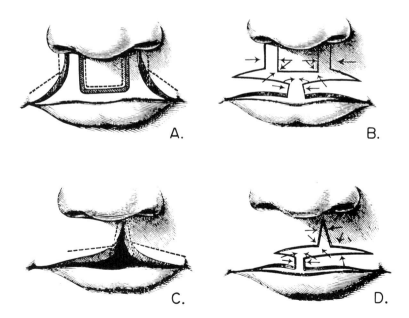

A.

B.

C.

D.

FIG. 1-7 *König (1881) devised what in essence was a quadrilateral flap technique. In the bilaterally cleft lip he erred in placing lip tissue beneath the prolabium, which foredooms the lip to excessive length due to growth.*

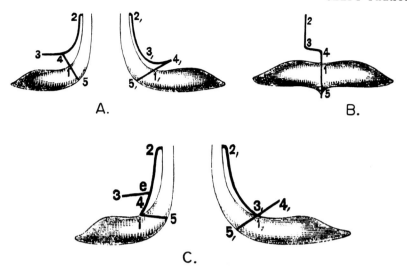

FIG. 1-8 *Hagedorn (1884) suggested the procedure which has formed the basis for LeMesurier's operation. C indicates later modification.*

wide undermining of the alar base. Blair and Brown, initially unmindful of Mirault's work, perfected this type of repair. They further emphasized correction of the nasal deformity and made great strides in cleft lip surgery. Their procedure is shown in Figure 1-9. These two master surgeons, who established the worth of Mirault's triangular flap method, issued a warning to others:

> Before adopting the more complex methods, the operator should make himself familiar with every detail of the operation and should

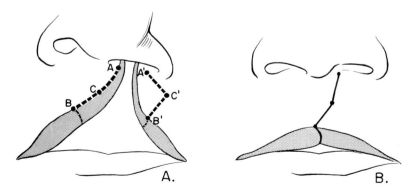

FIG. 1-9 *Schematic drawing of the Blair and Brown procedure, not unlike the principle of Mirault.*

understand the logic for doing it. As the operator acquires more skill he may feel justified in adopting a method that in earlier days he considered less feasible, but each modification will be like changing a golf stroke . . . not always free from immediate grief.

The Modern Period

The modern era of cleft lip surgery dates from 1949 when LeMesurier reported his cheiloplasty procedure based upon Hagedorn's method (1884). Photographs of a number of his patients have shown consistently good results. His reappraisal of the earlier procedure was received enthusiastically, and many plastic surgeons soon proposed modifications of the Hagedorn-LeMesurier technique. The LeMesurier and the original Hagedorn operations are shown in Figure 1-10. A quadrangular flap is taken from the cleft side and inserted into the normal medial side. Thus, LeMesurier was the first to attempt construction of the cupid's bow of the vermilion (Fig. 1-11). The shaded area on the uncleft medial side was rotated 90° to receive a rectangular flap from the cleft side. But as the vermilion of the unoperated lip does not have 90° torsion, overcorrection resulted.

Steffensen (1949) and Brauer (1953) excised a triangular segment of lip tissue above the mucocutaneous line to effect a more natural vermilion and cupid's bow. Their procedure, with LeMesurier's, appears in Figure 1-12.

With widespread adoption of the Hagedorn-LeMesurier operation, results of cleft lip surgery improved. But with the passage of time two distinct disadvantages of LeMesurier's technique became evident: (1) the scar in the midline of the upper lip is unnatural and therefore noticeable; (2) as the child grows, the lip on the cleft side becomes longer than on the normal side.

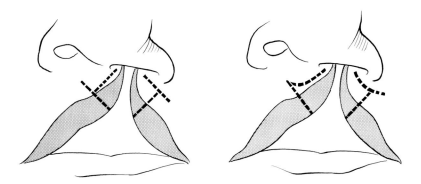

FIG. 1-10 *The LeMesurier (left) and the original Hagedorn (right) operations.*

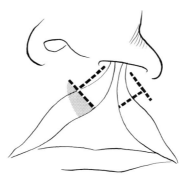

FIG. 1-11 *The shaded area on the uncleft medial side is rotated 90° in the LeMesurier operation, producing overcorrection.*

Tennison (1952) simplified LeMesurier's method, correcting one of its shortcomings while retaining all its advantages (Fig. 1-13). He measured the space from A to X (X equals height of the cupid's bow on the normal side) and divided it by 3. Each unit (AB, BC, CD) equals $AX/3$. A piece of wire the exact length of AX was then bent into a Z shape, with all limbs equal to $AX/3$, and used as a stencil. This triangular flap method was later modified by Skoog (1958) and Randall (1959).

Brauer, in 1959, concluded that Tennison's method is superior to LeMesurier's for repair of unilateral primary clefts for the following reasons: (1) it saves valuable tissue on the normal side of the cleft to form part of the cupid's bow for the cleft side, whereas this tissue is sacrificed by the LeMesurier operation; (2) it relieves vertical shortness of the lip on the cleft side in the body of the lip, rather

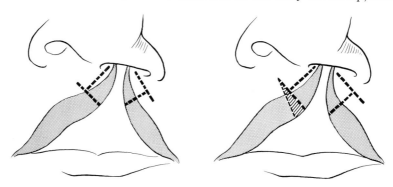

FIG. 1-12 *Steffensen (1949) and Brauer (1953) excised a triangular segment of lip tissue above the mucocutaneous line to produce a more natural vermilion and cupid's bow. Their modification (right) is shown vis-à-vis LeMesurier's.*

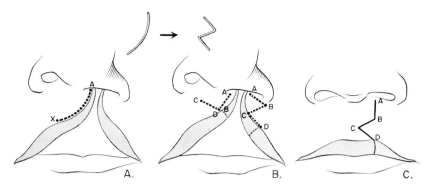

FIG. 1-13 *Tennison (1952) inserted a triangular flap from the cleft to the uncleft side, thus avoiding overcorrection. His method of marking out the proposed incisions, too, was an advance. He took a No. 30 steel wire and cut a length from A (base of the columella) to X (the peak of the cupid's bow upon the normal side). This he bent into the shape of a Z with all limbs of equal length. The stencil is placed upon the cleft side with one end of the Z where the ala meets the lip and the other end where the vermilion begins to thin. The lower limb of the Z is parallel to the vermilion. The wire stencil is shifted to the uncleft side. One end of the Z is at the columellar base, while the adjoining limb of the Z is parallel to the vermilion. The middle bar of the Z is approximately perpendicular to the vermilion. The lower limb is not used in the marking upon this side.*

than merely in the lower third; (3) the scar falls laterally, where it is far less noticeable than is a central scar which distorts the cupid's bow and displaces it laterally.

In 1958 Millard introduced the rotation advancement technique in cleft lip surgery. One of its major advantages is positioning the incision where it simulates the philtral ridge on the cleft side (Fig. 1-14). Long-term results of the Millard operation are eagerly awaited.

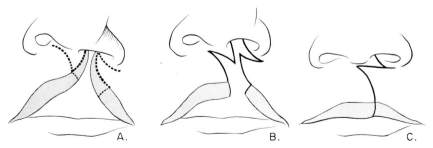

FIG. 1-14 *Millard (1958) introduced the principle of the rotational flap into the repair of the cleft lip. The suture line simulates the philtral ridge, one distinct advantage of the procedure. In addition, the interdigitation of flaps in the upper third of the repair has the dual advantage of elevating the columellar base and advancing the alar base medially.*

REPAIR OF BILATERAL COMPLETE CLEFT LIP WITH PROTRUDING PREMAXILLA

Unfortunately, there has been no such steady advance in repair of bilateral cleft lip as of unilateral, although important contributions have been made throughout the centuries.

Franco advocated complete excision of the prolabium and the premaxilla to facilitate lip repair in the midline, but most surgeons were more conservative, using the prolabium to form the central portion of the lip. Desault (1790) devised the technique shown in Figure 1-15.

A long controversy has revolved around repair of both clefts at the same operation or repair of the second cleft after healing of the first side. Desault, who repaired both at once, applied a compressive bandage over the projecting premaxilla for 11 days preoperatively to exert steady backward pressure and thus facilitate wound healing.

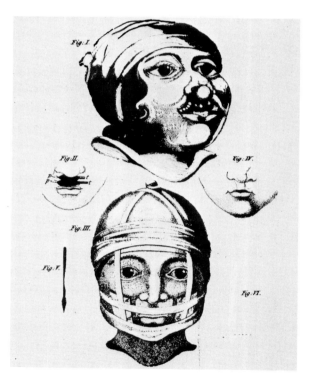

FIG. 1-15 *Desault (1790) advocated the preoperative backward compression of the protruding premaxilla in bilateral cleft lip, a forerunner of modern maxillary orthopedics. He eschewed removal of this intermaxillary structure for the sake of simplicity of closure. In addition, he closed both sides in a single operation.*

One of Desault's cases was a healthy 5-year-old girl, hospitalized on September 7, 1790, for correction of a bilateral complete cleft of the lip and palate. Chorin, a junior surgeon, described the preoperative bandage as follows:

> In order to bring the protuberance to a level with the lip, and to depress the projecting portion of the maxillary bones, M. Desault, who as the principal surgeon of the Hôtel Dieu, undertook the treatment of the case, had recourse to a linen bandage, which passed over the upper lip and was fixed at the back part of the neck. The good effects of this bandage in compressing the parts in question were so obvious, that its use was continued till the 18th day of September when the operation was performed.

Chorin strongly objected to excision of the prolabium or premaxilla, especially since the intermaxillary segment could be readily reduced to the level of the lateral lip elements by a compressive bandage. He also recognized that such excision resulted in a tight upper lip, a dish-face deformity, and relative prognathism:

> It can hardly fail to occasion inflammation of the neighboring parts; it will leave a considerable space between the maxillary bones; it will deprive the lip of its point of support at the place where it is divided; and if the reunion takes place, in spite of the disadvantages of such an arrangement, the action of the muscles will soon lessen the space between the maxillary bones, and the upper jaw will become contracted enough to fall within the under one, a circumstance which, at the same time that it renders mastication very difficult, will occasion a fresh deformity.

Gensoul seized the projecting premaxilla with strong forceps and forced it back to the perpendicular with a sufficient strength to fracture the vomer. In 1839, Dupuytren excised the projecting premaxilla and utilized the prolabium to construct the columella. Malgaigne combined Desault's preoperative retroposition of the premaxilla and Dupuytren's method of constructing the columella. In 1842, Blandin retroposed the premaxilla by resecting a triangular piece of bone with its mucosa from the vomer (Fig. 1-16).

J. Marion Sims—best known for repair of vesicovaginal fistula —successfully treated bilateral cleft of the lip, despite little experience in this field. His patient was a 21-year-old woman with "a most horrible case of harelip" (Fig. 1-17). On June 9, 1842, he removed the premaxilla, preserving the prolabium which he considered essential for proper repair. At a second operation 37 days later, he trimmed the lateral lip elements and prolabium with scissors and approximated the wound edges with a single through-and-through needle. The cephalic

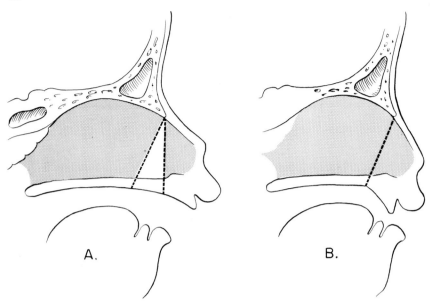

FIG. 1-16 *Blandin resected a triangular portion of vomer so as to retroposition the protruding premaxilla. Because the vomer contributes so much to the growth of the central part of the face, such a procedure may produce the dish-face deformity.*

aspect of each cleft was closed with an interrupted suture. The needle and the sutures were removed after 1 week. The patient wore an external "butterfly" support across the lip for a month. The result was described as good.

Von Bardeleben (1868) sectioned the vomer subperiosteally to

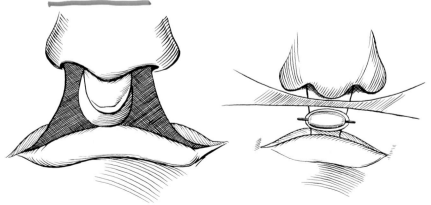

FIG. 1-17 *J. Marion Sims, founder of the specialty of gynecology and of the Woman's Hospital, New York, repaired a bilateral cleft lip in 1842.*

permit its backward displacement without sacrifice of any mucosa. In 1868, Guérin retroposed the premaxilla by subperiosteal resection of a triangular portion of the vomer, thereby combining Blandin's and von Bardeleben's method. Von Esmarch and Kowalzig held the bone in its new position by a rubber band attached to a head cap (Fig. 1-18).

As different flap-type cheiloplasty procedures were developed for unilateral cleft lip in the late nineteenth century, the same principles were applied in repair of bilateral cleft lip. Tissues from the lateral lip elements were inserted below the lower edge of the prolabium to increase its length, as seen in illustrations of the König, Hagedorn, and Owens operations. Rose, Thompson, Berry and Legg, Veau, Barsky, and Padgett and Stephenson were among others who developed techniques based on this concept. That the addition of tissues beneath the prolabium eventually produces an unduly long upper lip was not truly appreciated until the middle of the twentieth century.

Julius Wolff (1896) stressed the importance of using the entire prolabium for the full length of the central upper lip. He also shared the view that pressure from the united lip was sufficient to retropose the premaxilla. Vaughan (1946) used the prolabium to form the full vertical length of the lip. Schultz used lateral vermilion to construct the sulcus between lip and premaxilla (Fig. 1-19).

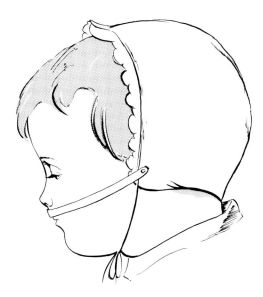

FIG. 1-18 *Retroposition of the premaxilla was accomplished by Von Esmarch and Kowalzig by means of a head cap to which was attached an elastic band.*

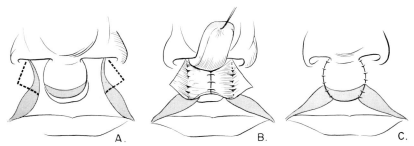

FIG. 1-19 *Schultz constructed the labioalveolar sulcus by elevating the prolabium and surfacing it with lateral turnover flaps of vermilion.*

The views now held by many surgeons doing bilateral lip repairs were summarized by Cronin in 1957:

1. The prolabium should be used to form the full vertical length of the middle of the lip.

2. The vermilion of the inferior margin of the prolabium should not be trimmed off.

3. The thin prolabial vermilion should be built up with vermilion flaps from the lateral lip tissue.

4. Symmetry is more easily attained when both sides of the lip are repaired at the same time.

5. Recession of the markedly protruding premaxilla, when properly done, results in bony union of the vomer at the site of resection and permits closure of the lip in one stage.

SECONDARY LIP REPAIR

COLUMELLAR ADVANCE

In 1833 Gensoul attempted to lengthen the short columella with a V-Y advancement flap in the midline (Fig. 1-20). A modification of the advancement principle was reported by Brown and McDowell in

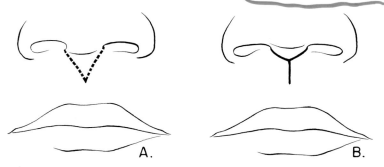

FIG. 1-20 *Gensoul proposed a median V-Y procedure to advance the columella.*

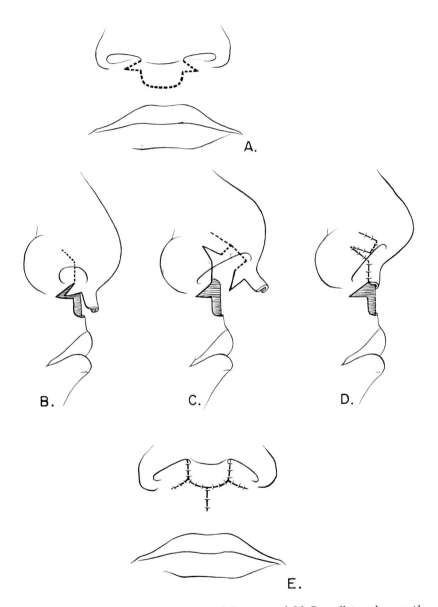

FIG. 1-21 *The fleur-de-lis procedure of Brown and McDowell to advance the columella.*

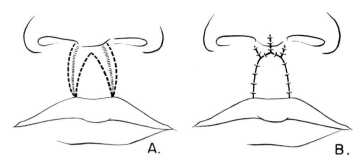

FIG. 1-22   *Millard advanced the columella by using a forked flap.*

1941 (Fig. 1-21). The advancement concept was further improved by Millard in 1958 and by Stark in 1962. Millard's forked-flap procedure consists of elevating two pointed flaps that join at the columellar base as a forked configuration. Two prongs of the fork are freed, advanced, and sutured in the midline to form the new columellar base. The two vertical scars following closure of the lip donor defects simulate the absent philtrum (Fig. 1-22).

SABATTINI-STEIN-ESTLANDER-ABBE FLAP

Sabattini in 1837 and Stein in 1848 switched flaps from the upper to the lower lip to close a defect following excision of a carcinomatous lesion of the lower lip. Estlander in 1877 utilized a single lip-switch flap to reconstruct a lower lip defect caused by typhoid fever. Abbe (1898) of St. Luke's Hospital, New York, was the first to advance a pedicle from the lower lip to correct a tight upper lip resulting from cheiloplasty for bilateral cleft lip (Fig. 1-23).

CORRECTION OF MISMATCHED VERMILION

Berry and Legg (1912) corrected mismatched vermilion, a fairly common deformity following cheiloplasty, by utilizing the Z plasty procedure (Fig. 1-24).

CORRECTION OF CUPID'S BOW

Gillies corrected asymmetrical or absent cupid's bow by carving the configuration in the skin of the upper lip, then advancing the labial mucous membrane (Fig. 1-25).

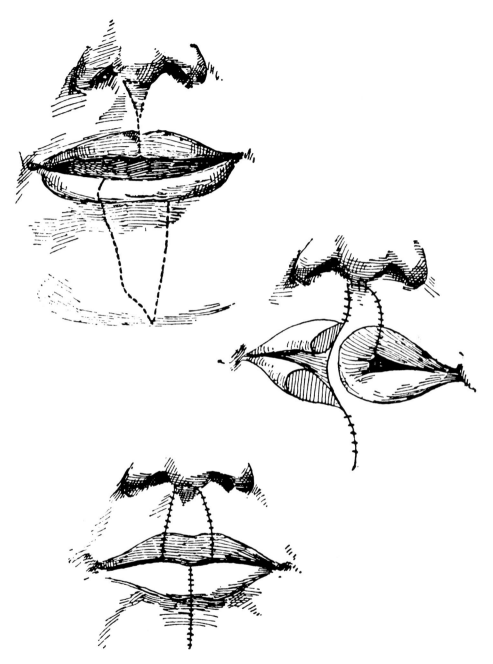

FIG. 1-23 *Original drawings of Abbe's flap from the protruding lower lip, which plumps out the tightness resulting from bilateral cleft lip.*

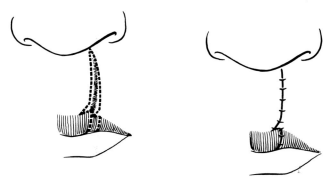

FIG. 1-24   *Z plasty used by Berry and Legg to correct the mismatched vermilion.*

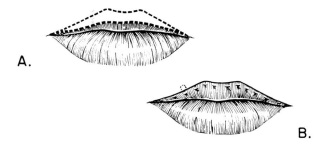

FIG. 1-25   *Gillies procedure to form a cupid's bow.*

CORRECTION OF UNDULY LONG UPPER LIP

Insertion of lateral lip flaps under the prolabium to increase the length of the central lip usually results in an unduly long upper lip. In 1940, Vaughn excised the scar with underlying muscle to correct this defect (Fig. 1-26).

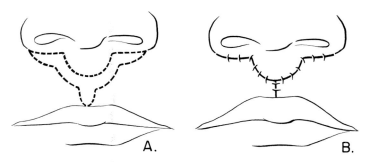

FIG. 1-26   *Vaughn's procedure to correct the unduly long lip produced by insertion of lateral lip flaps under the prolabium.*

CORRECTION OF UNSIGHTLY SCAR

Trusler (1952) suggested a zigzag or Z incision to revise a virtually straight scar when the lip is not tight (Fig. 1-27).

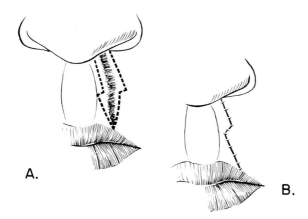

A.

B.

FIG. 1-27 *In revising a lip scar, the broken-line incision usually will be less obvious than the straight line.*

CHAPTER 2

History of
Cleft Palate
Surgery

DAVID E. SAUNDERS

Closure of a cleft palate to permit normal speech development without interfering with facial growth has been one of the surgeon's knottiest problems throughout medical history. New techniques for cleft palate closure have generally evolved when medical standards were high. The progress has been helped or hindered by religious beliefs, wars, and major medical discoveries such as anesthesia. Progress has depended upon isolated advances, many of which were preceded by alternative methods that were only occasionally successful. The earliest aim was simply to close the cleft; later, function became a goal.

The first records (600 B.C.) of plastic surgery are from the ancient Hindus and the Greeks (460–146 B.C.). Although cleft palate was known during this pre-Christian period, as shown by Smith's and Dawson's studies of Egyptian mummies, there were no medical reports of such defects. When medical knowledge spread to the Mediterranean countries, medical and surgical volumes were written by Hippocrates (460–370 B.C.) and Galen (A.D. 129–199), who discussed mutilated lips in detail, but did not mention cleft palate.

During the Dark Ages, when the Church proclaimed the ungodliness of surgical procedures, Rolando Capelluti of the school at Salerno was the first to mention cleft palate (twelfth century) which he called a "fissure of the palate."

The Renaissance brought new discoveries in medicine. Pierre Franco, a student of Ambroise Paré, was the first to recognize the congenital origin of cleft palate. In 1556, he described the anomaly in his articles "Lènvre fendu de nativité" (congenital split lip) and "Dents de lièvre" (hare teeth). The first description of suture of the soft palate was attributed to Jacques Houllier (1562) in Gurlt's *Geschichte der Chirurgie* (1898).

The patient's pain and bleeding as well as the surgeon's poor knowledge of functional anatomy led to crude prosthetic devices for closing the cleft even by the great Paré.

In the seventeenth century, the churches considered surgeons workers for the "Evil One." In fact, up to the early nineteenth century only isolated reports appeared on cleft palate. The nineteenth century, however, brought rapid progress in effective closure of the fissure.

A German, Carl Ferdinand von Graefe (1816), was the first to give a comprehensive description of closure (staphylorrhaphy) of a cleft of the soft palate (velum). Philibert-Joseph Roux (1819) of Paris soon popularized this procedure. Johann Dieffenbach (1826) of Germany was the first to close the cleft hard palate (uranoplasty) by mobilizing the soft tissues. In England, the first staphylorrhaphy was described by Thomas Alcock (1821) and the first in the United States was reported by Alexander Stevens (1827) of New York.

The next major advance in cleft palate surgery is credited to Sir Philip Crampton (1843) who, with Dr. James Cusack, suggested that after operation, instead of being starved, patients should be given a liberal amount of fluids.

In 1844, Sir William Fergusson dissected a cadaver with cleft palate and gave a detailed description of the palatal musculature. Fergusson originated the extensive muscle-cutting incisions that became modish in this period. This step, although unnecessarily extreme, helped to prevent disruption of the palatal wound. Even so, wounds still broke down with alarming regularity. Bernard von Langenbeck, realizing that hard palate mucosa was insufficient for successful closure, added the all-important periosteum (1859). This bilamellar mucoperiosteal layer at last provided a satisfactory method of performing uranoplasty.

Successful closure of palatal defects then became commonplace, and the aims of surgery began to change. Passavant (1862) noticed that successful closures were often followed by nasal speech. The length and function of the surgically closed palate was therefore subjected to scrutiny. Whitehead (1871) and Schoenborn (1875) added tissue to the velum, while Forbes (1875) lengthened the palate without adding to its mass.

During the nineteenth century many methods of palatal repair were tried. Dieffenbach first suggested osteal uranoplasty in 1826, used it in 1834, and reported his results in 1845. Montin's uranoplasty by compression (1836) was popularized by Brophy beginning in 1893.

In the meantime, new surgical possibilities had been opened by the introduction of anesthesia (1846) and replacement of Lister's antiseptic techniques by the aseptic methods of von Bergmann (1886). The problems of abdominal surgery were sufficiently challenging; operations undertaken purely for cosmetic improvement were looked on as frivolous.

World War I, during which thousands of soldiers received severe facial injuries, gave the first impetus for the use of plastic surgery. Plastic surgeons serving in the war, though few in number, sought new techniques for cleft palate closure after their return to civilian practice. The older concept of merely closuring the defect gave way to that of obtaining good function and speech. Ganzer performed the first push-back operation in 1920, and soon Ljovac, Veau, Wardill, Limberg, and Dorrance offered modifications.

From World War II came the first adequate supply of plastic surgeons properly trained to meet community needs. They soon suggested a bewildering variety of new ideas and modifications of old ones. After carefully examining large groups of patients followed for long periods, they realized that their responsibility did not end with simple closure, but extended to complete habilitation of the patient. The cleft palate team of mixed specialists was evolved thereafter.

THE EARLIEST METHODS OF CLEFT PALATE CLOSURE

The method attributed to Jacques Houllier (1562) consisted of suturing together the two edges of a traumatically split velum. No mention was made of denuding the edges; the statement, "if time does not cure the condition, it may be repeated, and if failure again occurs a prosthesis may be used," is significant.

Robert reported that in 1776 Le Monnier of Rouen had closed a complete cleft of the palate with sutures. Cautery of the edges produced inflammation and suppuration, which promoted union. Several other investigators reported a single case, but in general the experience was limited, owing largely to patients' reluctance. For example, Colombe sutured a split velum in a cadaver in 1813, but was unable, in 1815, to persuade a patient to undergo the traumatic and painful experience.

CLEFT PALATE SURGERY IN THE NINETEENTH CENTURY

Prior to Anesthesia

Carl Ferdinand von Graefe started the astonishing progress of the nineteenth century. His descriptions were the first to include methods, instruments, and results. His early attempts (1816) repeated eighteenth century methods: cauterizing the margins of the cleft velum with tincture of cantharides, then suturing the soft tissues. In a modification (1820), the edges were denuded with a uranotome, then sutured by a nut-and-bolt device. In 1827, von Graefe abandoned this device in favor of doubly knotted twine sutures.

Philibert-Joseph Roux greatly simplified staphylorrhaphy by first passing three sutures across the split velum, denuding the edges with a knife, and then tying the sutures. Roux's first patient was John Stevenson, a Canadian studying medicine in Edinburgh. The operation, which was called "velosynthesis" by Stevenson and "staphylorrhaphy" by Roux, was a success. Stevenson returned to Montreal, where he helped to found the Montreal Medical Institution (becoming the first professor of anatomy in 1832) and McGill University.

Surgeons from many countries began to report their methods, which differed mainly in placement of the sutures. Numerous special instruments were introduced. In a technique described by Ebel (1824), the palate was tickled prior to surgery to accustom the patient to instruments in the mouth so that he would find the actual procedure less objectionable.

The increasing number of successful closures pointed up various problems, of which wound tension was the principal one. Dieffenbach's staphylorrhaphy (1826) involved twisted wire sutures. Two years later, he made lateral relaxing incisions down to the bone to facilitate closure (Fig. 2-1). Mettauer (1837) made several small stab incisions for relaxation, counting on healing by granulation (Fig. 2-2).

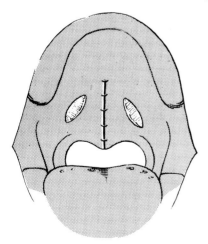

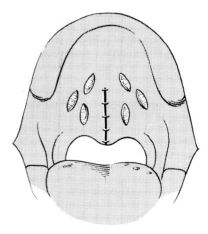

FIG. 2-1 *Dieffenbach made lateral relaxing incisions to release tension upon the midline palatal closure. As a result, the incidence of successful staphylorrhaphies increased.*

FIG. 2-2 *Mettauer made several stab incisions for relief of tension upon the new wound.*

Most repairs continued to reopen, however, owing to lateral pull of the muscles. To prevent wound disruption, the patients were starved postoperatively. After Sir William Fergusson's anatomical report had clarified the reason for failure, surgeons began to make extensive muscle-dividing, relaxing incisions. Fergusson divided the levator veli palatini bilaterally, the posterior pillar of the tonsillar fauces, and, if necessary, the anterior pillar. Liston (1846) divided the tensor veli palatini as well, and suggested that failures with Fergusson's procedure were due to this omission. Extensive lateral incisions remained in vogue for 50 years, until Billroth condemned their use in 1889.

Although it was possible to close the velum, the hard palate still presented many problems. Dieffenbach (1828) dissected off the mucosa to achieve closure; Jonathan Mason Warren (1843) "peeled off" the mucosa; and John Avery (1853) separated it from the fibrous tissue. The difficulties were reflected by Cloquet's report (1854) of closing clefts in 30 cases by repeated cauterization alone, using the electric cautery.

The solution to the uranoplasty problem was largely due to von Langenbeck, who realized the significance of elevating periosteum with the mucosa. His technique employing ice anesthesia was reported in 1861. However, he still relied on extensive myotomy, including the levator and palatopharyngeus muscles. The method of handling the mucoperiosteal flaps varied according to the case. Basically, von Langenbeck started the lateral relaxing incisions very close to the alveolar ridge and extended from his myotomy incision to the incisor teeth (1864). The flaps were then elevated, and the velum was freed from its attachment to the hard palate. If the bilateral bipedicle flaps met in the midline, they were sutured together.

Von Langenbeck's modification (1864) consisted of three methods according to the slope of the palatal shelves. When the palatal shelves appeared horizontal, he used the medial displacement technique described above. When one shelf was horizontal and the other vertical, he made a relaxing incision only on the horizontal side; a flap for the other side was derived from the nasal septum. To repair cases characterized by bilateral vertical shelves, he denuded the edges and united the flaps to the denuded septal edge. If this protruded into the oral cavity beneath the level of the palate, he drilled holes through the septum for passage of the sutures. Von Langenbeck performed this operation in one stage, but recommended a two-stage procedure.

Although surgeons were able more frequently to close total clefts successfully, significant strides were made only after the introduction of anesthesia. Buszard (1868) was the first to describe staphylorrhaphy under chloroform, but Collis is reported to have used this agent in 1867. Thomas Smith (1869) popularized the use of chloroform in cleft palate surgery.

After Anesthesia

With the advent of anesthesia, complete clefts of the palate were successfully closed by von Langenbeck's one-stage technique in an increasing percentage of cases. Efforts previously directed toward closure alone were broadened to include associated problems.

Passavant was the first to note that speech after closure still could be poor, with nasality and denasality often persisting. His idea that this was due to a shortened velum was to become the basis for many later operations. Despite this observation, most nineteenth century reports emphasized ways of ensuring closure without wound disruption. Even as late as 1926, Sprague described tension-relief pins which were passed the length of each mucoperiosteal flap and bound together.

Repairs varied from simple operations to two- or three-stage procedures with extensive myotomy. Annandale (1865), who condemned Fergusson's extensive myotomy, recommended a single-stage von Langenbeck procedure. Whitehead (1868) described uranostaphylorrhaphy in which the levator veli palatini, tensor veli palatini, and both pillars of the fauces were divided. Billroth in 1889 stated that extensive lateral incisions later interfered with velopharyngeal closure. He fractured the hamular process and suggested that removal of the fulcrum released the tension of the tensor veli palatini, producing the requisite relaxation.

Lannelongue (1872) first closed a cleft of the hard palate using a mucoperiosteal flap from the vomer, elevated from below upward and sutured to a lateral nasal flap (Fig. 2-3). This was used by Veau at the time of lip closure so as to avail himself of the exposure afforded by the cleft.

In 1897, Sir W. Arbuthnot Lane popularized a technique for

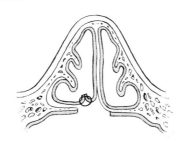

FIG. 2-3 *Lannelongue utilized vomerine mucoperichondrium to close the cleft in the hard palate.*

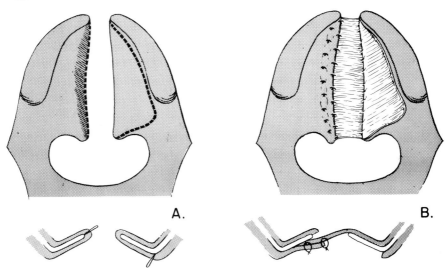

A.   B.

FIG. 2-4 *Krimer and then Lane popularized an eversion flap for cleft palate. Although there were many advocates of the method, the high incidence of necrosis and breakdown led to the abandonment of the procedure.*

closing palatal defects (either cleft or fistula) by basing a flap in a nearby area and turning it over or everting it into the defect, bringing the raw nasal surface into the mouth (Fig. 2-4). In 1827, Krimer had used a simpler method based on this concept; Nélaton (1836), Blandin (1836), Pancoast (1844), Botrel (1850), and Verneuil (1877) tried variations. Fitzgerald, in 1875, called it "a new operation for cleft palate." Davies-Colley (1890) combined flap eversion with medial displacement of flaps for cleft palate closure. Moszkowitz reported the same procedure in 1907.

Lane (1897) overlapped the edge of a large everted flap with a small flap from the opposite side of the cleft. He advocated surgery for cleft palate on the day of birth. In the absence of associated cleft lip, he split the normal lip to facilitate exposure. His mortality rate of nearly 10 per cent was comparable to Veau's (1900) for children up to 6 months undergoing surgery for cleft palate.

Flap eversion for cleft palate closure was followed by a high rate of early mortality and numerous necrotic flaps and postoperative fistulae. This difficult and unsatisfactory procedure has been virtually abandoned.

Brophy (1893) erroneously believed that a cleft palate was due to separation of two normal parts rather than a developmental tissue deficit. Uranoplasty, forcing the two segments together by compression, became widely known as the Brophy technique (Fig. 2-5) after his series of articles appeared: a preliminary report in 1893, and "A new operation for cleft palate" in 1896. Brophy in 1897 stated that "a theory in regard to palate operations has become a well-established practice." He had not abandoned this concept by 1923, when his book was published.

The various methods used for maxillary compression varied: external pressure on the cheeks to appose the segments, lateral pressure over the alveolar margins, and strong external pressure with the coapted margins held together by wires (Fig. 2-5).

Berry strongly criticized both the Krimer-Lane and the Brophy methods. Of the latter he said in 1905: "Violent operations upon the maxillary bones themselves, I think, may reasonably be left to those who prefer to overcome difficulties by force rather than craft." Berry and Legg wrote in 1912:

> Finally, it should be remembered that the complete clefts of the palate, the only ones suitable for Brophy's operation, are usually just those that can be closed without much difficulty by the ordinary operation. The cleft which is by far the most difficult to close satisfactorily by the ordinary means (a wide cleft of the soft palate and most of the hard palate with cleft alveolus) is one for which Brophy's wiring operation is quite useless.

Osteal uranoplasty, or lateral incision of the palatal bones with medial displacement (Fig. 2-6), was used by Dieffenbach (1834) and Wutzer (1834), and different combinations of methods were described

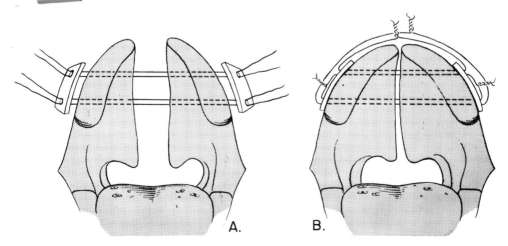

FIG. 2-5   *Brophy's uranoplasty by compression was popular in the early part of the twentieth century. Severe recession of the growth of the central third of the face resulted.*

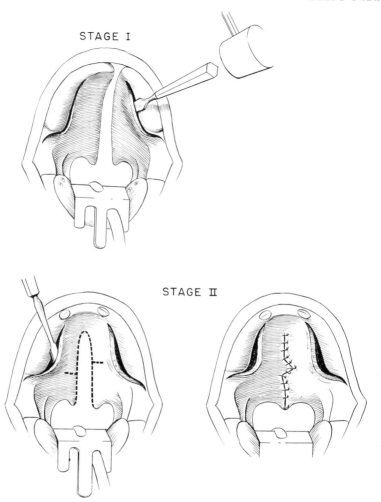

FIG. 2-6   *Dieffenbach in 1834 boldly made relaxing incisions not only through mucoperiosteum but also through the bone of the palatal shelves, leaving the blood supply of the hard palate undisturbed (Stage I). A second operation (Stage II) pared the mucous membrane of the cleft margin and sutured the soft tissues. Those who have brought the bone flap operation into the twentieth century (J. O. Roe, W. B. Davis, G. V. I. Brown, L. A. Peer) have added a Z plasty to provide additional palatal length.*

by Buehring (1850), Lowenhardt (1857), von Langenbeck (1861), Simon (1864), Fergusson (1873), Mason (1874), Lannelongue (1877), Goodwillie (1877), Woakes (1879), and Mears (1893).

The many different operations proposed during the second half of the nineteenth century reflect continuing problems in surgical closure, despite the higher percentage of successful results. These methods, however, were insignificant in comparison with Passavant's contribution. Besides considering final speech results after closure, he started a trend toward surgery designed to prevent or correct poor speech. In 1865, he outlined three methods to help overcome velopharyngeal insufficiency: (1) suturing the velum to the posterior pharyngeal wall; (2) uniting the palatopharyngeus muscles; and (3) an extension of the first method—dividing the velum from the hard palate and suturing it in retroposition to the pharyngeal wall (Fig. 2-7). The defect between hard and soft palates was closed later.

In 1878 Passavant described his earlier attempts and suggested construction of a ridge on the posterior pharyngeal wall, since named after him. He tried forming a shelf-like projection with a flap doubled on itself; he also used an obturator behind the pharyngeal muscles.

Simon (1864) suggested preventing the nasal escape of air by placing balloons in the nostril or pince-nez glasses on the ala nasi. He noted that the voice of the cleft palate patient lacked proper nasal resonance. Paul (1866) tried to increase the bulk of the velum by multiple lateral stab wounds that were left to heal by granulation. Mason (1869) divided the lateral attachments of the velum so that it hung freely like a big uvula. Whitehead (1871) added length to the velum by two flaps from the palatopharyngeus muscles. It was Schoenborn (1875) who first used a pharyngeal flap from the posterior wall to lengthen the velum.

Forbes lengthened the velum (1879) without adding tissue, by a

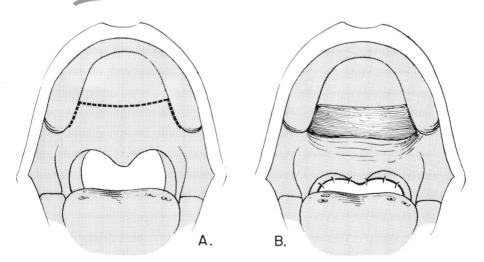

A.   B.

FIG. 2-7 *Passavant's operation for retroposition of the velum, which was sutured to the posterior pharynx.*

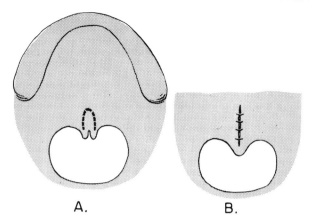

A.   B.

FIG. 2-8 *Forbes (1879) attempted to lengthen the velum in cases of bifid uvula.*

U-shaped incision which opened up to form a line (Fig. **2-8**). Muscle relaxing incisions to reduce tension on the velum were attempted by Billroth (1889) and Mears (1893).

In 1895 Smith reported primary retropositioning of the velum by separating it from the palate centrally, leaving lateral mucosal tissue that was medially displaced to fill the defect and, theoretically, maintain the velum in its new position.

CLEFT PALATE SURGERY IN THE TWENTIETH CENTURY

Prior to the Push-Back Operation

In the first two decades of the present century, known techniques held sway. Brophy continued his forceful compression of the maxillary segments; Girard, Berry, Peck, and Ombrédanne used modifications of the bilateral mucoperiosteal flap technique; Versany, Eckstein, Botrey, Perthes, and Pickerill devised methods to overcome velopharyngeal insufficiency; and Roberts modified the inverted Krimer-Lane flap method.

In his book *Oral Surgery* (1915), Brophy replied to critics who had deplored his "crushing" of the bones: "They are not broken but at a time in life when they are soft and flexible, they are bent and moved into correct position." Wires placed across the cleft from each alveolar margin were twisted until the segments came together. The edges of the cleft were denuded and united with horsehair. Wound tension was relieved by wire sutures tied over lead plates. Brophy did not favor lateral relaxing incisions. He closed the hard palate before the age of 3 months, leaving the lip open until later so as to facilitate surgery. The velum was closed at 12 to 18 months.

Girard (1901) advocated mucoperiosteal flaps with relaxing incisions described as reaching into the velum; in 1915 this was modified so that the incisions reached the pillars of the fauces. Berry (1905) believed relaxing incisions were less likely to interfere with function than myotomy.

In a later report, he and Legg proposed anti-tension, sutures and plates. In 1926 Berry said he first closed the velum when the cleft was wide to help narrow the cleft of the hard palate and hence facilitate uranoplasty. He thus anticipated the philosophy of Schweckendiek and of Slaughter and Pruzansky. Peck (1906) also preferred lateral relaxing incisions to myotomy.

Ombrédanne continued to rely on myotomy with medial displacement of the flaps. In a 1912 report, he described cutting the posterior pillars of the fauces, dividing the aponeurotic expansion of the tensor veli palatini, and suturing together the levator veli palatini muscles.

In an effort to advance the posterior pharyngeal wall, Gersuny (1900) injected liquid paraffin into the retropharyngeal space, and Eckstein (1902) used hard paraffin.

Botrey (1907) removed long vertical ellipses to narrow the pharyngeal wall. Attempts to narrow the velopharyngeal space included those of Morestin (1900) and Helbing (1912), who sutured the divided faucial pillars across the midline to add bulk to the velum.

Perthes (1912) is reported to have moved the mucoperiosteum and hence the velum posteriorly; he also implanted cartilage in the retropharyngeal wall extraorally. Pickerill (1912) converted the velum into a separate muscular bridge which was displaced posteriorly with a prosthesis.

The Push-Back Operation

Early in the twentieth century, most surgeons were still concentrating upon closure of palatal defects or secondary correction of velopharyngeal insufficiency. Roberts was the first to try to ensure adequate speech at the primary operation. His method for backward displacement of the velum was to make a curved incision across the hard palate at the level of the canine teeth and raise a mucoperiosteal flap based toward the velum. The velum was freed from its hard palate attachment and held posteriorly by suturing the tip of the mucoperiosteal flap to the posterior portion of the hard palate.

Two years later (1920), Ganzer pointed out that the von Langenbeck procedure produced a short velum. He suggested leaving a

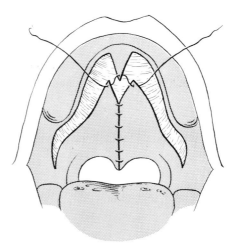

FIG. 2-9 *Ganzer's and Halle's W-shaped incision, sutured as a V to lengthen the palate.*

V-shaped segment of mucoperiosteum anteriorly, displacing the whole palate posteriorly and holding it in position by suturing the tips of the lateral flaps to the tip of the V—in effect a W-V modification of the V-Y principle (Fig. 2-9).

Gillies and Fry (1921), for the same reasons, made incisions into the velum parallel to and immediately behind the hard palate. The entire velum was pushed posteriorly. Its anterior edge was grafted and held back by an obturator which also occluded the unrepaired hard palate.

Veau and Ruppe (1922) believed the velum was shortened following closure because the raw surface on the nasal side of the mucoperiosteal flaps was allowed to heal by scarring. They therefore sutured the nasal mucoperiosteum separately across the bare area (Fig. 2-10).

Despite this new concept of preventing poor speech rather than attempting to cure it later, the problems of midline union remained. Sprague (1926) suggested tension-relief pins. Tschmarke (1927) reported that surgeons at the Leipzig Clinic relieved tension by blunt dissection of the tissues from the hamular process to relax the tensor veli palatini; blunt dissection of the soft palate tissues including the palatopharyngeal muscles up to the base of the skull to relax the levator veli palatini; and blunt dissection of the lateral and posterior pharyngeal walls to relax the pharyngeal constrictor muscles and thus produce circular narrowing of the pharynx.

Bunnell (1927) inserted a silver plate to protect the newly repaired palate from tongue movements. Monnier (1929) and Burdick (1930) placed metal strips around the mucoperiosteal flaps.

However, the trend was toward functional methods of primary palatal repair and secondary correction. Halle (1922) retrotransposed the palate, and Ernst (1925) attempted circular narrowing of the pharynx, which was reported by Halle in 1925 and became known as the Halle-Ernst method. It consisted of two main steps: lateral relaxing incisions to allow palatal closure were extended into the palatopharyngeus muscle; the superior constrictor muscle was then elevated from its lateral attachments and held in the new position by packing. The palate became retrotransposed as granulation tissue closed the wounds. This operation produced not only backward displacement of the velum but side-to-side narrowing of the pharynx. Halle also suggested using fascia in the retropharyngeal space, and reported on the method 3 years later.

Rosenthal (1924) proposed that speech disorders might be minimized by lateral relaxing incisions to close the hard palate and an inferiorly based pharyngeal flap to fill the middle portion of the cleft velum. In 1931, however, he favored Veau's method for children under 2 years, the Halle-Ernst method for children aged 2 to 4, and velopharyngoplasty for older children.

Kirschner (1925) employed the Veau-Ruppe palatoplasty with medial displacement of the pharyngeal walls. Von Gaza (1926) placed fat and fascia in the retropharyngeal space, via a neck incision to reduce the risk of infection.

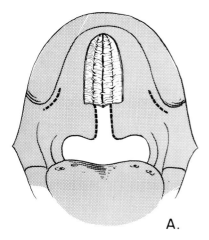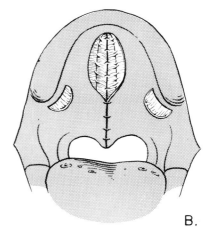

A.   B.

FIG. 2-10 *Veau and Ruppe (1922) pointed out that previous palatoplasties left a raw nasal surface. They were the first to insist upon closure of the mucoperiosteum on the nasal as well as the oral side to prevent palatal shortening by scarring.*

Limberg (1928) condemned division of the posterior palatine vessels and nerves in the Halle-Ernst technique. He relied on Ganzer's technique anteriorly and, when necessary, Ernst's incision in the velum, but resected the posterior wall of the greater palatine foramen to preserve the vessels and nerves. Interlaminar osteotomy of the internal pterygoid plate, allowing medial displacement of the plate with its hamular process, provided wound relaxation.

Changes in concepts and applications during this period are evident in a series of articles by Dorrance. His basic procedure for lengthening the soft palate in cleft palate operations (1925) consisted of making a curved incision through the hard palate behind the alveolar margin, elevating mucoperiosteal flaps, and relieving tension before the cleft margins were pared and sutured. He pointed out that the tensor veli palatini, when hooked around the hamular process, formed two sides of a triangle. It became the hypotenuse when freed from its attachment. He therefore sectioned the hamular process to relieve tension. His aim was to allow the velum to approach the superior constrictor muscle and obtain better velopharyngeal closure. By 1929 Dorrance had become concerned about the forward and lateral pull of the tensor palatini muscle in patients with cleft palate and corrected it by dividing the tendon. In 1931 and 1932 he described palatal insertion of the superior constrictor muscle to form a "palatopharyngeal sphincter." He later grafted skin on the nasal side of the mucoperiosteal flap to prevent scar contracture.

Freund (1927) combined Rosenthal's velopharyngoplasty with a form of staphylorrhaphy. In one case, the velar defect was closed by two everted turnover flaps, with the pharyngeal flap sutured on top of them. He subsequently suggested dividing the flap if it interfered with the palate's normal arch during speech.

Wardill (1927), combining pharyngoplasty with palatoplasty in a two-stage procedure, converted a horizontal muscle incision in the pharynx to a vertical suture line. He retrodisplaced the palate by the method of Ganzer.

Prior to World War II

Shortly before World War II, cleft palate surgery, aided by roentgenography and growth-pattern studies, was becoming limited to a few basic techniques. Embryological factors in cleft palate were discussed, and classifications were introduced. Pohlmann (1910) denied the existence of the classic facial processes described in the development of the face. Veau (1938), supporting this view, felt that the facial area was originally a hood of ectoderm which became invaded with mesoderm. These challenges to the classic concepts of human embryology were later reinforced by studies of Töndury and Stark.

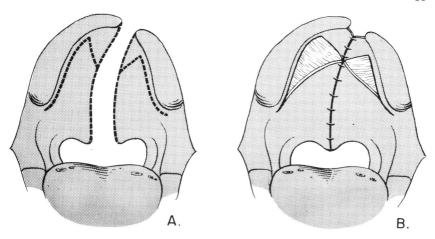

FIG. 2-11 *Wardill's (1937) four-flap operation to close the cleft in the anterior-most part of the hard palate.*

Peyton (1934) found no essential difference in palatal growth between normal children and those with cleft palate up to the age of 1 year, but his later studies revealed a developmental lag in the deformed children, indicating a tissue deficit.

Broadbent introduced cephalometric roentgenography in 1931, which Seiferth in 1935 found far superior to the blowing tests for evaluating velopharyngeal insufficiency. Significant modifications of basic methods were described in the literature.

Axhausen (1936) sutured the nasal and oral mucosa separately by Veau's method, bringing the mucoperiosteal flaps into contact with the nasal mucosa. His goal was to provide a good nasal lining and eliminate dead space.

Brown (1936) used Dorrance's push-back method, providing additional displacement by liberating vessels from the mucoperiosteal flaps. Wardill (1937) adopted Ganzer's W-shaped anterior incision with two lateral flaps for incomplete clefts, but introduced a four-flap method for complete clefts to ensure closure of the postalveolar cleft of the premaxilla (Fig. 2-11).

Classifications of cleft palate defects were introduced by Veau (1931) and by Davis and Ritchie (1922).

Present Concepts and Advances

Great strides have been made in the management of cleft palate since World War II. New examination techniques and discoveries in basic science, as well as carefully compiled statistical studies, have contributed to the recent advances. Treatment concepts have undergone a radical change. Total care of the cleft palate patient, who must be treated as an individual with multiple problems, has been shifted from the surgeon alone to a group of coordinated specialists. The past two decades have seen a large increase in the number of well-trained plastic surgeons as well as significant advances in audiology, speech therapy, orthodontics, and prosthodontics.

The first cleft palate team providing total rehabilitation was formed in 1939 by Herbert K. Cooper, an orthodontist of Lancaster, Pennsylvania. The Lancaster Cleft Palate Clinic was privately financed at the start, but in 1940 the State began to provide funds for families with a limited income. Cooper's team included specialists in general dentistry, orthodontics, prosthetic dentistry, speech therapy, psychology, surgery, and pediatrics, who examined each patient and helped plan his care. According to Ivy's report (1952), which included statistics on cleft lip and palate in Pennsylvania, the state had seven such clinics in that year and others have followed.

Long-term follow-up of a series of patients has helped the surgeon determine the best procedures available. According to Jolleys (1954), patients whose cleft palate was closed before the age of 2 had much better speech than those undergoing repair later. Glover's evaluation of 200 personal cases (1961) demonstrated that speech results were related to the type of anatomical cleft, the developmental characteristics, and the fidelity of the primary repair. Lindsay *et al.* (1962) evaluated palatal repairs in 618 of 1,453 patients treated over a 15-year period. Speech results were related to the presence of a bilateral cleft lip, the patient's intelligence, residual palatal defects, physical evidence of decreased velopharyngeal closure, and the surgeon's skill.

Consideration was also given to methods of improving residual speech defects. The most common method was to attach a posterior pharyngeal flap to the velum, an operation which was performed in so many ways that Webster *et al.* (1956) suggested a classification based on surgical techniques.

Pharyngeal flaps were not as well known in the United States as in Europe, where Rethie (1932), Precechtel (1932), and Meissner (1933) used them in different ways. Padgett popularized these flaps in the United States, reporting results in 1930, 1936, and 1947. Astoul and Blanchart (1947) employed a superiorly based pharyngeal flap first suggested by Sanvenero-Rossèlli (1935) with Veau's palate repair. In the same year Marino combined an inferiorly based flap with a Dorrance push-back operation. Moran presented cases in 1948, and in a report 3 years later stated that the operation helped patients with a congenitally short or paralyzed palate as well. Dunn (1951) also noted that patients with a pharyngeal flap required less speech therapy than those with other types of repair.

Other pharyngoplasties were introduced from time to time. Hynes (1950) increased the bulk of Passavant's ridge by converting two vertical flaps of the salpingopharyngeus muscles to a horizontal position. However, the pharyngeal flap alone or in combination with a secondary palatoplasty continued to be the secondary method of choice for residual poor speech, especially in the United States. Conway (1951) combined it with a push-back procedure. Stark elaborated further upon its use at the First International Congress of Plastic Surgeons in Stockholm in 1955.

Electromyographic studies by Broadbent and Swinyard (1959) revealed that the pharyngeal flap is a dynamic muscular bundle rather than a static post. They found no evidence to support Sercer's theory (1935) that the flap would regenerate the nerves in a paralyzed velum.

Genetic studies by Grunwald (1947), Adair (1930), and Fogh-Anderson (1942) indicated a familial link in inheritance of these defects. Fogh-Anderson concluded that cleft palate alone is due to a simple dominant gene with sex limitation to the female.

Stark's examination of embryos with cleft lip and palate (1954) reinforced earlier impressions that facial clefts were accompanied by a deficiency. Work by Töndury (1955) tends to bear out this concept. Kernahan and Stark (1959) suggested a new classification based on basic embryologic divisions.

With results of surgical techniques more thoroughly evaluated, the consensus was that closure of the cleft before the child begins to talk is most likely to ensure acceptable speech. Graber's cephalometric studies in cleft palate patients (1949) indicated that since the tissue deficit in the maxillary structures is more marked after early closure, surgery might have interfered with bony growth. In 1954, he was convinced that facial growth in patients with unoperated cleft palate was close to normal. He felt, however, that some of the more severe deficiencies observed in operated cases might be due to trauma from excessive manipulation, as with the Brophy technique. The controversy he started has not yet been resolved.

Slaughter and Brodie (1949), who also studied maxillary development, emphasized rapid development of the face until the fifth year, when it slows considerably. They believed that early operation on the hard palate covered its surface with scar tissue, resulting in loss of vascularity and thus interfering with development, and therefore felt that surgery on this structure should be deferred until after the fifth year. Waldron (1950) had similar qualms about certain operative procedures on the palate at a very early age because of possible interference with growth. Dunn (1952), who evidently had the same view, resorted to simple closure of the velum with minimal surgery to the hard palate to avoid interference with maxillary growth, even though prolonged orthodontia would be necessary later. He used vomerine flaps to the edge of the cleft and closed the defect between the hard and soft palates with very small mucoperiosteal flaps.

Slaughter and Pruzansky (1954) urged recognition of muscular forces in the palatal area and their role in the configuration. These surgeons closed the velum as a primary procedure, postponing work on the hard palate until after the age of 6. They recognized, however, that maxillary growth was normal in many cleft palate patients after surgery. Krogman in the same year stated that the only difference in the postnatal growth pattern of a cleft palate and a normal palate was the cleft itself. "As the face is cleft," he said, "so is growth inclined." Feeling that too-early surgery might interfere with growth, he gave 4 to 6 years as the optimum age.

Few plastic surgeons agree with this timing. Trusler et al. (1955) pointed out that the child would lose considerable potential for good speech. They felt that underdevelopment was due solely to poor surgical technique or the presence of a tight lip. Jolleys, who studied 254 children with clefts repaired at different ages by various methods, noted decreased maxillary growth in all of them. Swanson (1955) believed that reports varied widely because cleft palate patients were being judged by an "ideal profile"; if they were instead compared with a random sample of children, the resemblance would be close. He again emphasized that children with cleft palate have the same differences in growth potential as normal children; since the results were so good, surgery should not be postponed.

Bill et al. (1956) also felt that the type of surgery was related to growth. In a study of 41 cases they found no interference with growth following von Langenback's method. Coupe and Subtelny (1960) have indicated an actual tissue deficit in cleft palate cases. Coccaro's studies of soft palate growth (1960) seem to show that with good surgical repair it equals that of normal children. This and other reports on growth potentialities of the velopharyngeal areas, especially following a pharyngeal flap procedure, reflect the continuing trend toward evaluation of results—vital to optimal total treatment.

Although some surgeons still delay hard palate repair pending full maxillary growth, others believe the main goal of palatoplasty is to obtain the best speech results. Opinion is divided as to the relative merits of a push-back method, resurfacing of the nasal side of the flaps to prevent subsequent shortening of the palate, osteouranoplasty, and primary pharyngoplasty with palatoplasty.

Dorrance (1946) reported 20-year results with the push-back

operation in which the nasal side was lined with a skin graft, considered necessary to prevent scarring and yield a soft, resilient palate. Baxter (1942) employed a skin graft placed by means of a stent. Cronin (1957) used the nasal mucosa for a lining, and Millard (1962) used an island flap from the oral mucosa.

Warren Davis reintroduced osteoperiosteal flaps in 1940; Hyslop and Wynn (1952) were convinced the mucoperiosteal flaps interfere with maxillary growth and pointed out the superiority of osteomucoperiosteal flaps which move the parts without such interference.

Kilner (1950) suggested Z plasties on the mucous membrane of the repaired palate. Cuthbert (1951) advocated transposed flaps to improve the push-back operation as a primary procedure. Other surgeons have refined these original methods in various ways to increase the effectiveness of the push-back. Brown's method of freeing the greater palatine vessels from the foramina without cutting them (1936) was adopted by Marino (1944) and Conway (1947). Edgerton's sharp dissection of the vessels from the palatal flaps, liberating without cutting them, was an improvement.

Primary pharyngoplasty has been suggested as a means of preventing the residual poor speech that commonly follows standard push-back operations. In 1960, Stark and De Haan reported on the use of a pharyngeal flap with von Langenbeck closure as a primary procedure for 1-year-old children. There were no poor results in those who had begun to speak. Cox and Silverstein (1961), noting the excellent results of a secondary pharyngeal flap, employed a primary flap after the onset of speech. Results were gauged by the children's ability to produce normal sounds after stimulation; final speech evaluation is impossible until they are older.

Intensive studies are under way in an effort to obtain more normal maxillary growth and positioning of the component parts. Early orthodontia without surgical interference was reported by McNeil (1956), who used a dental appliance before the palate was repaired. Burston (1958) described a similar method. Another aspect of this new concept of orthodontic care in infants is bone grafting to stabilize the maxillary parts in the desired position.

Schmid is credited with the first use of bone grafts to stabilize the alveolar segments (1952), publishing his findings in 1960. Schrudde and Stellmach (1959) found that such a graft does not prevent molding of the alveolar arch by the force of the repaired lip but reduces the rate of molding. Schuchardt (1960) and Derichsweiler (1958) have used the same technique.

Brauer et al. (1962) have combined orthodontia and bone grafting in an attempt to correct malpositioning in children of 3 years or slightly older when the maxillary segments still move with relative ease. Bone grafting, however, does not maintain the new position; indeed, there have been reports of recollapse of maxillary segments following primary bone grafting (Johanson, 1955).

Primary pharyngoplasty, early orthodontia, and bone grafting must still stand the test of time. The full effects on maxillary growth, speech, and orthodontics can be assessed only when the treated children reach maturity. Cinefluorography is an invaluable aid in both the pre- and postoperative assessment of various components of cleft palate treatment.

With increasing knowledge of the individual problems and its spread from one specialty to another, Curtin's statement—that the cleft palate team will eventually make itself unnecessary—may well be borne out.

CHAPTER 3

Congenital Defects

RICHARD B. STARK

ETIOLOGY OF CONGENITAL DEFECTS

The world's "abnormal" children have been sometimes worshipped, sometimes ridiculed, sometimes depicted artistically, and sometimes destroyed, but people have always been curious about them and the reasons for their abnormalities. For centuries it was believed that thoughts, dreams, wishes, and desires conceived within the pregnant woman's cranial "camera" left a positive imprint on the unborn. She therefore went through a period of religious and cultural preparation for the birth. Then in the last half of the nineteenth century came Mendel's law explaining the inheritance of certain parental traits and characteristics.

In the twentieth century, the experimental embryology of Spemann and Harrison; the research of Stockard, Hale, and Warkany; the clinical observations of Gregg; the chromosomal findings of Tjio and the discovery of the chromatin configuration by Barr; and radiation effects reported by Muller, Morgan, and Snell have been rich contributions to the new field of experimental teratology.

In some species of laboratory animals there is a period during which the cell is for a brief time multipotential. The moment when multipotentiality suddenly ceases is the moment of determination. The preceding period corresponds to organogenesis in the first trimester of human gestation. Because of the early pleopotentiality of cells in certain species, heterotopically transplanted cells assume characteristics of the recipient site. These findings have been very helpful to the science of teratology.

Developmental changes are triggered by inductors, enzymes synthesized by metabolites. Development of body parts is usually sequential, an early structure influencing the development of a later one. For example, an enzymatic inductor is responsible for tubulation of the neural crest with cephalic development of the brain. The forebrain triggers formation of the optic cup, which dictates formation of the lens. The lens, in turn, clears tissue superficial to it, thereby producing the cornea. In this rapid sequence of organogenetic events, defective genes or toxic environmental factors may inhibit one phase of development and thus break the chain of normal subsequent development. Thus, introduction of a toxic factor at the time the optic cup is normally formed would preclude later development of the lens and cornea, resulting in an anophthalmic infant.

Hereditary Factors

According to Fraser, 10 per cent of anomalies have a clear-cut genetic basis. Dominant genes are expressed in the offspring (F_1 hybrids) in the ratio of 3:1, i.e., three offspring bearing the characteristics of this gene to one without them. Only the dominant one of the pair of genes (heterozygous) manifests itself. This is true of children with polydactylia, syndactylia, ectrodactylia, brachyphalangia, Marfan's syndrome, achondroplasia, and acrocephalia. The last three conditions are seldom transmitted because affected individuals rarely procreate.

Recessive genes manifest themselves if present in both parents. This is especially likely in cases of consanguineous marriage where the "ubiquitous heterozygote" may be matched with another heterozygote bearing the same recessive gene.

Certain characteristics are sex-linked, passed on by a carrier and manifested in the offspring; others are sex-limited, generally showing up in one sex only. Fundamentally, cleft lip is an anomaly of the male and cleft palate an anomaly of the female, although the two together occur in the same proportion of males and females.

Genes are responsible for the production of inductors and also for the hormonal secretions that later have a marked effect on the physique as well as the activities of various organs.

In 1955 Barr stained cell scrapings from buccal or vaginal mucosa by Papanicolaou's technique and found a small chromatin blob on the inner side of the nuclear membrane in over 90 per cent of female cells and only 4 per cent of male cells. In the next year Tjio and Levan found that man does not have 48 chromosomes but 46—22 pairs of autosomes and 1 pair of sex chromosomes (XY in males and XX in females). Using a squash technique with bone marrow or peripheral blood, they produced an idiogram (diagram of the chromosomal constitution) which revealed more than the usual number of autosomes in some individuals. For example, a few mongoloids had an extra (third) chromosome in diploidal positions 17 and 21—a condition termed trisomy. The technique also revealed an abnormal number of sex chromosomes in certain aberrant sexual conditions. In Klinefelter's syndrome, affecting only males, the principal characteristics are underdeveloped sex glands, enlarged breasts, and sometimes mental retardation. Most of these patients showed Barr bodies in cells from the buccal mucosa and "drumsticks" in the polymorphonuclear leukocytes, indicative of the female sex. They had a total of 47 chromosomes, one extra X (XXY).

Females with Turner's syndrome are usually very short, have tiny ovaries, and do not develop the usual sexual characteristics noted at puberty. No Barr bodies are found in the buccal mucosa and no drumsticks in the blood cells. Their chromosome count is only 45, one sex chromosome (X) instead of the usual two (XX).

It has recently been established that certain women, often retarded mentally but without any distinct clinical condition, have three X chromosomes—a total of 47. Their cells show two Barr bodies instead of one. This is also true of a few men who have three X chromosomes and one Y, with characteristics of Klinefelter's disease. Still more rare are males with XXXXY chromosome configuration and females with XXXX. Whether from males or females, cells with four X chromosomes have a maximum of three Barr bodies.

Females with a single X chromosome are not normal. No persons have been found with a Y chromosome but no X. It is therefore believed that at least one X chromosome is essential to functioning; embryos lacking an X fail to develop. A missing autosomal chromosome is usually incompatible with life. This abnormality may be due to nondisjunction or the chromosome's failure to divide at the first miotic phase of gametogenesis. Segments of chromosomes split off the centromere, then may be exchanged for other loose segments by the process of translocation. Also, chromosomes may suffer from the upside-down position (inversion).

The reasons for genetic predisposition to cleft lip and palate, as well as to congenital heart disease and anencephalia, are not yet well understood. The maternal age tends to be higher than average in cases of mongolism (Down's disease), however, and the paternal age appears to be higher in cases of achondroplasia and acrocephalosyndactylia (Apert's syndrome).

Environmental Factors

METABOLIC DEFICIENCY

Teratogenic or deficiency diets have produced phenotypic malformations in animals. These so-called phenocopies (Goldsmith) have resulted from too little vitamin A in the maternal diet (Hale) and from too much of the same vitamin (Cohlan). Warkany demonstrated that riboflavin is necessary for organogenesis, since a diet lacking this metabolite produced offspring with anomalies. Without riboflavin, folic acid cannot be stored by the liver as the citrovorum factor. Karnofsky showed that the absence of folic acid influences teratogenesis. Other metabolites necessary for normal organogenesis are magnesium, pantothenic acid, and vitamin E. Logically enough, starvation produced numerous congenital defects in animals, as demonstrated by the studies of Runner and of Kalter.

During a time of starvation conditions in Leningrad (1944) and in the Netherlands (1944–1945), when women suffered from amenorrhea and diminished fertility, premature births as well as stillbirths increased. The incidence of congenital defects did not rise, however, indicating that although dietary deficiencies may give rise to anomalies in animals, human beings are not necessarily affected similarly. In fact, this is but another illustration of the folly of extrapolating findings in laboratory animals to man.

PRESENCE OF ANTIMETABOLITES

There is explosive activity during organogenesis. In the mouse, the most extensively studied animal teratologically, this takes place in the first 2 weeks of a 20-day gestation; although dietary deficiencies are revealing during this period, antimetabolites offer more precise evidence of the specific role of metabolites in development. These compounds, structural analogues (mirror images) of known metabolites, act by blocking enzymatic or inductor action, by inhibiting substrate, or by forming foreign nuclear proteins, all of which interfere with DNA synthesis. Antimetabolites found to be teratogenic are aminopterin, a folic acid antagonist; galactoflavin, a riboflavin inhibitor; 6-mercaptopurine, an adenine inhibitor; azaserine, a glutamine antagonist; 5-fluorodeoxyuridine (FUDR), a thymidine analogue; and aminonicotinamide, a nicotinamide antagonist.

RADIATION

Radiation is particularly devastating since it may cause chromosomal mutation during organogenesis. This environmental factor influences the genes themselves, before or after conception. Whole chromosomal segments may be lost or transferred (translocation). Brent's radiation studies involving differential shielding revealed that shielding protected pregnant animals and their litters, but radiation applied directly to the embryo caused anomalies.

HYPOXIA

Ingalls and Philbrook reported that a high percentage of the offspring of animals subjected to reduced oxygen tension (in a chamber simulating an altitude of at least 20,000 feet) had anomalies. The toxic effects of vascular deficiency have caused similar reactions. Trasler showed that anomalies occurred more frequently in rabbits carried in the least vascular (most lateral) portion of the uterine horn. Brent and Franklin clamped a uterine horn in rabbits with a hemostat for a period of time and found that the resulting ischemia caused marked anomalies in the offspring.

Toxic Factors

GROWTH INHIBITORS

Tumor-inhibiting drugs, of which nitrogen mustard is the prototype, are particularly teratogenic (Danforth and Center). Alkylating agents, such as chlorambucil, triethylamine melamine (TEM), and thio-TEPA, affect DNA in much the same way as radiation.

Many drugs have proved to be teratogenic. In general, smaller litters of test animals may be a valuable teratogenic index since many agents in the given doses are lethal to the embryo; in lesser amounts, however, they may well be teratogenic. Pregnant animals treated with such drugs as boric acid, salicylic acid, colchicine, and selenium have produced anomalous offspring.

The tragic discovery that thalidomide (alpha glutarimide), which was extensively tested in animals, causes serious deformities in man points up once again that teratogenic data are not interchangeable between the two species. In early tests, thalidomide appeared to be an ideal sedative. No LD_{50} could be found, and therefore it could not be a lethal agent. It provoked no respiratory or cardiac symptoms. Yet this drug, discovered in 1953 and marketed in 1957, received worldwide publicity in 1961 because of its link with grotesque abnormalities of the extremities and, in a few cases, of cleft palate.

INJECTION OF HOMOLOGOUS TISSUES

Injections of homologous brain tissue have produced abnormalities in the offspring of the mouse (Langman), and human heterologous carcinoma cells have produced mongoloid-type offspring in hamsters (Toolan).

VIRUS INFECTIONS

The most notorious virus infection in human teratogenesis is rubella. Gregg studied 74 infants born to women who had had severe rubella in the first trimester of pregnancy or even prior to conception. Most of the offspring had congenital cataracts; some had cardiac malformations. Hog cholera and blue tongue virus have caused anomalies in lower animals.

PARASITIC INFECTIONS

We have seen one infant with cleft lip and palate as well as congenital heart disease born to a woman who had had toxoplasmosis in the first trimester.

Hormonal Factors

SEX HORMONES

Testosterone, progesterone, and diethylstilbestrol pass the placental barrier and may act upon the genital eminence, which early in embryonic life is sexually bipotential, producing masculinization in a genetically female embryo or feminization of a male embryo. A similar effect may occur with virilizing tumors of the adrenal.

THYROID HORMONE

Thyroidectomy in animals prior to pregnancy has caused anomalies in subsequent offspring (Langman and Van Fassen, 1955). Propylthiouracil or iodine compounds may produce congenital goiter, but the condition usually regresses spontaneously. Trypan blue displaces thyroxin from the plasma protein and thus makes it unavailable to the embryo. Gilbert and Gillman have shown that this azo dye causes anomalies in offspring in much the same way as does thyroidectomy.

STEROIDS

Large doses of cortisone in pregnant animals have produced cleft palate in the offspring. Steroids inhibit elevation of the palatal shelves above the tongue so they can grow and fuse in the midline. Their action is possibly to interfere with sulfation of the ground substance.

PANCREATIC HORMONES

Smithberg and Dixit have demonstrated that Tolbutamide (Orinase) inhibits the uptake of glucose, causing anomalies in the offspring of fish so treated. The higher-than-normal incidence of congenital defects among children of diabetic mothers is well known.

ADRENAL HORMONES

Adrenalectomized women frequently have offspring with anomalies of the central nervous system.

Mechanical Factors

Hydramnios and oligohydramnios have both been associated with anomalies. In oligohydramnios, grayish nodules appear on the placental surface (amnion nodosum); hyperflexion of the head fold results, producing a small jaw (micrognathia). The small jaw pushes the normal tongue upward, impeding fusion of the palatal shelves. Since the head is turned to the right by the enlarging heart, the left side of the lip is inferior and pressed against the chest, often resulting in cleft lip and palate on that side.

Javert has shown that many abnormalities of the cord and of implantation of the placenta may be responsible for congenital defects or spontaneous abortion.

PATHOGENESIS OF CLEFT LIP AND PALATE

The lip structures—prolabium, premaxilla, and cartilaginous septum—are formed between the fourth and seventh weeks of intrauterine life in a different manner from the palate, which is formed between the seventh and twelfth weeks. Imperfect development of either results in a separate cleft deformity. An infant may be born with a cleft in each area (i.e., cleft lip and cleft palate), presumably due to one or more deleterious influences prevailing for a prolonged time during organogenesis (4 to 12 weeks).

Because "lip" is not a sufficiently inclusive term for the three contiguous structures developing as a unit, embryologists have suggested the term "primary palate," since (these structures develop first chronologically). Since the hard and soft palates develop as a unit later, they have been called the "secondary palate." The two are divided by the incisive foramen, located behind the upper central incisor teeth.

The Primary Palate

Embryology of the lip and allied structures (primary palate) described by the German anatomists Dursy (1869) and His (1874) has been perpetuated in textbooks to this day. In their view, the central third of the face developed by a series of facial processes—mesodermal projections surfaced with ectoderm and surrounded by open spaces or clefts. Normally, the processes grew until they met and fused, whereupon the ectoderm at contact points slowly disappeared (Patter called this "merging"), leaving a solid mesodermal union. In the event of interruption in growth of a facial process, the persisting space would be manifest as a congenital facial cleft. A re-examination of the pathogenesis of facial clefts appears to be long overdue for several reasons: Dursy and His failed to explain the rare clinical entity of a true median cleft of the primary palate; their optical instruments and microtechniques were primitive by today's standards; and their studies were based solely on animal specimens.

Recent studies of human embryos with facial clefts have led to several different theories. Although Maurer and Hoepke (1936) considered Dursy's and His classic concepts adequate, they believed the human embryo could heal a formed cleft, since serial section of their specimen showed a Simonart's band across the cleft. Patten (1961) also holds essentially with the classic concepts, suggesting that once the facial processes have met, ingrowth of mesoderm gradually elevates the depressed lines of juncture and reinforces the union (mesodermal merging).

According to Steininger (1939), cleft lip is due to inclusion cysts, apparently caused by burial of ectoderm at the fusion site. Kraus (1965) and others suggest that epithelial "pearls" found along the cleft margins are evidence of postfusion rupture.

Hochstetter (1891), after studying two human embryos with facial clefts, concluded that the upper lip and premaxilla appear originally as an "epithelial wall' and that their normal development depends on reinforcement of this wall by migrating mesoderm—a view fully supported by Veau (1937). Töndury (1955) suggested that the epithelial wall develops from the lateral aspect of the olfactory placodes, the paired umbilicated discs above the primitive lip representing the nasal primordium.

The theory that mesoderm must penetrate a pre-existing epithelial structure for normal development of the prolabial musculature, septal cartilage, and premaxillary bone and teeth was further supported by Stark's study of six human embryos (1954). He agrees with Hochstetter that the epithelial wall is formed as follows.

At the third week of intrauterine life (Fig. 3-1), the human embryo develops a head and a tail fold. Below the bulging forebrain is an invagination or dimpling of the oral pit, at the bottom of which is the stomadeum or oral plate dividing oral ectoderm from gastrointestinal entoderm. Because of infolding of the oral pit, the upper lip region forms as a bilamellar structure with each layer consisting of ectodermal cells—the "epithelial wall" described by Hochstetter. Mesoderm migrates into this wall from its former location and composition as dorsal neuroectoderm (Fig. 3-2). Johnson (1964) tagged neuroectoderm with tritiated thymidine in chicks, using a radioautograph technique, and followed this migration to the anterior face and lip areas.

Stark's study included planimetric determinations of the meso-

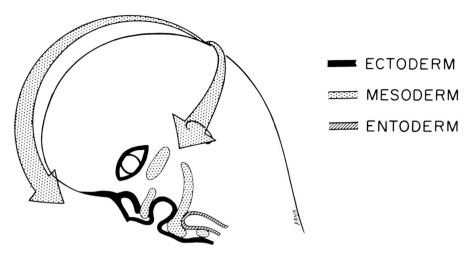

ECTODERM

MESODERM

ENTODERM

FIG. 3-1 *At the third week of intrauterine life, the human embryo develops a head and tail fold. Below the bulging forebrain is an invagination or a dimpling of the oral pit, at the bottom of which is the stomadeum. Because of the invagination of the oral pit, the region of the upper lip forms as a bilamellar membrane, consisting of an outer as well as an inner layer of epidermal cells. The upper lip anlage has been termed the epithelial wall. Into this epithelial branchial membrane, neuroectoderm (in the form of mesoderm) migrates to reinforce the membrane of the lip if it is to develop normally.*

Between the stomadeum and the heart are the branchial arches. Once the stomadeum ruptures and the oral pit joins the primitive gut, in the mentocervical region, the embryo then has an outer layer of ectoderm and an inner layer of entoderm. Such bilamellar membranes are termed branchial membranes. Into this branchial membrane, as in the upper lip, mesoderm will migrate from the dorsum.

There is mesodermal migration normally into the maxillary region forming the zygomatico-maxillary complex; similarly there is mesodermal penetration into the mandibular region forming the first branchial arch of which Meckel's cartilage makes up the greatest part. This arch will form the malleus, the incus, and a portion of the stapes, as well as the muscles of mastication and the trigeminal nerve. The branchial cleft between the first and second forms the external auditory canal; and the bilamellar membrane persists as the tympanic membrane. The first pouch forms the eustachian tube. The second branchial or hyoid arch depends upon migration of mesoderm to form the remainder of the external ear as well as portions of the hyoid arch. The second gives up the muscles of facial expression and the facial nerve.

If the relative lack or absence of mesoderm is in the zygomatic region, Treacher-Collins or palpebral-zygomatic syndrome will result.

If the first arch is deficient, there will be a distortion of the helical crus, preauricular tabs, minignathia, and macrostomia (first branchial arch syndrome). Relative hypoplasia of the first branchial arch will produce Pierre Robin syndrome. Absence of the second arch will result in distortion of the lower portion of the auricle and facial paralysis. If the deficiency of mesoderm is in the first and second arch regions, the patient will exhibit hemignathia and microtia.

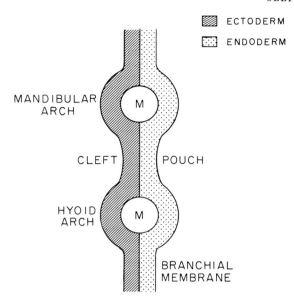

FIG. 3-2 *In the area of the mandible and neck there is migration into several areas, forming surface elevations or branchial arches. These arches are mesoderm, surfaced on either side by epithelium. Between the arches are branchial membranes, bilamellar structures, which, if not adequately supported above or below, may pull apart, forming clefts or cervical fistulae. Behind the convex arches are concavities or pouches which give rise to well-known adult structures.*

dermal volume of each serial coronal section from the six human embryos, three of which had bilateral clefts—a total of nine clefts. Absence of mesoderm on the cleft side, an invariable finding, led to the conclusion that the primary palate is originally an epithelial structure and requires reinforcement from three migrating mesodermal masses, two lateral and one medial (Fig. 3-3). Deficiency or absence of one or two of these masses leaves an epithelial wall that will pull apart and result in a cleft or clefts. The character of the clefts is determined by the degree of mesoderm present: slight deficiency, incomplete clefts; great deficiency, complete clefts.

As mentioned above, the prolabium, premaxilla, and cartilaginous septum are formed conjointly because the nasal structures develop immediately cephalad. At the fourth week, the olfactory placode appears as two discs with central umbilications. Töndury's theory that the placode's lateral rims form the epithelial primordium of the lip (epithelial wall) is invalidated, however, by occasional clinical cases in which the lip is intact and the nose absent.

The nasal umbilications deepen into burrowing pits which, at

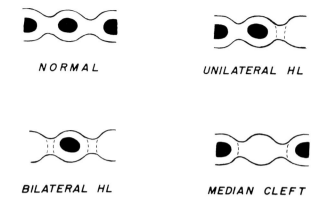

NORMAL   UNILATERAL HL

BILATERAL HL   MEDIAN CLEFT

FIG. 3-3   *Mesoderm migrates into the bilamellar upper lip membrane in three areas: one medially placed mass of mesoderm and two laterally placed masses. If any of these masses are absent or in short supply, the epithelial wall (branchial membrane) will pull apart and a cleft will develop. The amount of mesoderm that is present may be great or small. If it is small, an incomplete cleft will develop; if great, the cleft will be total or complete. A paucity of upper lip mesoderm, depending upon its locus, will lead to the formation of a unilateral, bilateral, or median cleft of the lip.*

the fifth week, rupture into the oral cavity as oral-nasal membranes, forming the primitive nasal choanae (Fig. 3-4). The nasal pits then curve above, encircle, and partially isolate the primary palatal structures.

Monie (1962) showed that the philtrum is formed of vertically

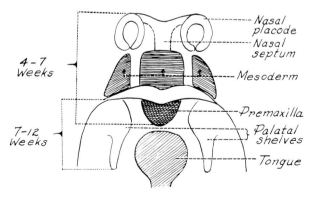

Nasal placode
Nasal septum
4-7 Weeks
Mesoderm
Premaxilla
7-12 Weeks
Palatal shelves
Tongue

FIG. 3-4   *The umbilications of the nasal placodes deepen at the fifth week and break through the oral-nasal membrane to isolate the primary palatal structures (prolabium, anterior nasal septum and columella, and premaxilla). The primary palate forms from the fourth to the seventh week. At this time the two palatal shelves hang downward alongside the tongue.*

positioned connective tissue from the third to the fourth month, after the lip has developed.

The Secondary Palate

The hard and soft palates develop later than the primary palate and differently, illustrating the classic development of processes by fusion. The palatal shelves, mesodermal processes surfaced by ectoderm, initially hang downward on each side of the tongue, and after the seventh week swing upward above the tongue through an arc exceeding 90° (Fig. 3-5). The positional change begins posteriorly and ends anteriorly, behind the premaxilla. With the shelves nearly approximated, they fuse anteroposteriorly starting with the premaxilla and finishing in the uvular region. The premaxilla becomes the keystone of the hard palate, producing the alveolus with the four central incisors. With palatal fusion, the oral cavity cedes considerable space to the nasal airways, thus moving the nasal choanae posteriorly.

Contrary to earlier classifications, the primary and secondary palates join at the incisive foramen, not at the alveolus—the core of our classification at St. Luke's (Fig. 3-6). Clefts of the primary palate occur because the epithelial primordium of the upper lip (the bilamellar branchial membrane) is insufficiently reinforced by mesoderm. A true median cleft is due to absence of the central mesodermal mass. A pseudomedian cleft occurs when only a minute amount of this mesoderm is present. If a mesodermal mass is absent on one side, a unilateral cleft occurs; if the two lateral masses are absent, a bilateral cleft results.

Clefts of the secondary palate occur when the palatal shelves

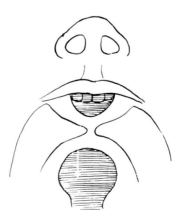

FIG. 3-5 *Once the primary palate has formed, the palatal shelves elevate over the dorsum of the tongue in a wave-like motion, the velum rising before the region of the hard palate.*

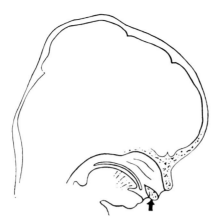

FIG. 3-6 *Sagittal view, with arrow pointing to the intermaxillary segment (premaxilla); behind it is the incisive foramen. Immediately behind the incisive foramen are the palatal shelves.*

fail to fuse, due to (1) insufficient mesoderm to elevate them in time to unite before the pre-existing cleft is widened by transverse growth of the skull; (2) inability of normal palatal shelves to bridge the skull's abnormal width (oxycephalia); or (3) interposition of the tongue in an overcrowded oral cavity (micrognathia with Pierre-Robin syndrome) (Fig. 3-7).

In our classification, based on the embryological data presented, the two anomalies are separated into clefts of the primary palate (prolabium, premaxilla, columella, and anterior nasal septum), and clefts of the secondary palate (hard and soft palate) with the incisive

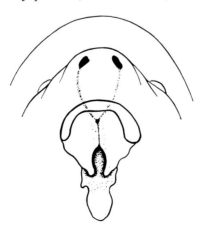

FIG. 3-7 *Once the palatal shelves have elevated, they meet and fuse, this time in an anterior to posterior direction.*

TABLE 3-1. INCIDENCE OF CLEFT LIP AND PALATE

Year	Investigator	Source	No.:Total Patients	Incidence
1833–63	Fröbelius	St. Petersburg, Russia	118:180,000	1:1525
1908	Rischbieth	London	39:67,945	1:1742
1924	Davis	Baltimore	24:28,085	1:1170
1929	Péron	Paris	106:100,889	1:942
1931	Schröder	Münster, Germany	28:34,000	1:1214
1931	Günther	Leipzig, Germany	102:102,834	1:1000
1933	Sanders	Leiden, Rotterdam, Groningen, Holland	16:15,270	1:954
1934	Grothkopp	Hamburg, Germany	74:47,200	1:638
1934	Faltin	Finland		1:950
1934	Sanvenero-Roselli	Italy		1:1000 1:1500
1939	Edberg	Göteborg, Sweden	28:27,000	1:960
1939	Fogh-Anderson	Copenhagen, Denmark	193:128,306	1:665
1940	Conway	New York City	32:22,513	1:700
1940	Henderson	Hawaii	35:18,024	1:550
1942	Grace	Pennsylvania	250:202,501	1:800
1935–44	Mueller	Wisconsin	736:567,504	1:770
1946	Hanhart	Switzerland		1:1250
1947	Phair	Wisconsin		1:770
1949	Oldfield	England		1:600
1949	Hixon	Ontario, Canada	695:655,332	1:943
1950	Ivy	Pennsylvania	766:583,690	1:762
1951	Wallace *et al.*	New York City		1:1265
1953	Wallace *et al.*	New York City		1:1202
1950–54	Douglas	Tennessee		1:1694
1955	Lending *et al.*	New York City		1:1342
1960	Sesgin and Stark	New York City	21:27,087	1:1289
1960	Rank and Thomson	Tasmania		1:602
1955–61	Tretsven	Montana	229:123,114	1:538
1963	Robertson	Trinidad, W. Indies		1:500 East Indian Population); 1:600 (Other population)
1960	Broadbent	Utah	89:59,000	1:662
1964	Soivio	Finland		1:543
1964	Fogh-Anderson	Denmark		1:549
1964	Longenecker *et al.*	New Orleans	154:199,109	1:1221
1964	Conway and Wagner	New York City	1457:1,823,244	1:1260

foramen as the point of division. Classification is further clarified by reference to unilateral, bilateral, and median as well as complete and incomplete clefts. In essence, this classification was adopted by the International Confederation for Plastic Surgery in 1967.

INCIDENCE OF CLEFT LIP AND CLEFT PALATE

Statistics on the occurrence of facial clefts, kept only in the last century, suggest an increasing incidence (Table 3-1). These anomalies are appearing more frequently in certain parts of the world, but less frequently in certain racial groups. Consanguineous marriages may account for the high incidence in the small countries of Denmark, Finland, and Greenland. The reason for an increased incidence in Hawaii and the Philippines is not clear, although it may be traceable to racial and/or dietary factors.

Reports by Davis (1924), Douglas (1950–1954), Shapiro, Eddy, Fitzgibbon, and O'Brien (1958), Sesgin and Stark (1960), Ivy (1962), and Longenecker, Ryan, and Vincent (1964) show that more clefts of the lip and palate occur in the United States white population than in the United States Negro population (a five times higher incidence according to Ivy, and a three times higher incidence according to Longenecker *et al.*).

It is unfortunate that most reports give combined statistics on cleft lip and palate, since they are separate entities developing differently and at different times in embryonic life. Our 1960 research revealed the following incidence: cleft palate, 1:2709; cleft lip and palate, 1:3386; and cleft lip, 1:9029.

CHAPTER **4**

Classification

DESMOND A. KERNAHAN

Interest in the embryology of cleft lip and palate at St. Luke's Cleft Palate Clinic led, in 1958, to a new classification of these deformities, formulated after study of the hospital's collected embryological material (Stark, 1954). The classification was based on the evolution and mode of growth of tissues forming the primary and secondary palates. Briefly, the primary palate—comprising the central portion of the upper lip, premaxilla, upper incisors, and anterior nasal septum—forms between the fourth and seventh weeks of intrauterine life and extends to the nasopalatine canal, site of the incisive foramen. The secondary palate—comprising the remainder of the hard palate and the soft palate posterior to the incisive foramen—forms between the seventh and twelfth weeks as a pair of shelves that grow toward the midline and fuse in a normally developing embryo.

In view of these findings, the genesis of both rare and common lip and palate deformities becomes obvious. Either the primary or secondary palate or both may be involved, resulting in any degree of malformation from a submucous palatal cleft or a vermilion notch to a bilateral cleft involving all dimensions of both palates.

Since the secondary palate fuses anteroposteriorly, the uvula alone may be cleft, but an isolated fistula of the hard palate does not occur as a cleft. Similarly, mesoderm may penetrate the primary palate region dorsoventrally, causing slight notching of the free border of the upper lip but no isolated fistula of the floor of the nasal vestibule.

The original classification of Kernahan and Stark (Fig. 4-1), which is still considered valid and reasonable, clearly relates the congenital deformity to embryological development and in each case indicates the degree of difference from the embryological norm. It

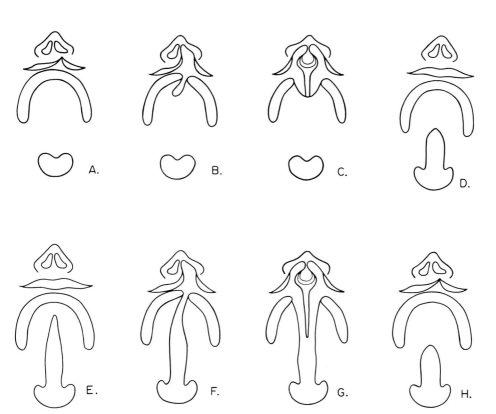

FIG. 4-1 *This classification, published by Kernahan and Stark in 1958, relates to embryological development. The incisive foramen divides the separate anomalies of cleft lip from cleft palate. Cleft lip, however, is not an inclusive enough term, since such a cleft may affect not only lip but anterior nasal septum, columella, and premaxilla. Therefore, we have elected to term such anomalies "clefts of the primary palate," since they occur chronologically earlier (at 4 to 7 weeks of embryonic life) than fissures in the hard and soft palates posterior to the incisive foramen; the latter (which occur at 7 to 12 weeks), we term "clefts of the secondary palate."*

A. *Left unilateral incomplete cleft of the primary palate.*
B. *Left complete cleft of the primary palate, ending at the incisive foramen.*
C. *Bilateral complete cleft of the primary palate.*
D. *Incomplete cleft of the secondary palate (when alone).*
E. *Complete cleft of the secondary palate (soft and hard palates).*
F. *Left complete cleft of the primary and secondary palates.*
G. *Bilateral complete cleft of the primary and secondary palates.*
H. *Left incomplete cleft of the primary palate and incomplete cleft of the secondary palate.*

This classification was adopted by the International Confederation for Plastic Surgery in 1967.

may be compared to the classification of cerebral tumors by Bailey and Cushing, (1926) based on the degree to which their cellular pattern differs from that of normal, mature cerebral tissue.

EARLY CLASSIFICATIONS

Before considering how best to adapt the embryological concept to clinical necessity, it may be of interest to trace the successive, increasingly complex classifications of cleft lip and cleft palate defects.

Many descriptions throughout the world, such as *harelip* in English, *bec de lièvre* in French, *Hasenschatte* (harelip) and *Wolfsrachen* (wolf's throat) in German, and *lábio leporino* (harelip) in Spanish suggest lower animals. Though still widely used, lamentably even by clinicians, such terms should be relegated to the realm of folk medicine.

The first serious attempt at scientific classification was that of Veau (1931) (Fig. 4-2). He indicated degrees of deformity by a numerical scale of I to IV, much like the Wassermann reaction or Broders' index of the characteristics of malignant cells: the higher the number, the greater the variation from the norm. While Veau covered different types of cleft palate, with or without cleft lip, he ignored cases of cleft lip and alveolus without a palatal cleft—the important group which we call clefts of the primary palate. Inasmuch as he was as interested and experienced in treating lip clefts as in treating palatal clefts, this omission is difficult to understand, though not without precedent in medicine. Unfortunately, it leaves his classification incomplete, despite the sound underlying idea.

By far the most carefully considered and useful of the earlier classifications was proposed by Davis and Ritchie (1922) at the American Medical Association's annual meeting in that year. Assembled in St. Louis were many of the leading experts in cleft lip and palate rehabilitation, including James E. Thompson of Galveston, Vilray P. Blair of St. Louis, and Truman Brophy of Chicago. Some of their classifications are shown in Table 4-1, along with that of Davis and Ritchie.

After Ritchie had reviewed previous classifications in detail, he urged adoption of the new classification for the sake of uniformity, to facilitate communication and comparison. Recognizing the three major types of deformity—cleft lip, cleft palate, and the two combined—he suggested that they be designated Groups I, II, and III, respectively (Fig. 4-3). Unilateral, bilateral, and median variants of the principal groups could be indicated by adding further numerals. These surgeons, believing that the alveolus decisively separates clefts of the lip alone from those of the palate, stressed its importance in distinguishing the three groups. In the subsequent discussion, Blair admitted that if with further developments in cleft palate surgery the alveolus proved of lesser importance, the classification would be based on an anatomical concept that had not stood the test of time.

The Davis and Ritchie classification has always posed certain difficulties. Some surgeons place unilateral and bilateral total clefts of the primary palate alone in Group I, adding "with cleft alveolus." Others, following the authors' suggestion, place them in Group III along with a cleft palate and cleft (alveolar) process "if they occur." We believe that such clefts (i.e., cleft palate and cleft alveolus without cleft lip) do not occur because of differences in time of appearance,

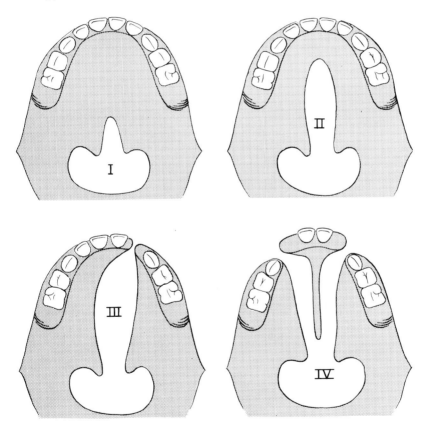

FIG. 4-2 *In his 1931 classification, Veau omitted clefts of the lip with or without alveolar clefts (clefts of the primary palate). He termed clefts of the velum Group I; clefts of the hard and soft palates (secondary palate), Group II; unilateral complete clefts of alveolus and secondary palate, Group III; and bilateral complete clefts of alveolus and secondary palate, Group IV.*

TABLE 4-1   CLASSIFICATIONS OF RITCHIE AND DAVIS, VEAU, BROPHY, SHERMAN, AND THOMPSON

	Ritchie and Davis	Veau	Brophy	Sherman	Thompson
Clefts of lip alone			Not in-		Not in-
Unilateral	Group 1	1.1	cluded	Group 1	cluded
Median		1.2			
Bilateral		1.3	9 Groups		
Clefts of palate alone					
Uvula		⅓	Groups		
Soft palate ⅓		⅔	Group 1 1, 2, 3,		
⅔	Group 2	⅗	4, 9, 14	Group 2	Group 3
⅗		⅓	Group 2 5, 6		
Hard palate ⅓		⅔			
⅔		⅗			
⅗					
Clefts of lip, alveolus, hard and soft palates					
Unilateral	Group 3	3.1	Group 3 Groups 7, 13	Group 3	Group 1
Median		3.2	Group 15		
Bilateral		3.3	Group 4 Group 8	Group 4	Group 2

Courtesy of *Plast. Reconstr. Surg.* *29*:551, 1962.

extent, and formation of the primary and secondary palates. If the demarcation point were moved backward from the alveolus to the incisive foramen, the Davis and Ritchie classification would be comprehensive, embryologically correct, and surgically acceptable. Its one drawback, a numerical code, might be justified for brevity's sake.

The classification of Kernahan and Stark (1958) is similar to that of Fogh-Anderson (1942).

RECENT CLASSIFICATIONS

An interesting system (Fig. 4-4) described by the Spanish plastic surgeon Vilar-Sancho (1962) differs in two respects from other classifications in general use in the English-speaking world: all clefts are classified as incomplete or complete, and the location is indicated

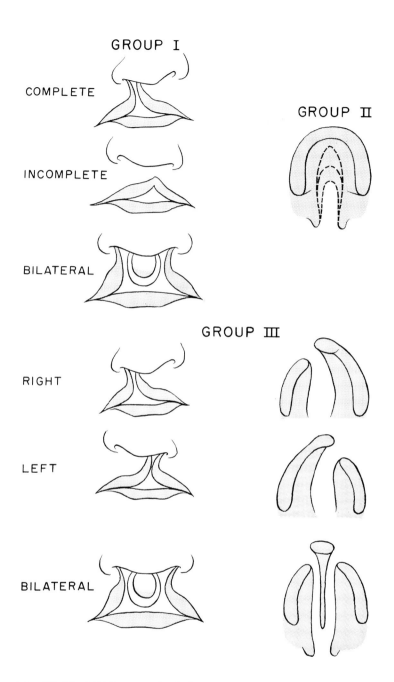

FIG. 4-3 *Ritchie (1922) recognized three major types of deformity: cleft lip, cleft palate, and the two clefts combined. Cleft lip he designated as Group I, cleft palate as Group II, and the combined anomalies as Group III. Unilateral, bilateral, and median variants were indicated by the addition of other numerals.*

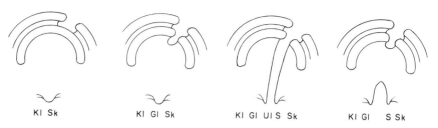

KI Sk   KI GI Sk   KI GI UI S Sk   KI GI   S Sk

FIG. 4-4 *Vilar-Sancho (1962) classifies all clefts (Sk) as incomplete (small letter) or complete (capital) using the appropriate letter of the Greek word for the structure involved (K for lip, G for maxilla, U for hard palate, and S for velum), depending upon the location of the anomaly. After the letter of location and cleft extent, he indicated the side affected (d for right, l for left, and s for bilateral). Several examples of this classification are shown here.*

by the first letter or letters of certain Greek words rather than by numerals: K for *kilos* (lip), G for *gnato* (maxilla), U for *urano* (sky), S for *stafilos* (bunch), Sk for *skisis* (cleft).

Greek derivations were frequently noted in the early literature on cleft lip and palate and still appear as synonyms in the latest classification prepared by the Nomenclature Committee appointed by the American Cleft Palate Association. They are seldom used in everyday surgical practice, however, and, with the declining popularity of classical languages in the Western world, would seem on the way out.

Harkins *et al.* (1962), who were appointed to the Nomenclature Committee of the American Cleft Palate Association after Kernahan and Stark proposed their new classification, have now published their report (Fig. 4-5). In addition to the usual three major groups, they propose a fourth group covering facial clefts other than those of the lip and palate, and suggest "prepalate" as a synonym for primary palate. The classification also delineates the extent of clefts (in thirds of the region involved), their width, and the degree of premaxillary protrusion. Inclusion of these details makes the classification seem rather cumbersome. Such distinct clinical conditions as rare facial clefts and mucous pits of the lower lip do not logically come under the heading of cleft lip and palate, nor does it seem necessary to note which palatal process is attached to the vomer. These data should be recorded in the clinical chart and accompanying diagram to furnish a complete record and indicate differing incidence in comprehensive case reviews. The underlying mechanism is the same, i.e., failure of fusion of the palatal shelves, and all that is required in a classification system.

CLEFTS OF PREPALATE (CHEILO-ALVEOLOSCHISIS)

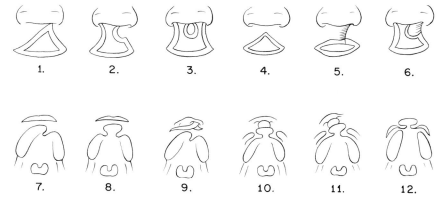

1.   2.   3.   4.   5.   6.

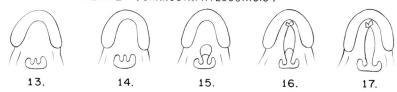

7.   8.   9.   10.   11.   12.

CLEFTS OF PALATE (URANOSTAPHYLOSCHISIS)

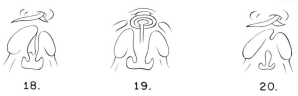

13.   14.   15.   16.   17.

CLEFTS OF PREPALATE AND PALATE (ALVEOLOCHEILOPALATOSCHISIS)

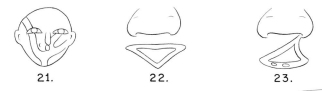

18.   19.   20.

FACIAL CLEFTS OTHER THAN PREPALATAL AND PALATAL (RARE)

21.   22.   23.

FIG. 4-5 *A visual symbol in the shape of a pentagon, as advocated by the Northwest German Jaw Clinic, Hamburg, facilitates cataloguing of cases.*

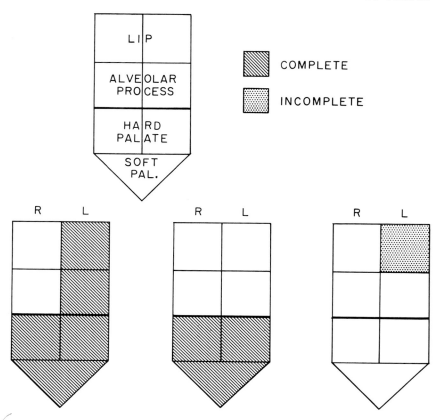

FIG. 4-6 *The Nomenclature Committee of the American Cleft Palate Association has suggested a classification which includes clefts other than those of lip and palate. The gradation of the cleft (in thirds of the area involved), its width, and the degree of premaxillary protrusion all are added, and generally obscure rather than simplify the classification.*

A visual symbol to facilitate indexing of cleft lip and palate cases has been advanced by Professor Schuchardt's Northwest German Jaw Clinic in Hamburg (1964). The figure is in the shape of a pentagon, and its various parts indicate the severity of the defect (Fig. 4-6).

Why have none of the many systems found universal acceptance? The inertia that works against change in any one clinic is strong indeed, but the treatment of cleft lip and palate has now extended beyond the confines of surgery. Workers in this field must now understand the early use of maxillary orthopedics and speech therapy, the underlying genetic factors (e.g., the occurrence of severe forms associated with **17-18** and **13-15** trisomy), as well as the teratogenic factors revealed in both experimental and clinical research.

Taking into account these expanding horizons, the St. Luke's group has based its classification on recent embryological developments which now strongly indicate the possibility of assigning all types of cleft lip and palate to one of three main groups. This can be done by anyone thoroughly familiar with embryology.

CHAPTER 5

The Operation
of a Cleft Palate
Clinic

R. C. A. WEATHERLEY-WHITE

An important development in medicine is the concept of a team approach for treating the child with cleft palate. His complex problem will undoubtedly call for the services, early in his life, of members of different medical and paramedical specialties. For young parents already deeply disturbed by their infant's deformity, constant referrals merely add bewilderment. In rural areas where the medical center may be a full day's journey from the patient's home, there may be a genuine economic burden.

For these and other reasons, many cleft palate clinics have been established over the past 20 years where a child can be treated by the entire team. The latest directory of the American Cleft Palate Association lists 72 clinics located in 33 states and 4 Canadian provinces.

Acceptance of the team concept came slowly, after considerable controversy over the wisdom of sharing responsibility for a medical problem with nonmedical team members trained in widely differing fields. In general, however, surgeons on a cleft palate team have found the care provided through this approach superior to purely individual care.

Material submitted for review by representative clinics in the United States and Canada reveals a wide spectrum of interests and activities. Some clinics are primarily community-oriented, maintaining a close liaison with the local department of handicapped children, or its equivalent. Then there are clinics with the emphasis on making individual care available to all relevant children within the district. Other clinics, particularly those associated with large medical centers, may see only patients with unusual problems. Since clinical investigation plays an important role, the type and quantity of information gathered depend on available finances as well as on orientation of the key personnel. The purpose of all cleft palate clinics is to improve care of individual patients and at the same time enhance and enrich the teams members' postgraduate education.

St. Luke's Cleft Palate Clinic is relatively small. Its aim is to provide maximal care and investigative material with minimal administrative and clerical work. Founded in 1956 under the direction of Richard B. Stark, it was shortly thereafter approved for support of child care by the Department of Health of the City of New York. Staff conferences to present patients and discuss phases of treatment have been held monthly from the outset. Several reports on various aspects of cleft palate repair were based on material from these conferences (Fig. 5-1). Approximately half the clients are private patients of the clinic's plastic surgeons, and the other half are ward patients referred from St. Luke's Pediatric Clinic or the Obstetrical Service of its Woman's Hospital Division. The cost of care for the latter group is borne by the New York Bureau for Handicapped Children.

The referred patient is first seen in the Plastic Surgery Clinic, where the resident takes the routine clinical history, conducts the physical examination, and fills out a "routing sheet" (Fig. 5-2).

The routing sheet consists of a brief description of the birth

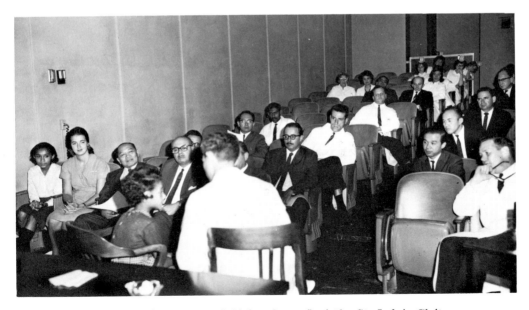

FIG. 5-1 *Monthly conferences are held by the staff of the St. Luke's Cleft Palate Clinic. Two or three private and ward patients are presented for discussion of diagnosis and treatment. Visitors are invited to participate in the discussions.*

ST. LUKE'S HOSPITAL
NEW YORK CITY
CLEFT PALATE CLINIC

HOSP NO. 50-35-71

NAME _____ N. _____ R. _____   SERVICE _____ Plastic Surgery _____
         Last   First

MAKE APPT. FOR	TESTS AND CLINICS	DATE	SIGNATURE OF RESPONSIBLE PERSON
X	1. INITIAL VISIT CLEFT PALATE CLINIC		
	2. REGISTRAR		
X	3. SOCIAL SERVICE (ANOMALY QUESTIONNAIRE)		
X	4. AUDIOMETRIC		
X	5. SPEECH EVALUATION		
	6. PSYCHOMETRIC		
X	7. DENTAL EVALUATION		
X	8. PHOTOGRAPHY		
	9. PROSTHODONTIC		
	10. CLEFT PALATE CLINIC REVISIT		

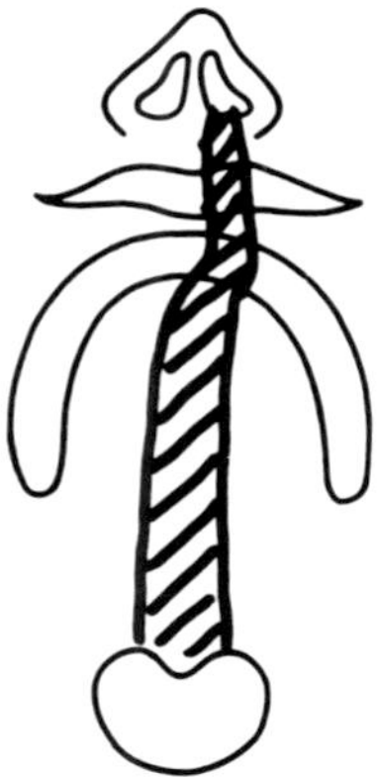

REMARKS:
29 year old Brazilian dancer

Born with total unilateral cleft of lip and palate

6 operations on palate   All in Brazil
19 operations on lip and nose

Now has:
1) Markedly defective speech
   short, scarred palate
   incomplete velopharyngeal closure
2) Thick transverse scars across lip
3) Asymmetry of nose with depressed left ala
4) Moderate cross-bite.

R.C.A. Weatherley-White, M.[

FIG. 5-2 *In most cleft palate organizations, the individual specialty clinics are scattered throughout the hospital. To facilitate the work-up, a routing sheet has helped our organization. This contains a brief description of the anomaly and the past treatment, and a cursory summary of the extant problems. The patient is then routed through all clinics whose examination, diagnosis, and treatment are pertinent to the case. All such clinic visits are completed within a month. The patient is then presented to the monthly conference.*

and maternal history, a diagram showing the extent of the defect, and a checklist of clinics that may be involved in the treatment.

All parents are referred to the Social Service Department where the St. Luke's Anomaly Questionnaire (discussed in Chapter 23) is completed. Appointments are scheduled within 1 month. The patient is then returned to the Plastic Surgery Clinic. The resident ascertains that all services eventually to be involved in care have made their own evaluation of the problems, and then arranges for presentation of the case at a monthly staff conference, usually about a month after the first clinic visit. Private patients are similarly but less formally routed; consultations are subsituted for referrals, but the same type of information is obtained.

The two or three new patients presented at each monthly conference are examined and discussed by members of the Cleft Palate Clinic, who make recommendations based on their specialized knowledge. The ultimate responsibility for deciding whether to take a new patient for intensive treatment and for determining the long-range management of patients already under care rests with the plastic surgeon, over-all director of the team. Brief follow-up reports on current cases are followed by a general discussion. Visitors may also examine the patients.

Excerpts from a typical conference follow:

72ND CLEFT PALATE CONFERENCE: NOVEMBER 4, 1963

Guests were Dr. Donald Robinson of Adelaide and Dr. John Snell of Melbourne (Australia) and Dr. Peter Zellner of West Berlin, all of whom had attended the Third International Congress of Plastic Surgeons in Washington, D.C.

A progress report on the book *Cleft Palate* by members of the clinic showed that 10 chapters have been completed. It was announced that Dr. Daphne Trusler of McGill University, Montreal, would speak on embryology of the cleft palate at the next meeting.

Dr. Stark discussed secondary deformities of bilateral cleft lip. Following lip repair in infancy, children commonly have a rather flat lip, a tight snub nose with an inadequate columellar-labial angle, and a wide prolabium lacking a philtrum and often a cupid's bow as well. It is as important to correct these features as to achieve a good primary repair of the lip itself. Of several procedures designed to achieve a satisfactory lip-nose complex in this situation, our clinic prefers a forked-flap columellar advance, using the wide prolabium. Narrowing of the alar bases at the same time creates a high and pointed nasal apex. A movie of the operation was shown, with slides of several children so treated.

Patients Presented

J. S. (43-00-13), a 3-year-old boy with total bilateral cleft lip and cleft palate, had undergone lip repair at St. Luke's shortly after birth. Although the cupid's bow was good, the characteristic triad of secondary deformities mentioned by Dr. Stark had developed. A forked-flap columellar advance was therefore formed 3 weeks earlier (with surgery viewed by team members over closed-circuit television) and the child was presented to show the immediate postoperative appearance. Although the lip was still erythematous and indurated, his appearance was strikingly improved when compared with preoperative photographs.

On examining the boy, Dr. Vollmer suggested starting orthodontia at the age of 4 to expand the lateral alveolar segments. The speech patterns were insufficiently developed to permit a determinate evaluation.

Dr. Snell commented on Dr. Burston's impressive work in very early orthodontia. The Liverpool orthodontist takes impressions soon after birth, inserts an acrylic splint at 2 weeks and begins expansion. Lip surgery is deferred pending alignment of the premaxilla with the lateral segments. Dr. Stark questioned the permanent results of orthopedic correction without the support and immobilization afforded by a bone graft, which all agreed was still in its infancy.

A. G. (316-289), an 18-year-old Spanish-American girl, was the second patient. She had been aware of her speech abnormality but it was diagnosed only when she was seen at St. Luke's Emergency Room.

On referral to our speech therapist, Mr. Burgess, she was found to have hypernasality, considerable nasal emission, and many high-frequency articulatory omissions. Following speech evaluation and a clinical examination, he made a presumptive diagnosis of submucous cleft of the secondary palate. When the clinic members examined A. G., they noted her abnormally deep pharynx with no velopharyngeal closure. The soft palate was thin and moved poorly, the uvula was notched, and a large bony cleft was palpable in the hard palate. It was planned to admit her for a thorough work-up, including audiometric evaluation and cinefluorography of the palate before scheduling palatoplasty with pharyngeal flap.

After a discussion of various problems relating to learned language and speech therapy, the meeting was adjourned.

Immediate consultation in the conference setting, the most obvious advantage of the cleft palate clinic, must be supported by simple, accurate documentation. Detailed minutes of the conference are compiled by the plastic surgery resident, approved by the director of the clinic, duplicated, and distributed. One copy of the section pertaining to each patient goes into his hospital chart; another is edited and sent to the parents. A third copy is kept in a special file under the patient's name, along with similar material on his case from previous conferences (Fig. 5-3).

Following are excerpts from the record of one patient, W. M., over several years:

35TH CLEFT PALATE CONFERENCE: JANUARY 4, 1960

Dr. James W. Smith of New York Hospital was a guest.

W. M. (40-58-48) is a 4-year-old Puerto Rican boy with a total bilateral cleft of the primary palate (lip, anterior nasal septum, and premaxilla) and secondary palate. The lip was repaired on the 3-month-old infant in Puerto Rico, and the soft palate alone was repaired at $2\frac{1}{2}$ years in New York by Dr. Theodore Capecci. No further surgery was attempted until Dr. Capecci made the referral to St. Luke's. He felt that tension exerted by the closed soft palate might bring the lateral dental arches closer together, facilitating secondary closure of the very wide cleft of the hard palate (Schweckendiek procedure). Examination by team members bore out this impression.

W. M. was cooperative during the physical examination, which revealed moderate scarring of the upper lip and a broad flat nose with a snub tip and short columella. A wide defect extended through the alveolar ridge and hard palate. The repaired soft palate was short and relatively immobile. The premaxilla, in fairly good position, was moderately stable.

Otolaryngological examination by Dr. Kirkbright showed slight retraction of both tympanic membranes but no evidence of chronic infection. No history of otitis media was elicited. He felt that there was no immediate indication for removing of either the enlarged tonsils or small adenoids.

Mr. Stennerson's audiometric examination was incomplete because of limited time, but he gained the impression that W. M. has normal or only slightly impaired hearing.

Plans were made to admit the child to the hospital soon for

further evaluation and repair of the hard palate plus pharyngeal flap.

Dr. Stark, in discussing initial surgery for bilateral cleft lip, pointed out that use of the lateral lip elements to form the lip's central lower half makes it overly long, a defect difficult to correct later.

Dr. Smith of New York Hospital stated that in his opinion it is better to repair the hard and soft palates together than the soft palate alone.

36TH CLEFT PALATE CONFERENCE: FEBRUARY 1, 1960

A palatoplasty (von Langenbeck) with a superiorly based pharyngeal flap was performed on W. M. on January 28, 1960. The postoperative course was uneventful. W. M. was quite willing to have the team examine his palate, which was healing satisfactorily with minimal inflammatory reaction.

A speech recording, taken when he was uncooperative, could not be interpreted properly. Further recordings will be made. Early initiation of speech training was the only recommendation made at this time.

Mr. Stennerson reported that W. M. has normal hearing. A complete otolaryngological examination was recommended before his discharge from the hospital.

A cousin of W. M.'s mother had had surgery for correction of a speech defect. W. M.'s mother described her pregnancy as normal except for a pelvic infection during the sixth month.

38TH CLEFT PALATE CONFERENCE: APRIL 4, 1960

Mr. John Barron, a surgeon of Salisbury, England, was a guest.

On examination, W. M. was found to have a flattened and asymmetric nose, lip scarring, and a large oronasal fistula. The hard and soft palates were solidly healed. The superiorly based pharyngeal flap formed late in January was intact although somewhat narrow. All team members were able to examine the palate and flap.

Mr. Barron emphasized the importance of utilizing the prolabium to form the entire central element of the lip at the time of primary repair; if the lateral elements are used initially to lengthen the prolabium, the lip will ultimately be much too long. He agreed with our group that bilateral repair of the lip at one operation is preferable to a two-stage procedure.

Dr. Stark commented that correction of a bilateral cleft of

the primary palate is still not completely satisfactory. He and
Mr. Barron discussed growth of the central portion of the lip
and palate. Attempts to evaluate W. M.'s speech since surgery
have not been successful, but according to his father, he talks a
great deal at home and has improved considerably.

CLEFT PALATE PROGRAM

PATIENT: S.,J.

GUARDIAN:

ADDRESS:

FINANCIAL ARRANGEMENT

48-78-80

HOSPITAL NO.   374-976

TELEPHONE   _____

DATE OF BIRTH   9/28/47   _____

PVT. ( )   NYC (X)   STATE ( )

ANOMALY:

    Harelip, Complete Bilateral
    Cleft Palate, Complete

SURGICAL PROCEDURES:

    Cheiloplasty (2 stages). Age: 7 weeks,6 months
    Palatoplasty (2 stages). Age: 14 months, 2 years
    Abbe Flap to Upper Lip. Age: 8 years
    Secondary Cheiloplasty. 2/10/59
    Rhinoplasty. 7/30/63

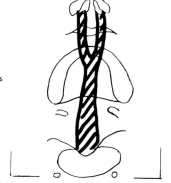

SOCIAL SERVICE INTERVIEW:
Findings:

Questionnaire: Complete   (X)
                Incomplete ( )

    Persistent morning sickness throughout pregnancy

PEDIATRIC EVALUATION:
Findings:

    Rheumatic Heart Disease, Inactive

Recommendations:

    None

ENT EVALUATION:
  Findings: Large Tonsils; Small adenoids
            Ears Negative
  Recommendations: Deviation (rt) of nasal septum
            None
            Re-evaluation in one month

FIG. 5-3   *The Composite Patient Record Book contains a capsule chart of all
patients being followed by the Cleft Palate Clinic. This page contains a
description and a diagram of the anomalies, information regarding past
surgery and social problems, and evaluations by the pediatric and otolaryn-
gology services.*

49TH CLEFT PALATE CONFERENCE: MAY 1, 1961

On April 25, 1961, a secondary cheiloplasty was performed on W. M., now 6 years old. Kodachrome slides demonstrated the long lower lip before surgery. The immediate postoperative result was demonstrated. The lateral elements above the vermilion were removed together with ellipses from the nostril floor. This has made the lip shorter and more natural looking.

CLEFT PALATE PROGRAM

AUDIOMETRIC EVALUATION: 12/18/58

FINDINGS: Mild conductive deafness probably due to cerumen
                 1/23/59 Normal hearing bilaterally

RECOMMENDATIONS: Thorough cleansing of ears
                    Repeat audiometric examination

SPEECH EVALUATION:

DATE RECORDING	FINDINGS	RECOMMENDATIONS
2/15/58	Hyponasality without nasal emission Articulation fair	Speech therapy
3/17/59	Shy, quiet; Voice breathy and weak Rate rapid with omissions and distortions	Speech therapy

PSYCHOMETRIC EVALUATION:

FINDINGS:

RECOMMENDATIONS:

DENTAL EVALUATION: 1/9/58

FINDINGS: Absent teeth
             Delayed eruption of permanent dentition
             Mal position of teeth

RECOMMENDATIONS: Delay treatment until upper teeth erupt
                    Remove supernumerary tooth from palate

PHOTOGRAPHY:

DATE	VIEW	B&W	COLOR
12/12/58	Frontal and lateral		
7/30/63	Front, side, and oblique Face	X	

ORTHODONTIC TYPING:

TREATMENT: Delay orthodontia until upper teeth erupt
4/23/59 – Findings: Upper dental arch in state of mutilation, retardation, and
                     collapse. Mandible extremely prognathic. Prognosis orthodontically
                     exceedingly unfavorable and unpredictable.
           Recommendations : No immediate therapy
3/23/60 Type 8 – Recommend: Remove rt. lower (septic) deciduous molar now.
                            Do not attempt to correct upper central incisors.
                            Remove upper incisors before beginning prosthodontic
                            therapy. No orthodontia indicated because of severity of
                            condition.

FIG. 5-4 *Page two of the Composite Patient Record Book contains information about the patient's hearing and speech, plus psychometric, dental, and orthodontic evaluations. The photographic views and the film types are recorded.*

73RD CLEFT PALATE CONFERENCE: DECEMBER 2, 1963

Since W. M. still has a somewhat tight upper lip in comparison with the lower one, and a receding premaxilla, he was brought into the clinic. His speech and hearing had not been tested for over a year, so appointments were scheduled. Dr. Vollmer, orthodontist, considers his premaxilla in fairly good position and quite stable. According to Dr. Stark, there is no indication now for an Abbe flap to add tissue to the upper lip.

A file of this kind is useful to check previous discussions and recommendations on each patient who is to be presented at a conference. Complete copies of the minutes are bound and distributed to the clinic staff and supporting agencies.

The final and most important log of each child's progress, which appears in the Composite Patient Record Book, is the resident's record including the initial evaluation, details of all operative procedures, and abstracts of later diagnostic evaluations by all departments participating in the clinic. A regular review of this up-to-date capsule chart makes it easy to discover needs, e.g., for follow-up studies, or to set the optimal time for further surgery (Figs. 5-3, 5-4, 5-5).

In our clinic, unlike others, much of the administrative and clerical detail falls to the plastic surgery resident and to the director of the clinic, rather than to a lay coordinator. Under this strict policy, the exact current details of each patient's progress are best known to those responsible for his care. Table 5-1 outlines the responsibilities of each of the services associated with the Cleft Palate Clinic.

CLEFT PALATE PROGRAM

PROSTHODONTIC TREATMENT: Delay insertion of tooth-bearing "plumping" device for upper lip
Oct. '63   Bicuspids crowned

CLEFT PALATE CONFERENCE:
DATE	RECOMMENDATION:
1/5/59	Speech therapy
	Repeat audiogram
	Delay insertion of expansion device in upper dental arch until anterior teeth erupt
	Insert tooth-bearing "plumping" device for upper lip (delay)
	Cheiloplasty
3/17/59	Repeat audiogram - speech therapy
COMMENTS:	Referred to Dr. Eby for opinion re orthodontia
	No further palatal surgery

FIG. 5-5 *Page three records prosthodontic data and enumerates the recommendations of the group made at the monthly cleft palate conference.*

TABLE 5-1. DUTIES OF THE VARIOUS MEDICAL AND PARAMEDICAL PERSONNEL

Age of patient	pediatrician	Plastic surgeon	Social service	Nursing service	Prophylactic dentistry service	Orthodontic service
0–2 weeks	Rule out associated anomaly or other condition which would interdict surgery	Discuss infant's future with parents: perform cheiloplasty	Fill out anomaly questionnaire	Attend to special feeding, care for lip wound		
1 year	Rule out sepsis which may interdict surgery	Perform palatoplasty and primary pharyngeal flap	Maintain personal contact with family to assure follow-up visits	Attend to special feeding		
3 years	Follow and, when necessary, treat the whole child	Follow-up every 6 months			Teach oral hygiene, treat caries	Perform orthodontic typing
4 years					Teach oral hygiene, treat caries	Begin orthodontia to correct loss of incisor teeth, ectopic teeth, dental arch collapse
5 years		Correct mismatched vermilion, dermabrade lip scar, close oronasal fistula, advance columella			Teach oral hygiene, treat caries	

ASSOCIATED WITH ST. LUKE'S CLEFT PALATE CLINIC, ACCORDING TO AGE OF PATIENT

Prosthodontic service	Oral surgeon	ENT service	Psychology service	Anesthesia service	Audiology service	Speech therapy service
				Skilled anesthesiologist monitors sedated child during operation under local anesthesia		
		Treat URI or OM if necessary		Skilled anesthesiologist administers general endotracheal anesthesia		
	Remove ectopic teeth		Perform psychometric examination if indicated		Perform PGSR hearing evaluation	Mother encouraged to teach child miming verses from TV or radio
						If needed, begin speech therapy
Provide temporary prosthesis, speech bulb if indicated		Perform adenoidectomy if needed to correct hearing deficit			Perform audiometric studies	

TABLE 5-1. DUTIES OF THE VARIOUS MEDICAL AND PARAMEDICAL PERSONNEL
(continued)

Age of patient	pediatrician	Plastic surgeon	Social service	Nursing service	Prophylactic dentistry service	Orthodontic service
6 years		Perform pharyngeal flap on palate closed elsewhere if speech deficient after 1 year of speech therapy			Teach oral hygiene, treat caries	Obtain dental arch alignment, ready for bone graft to cleft alveolus
8–10 years					Teach oral hygiene, treat caries	
Adolescence		Perform rhinoplasty, Abbe flap				

ASSOCIATED WITH ST. LUKE'S CLEFT PALATE CLINIC, ACCORDING TO AGE OF PATIENT

Prosthodontic service	Oral surgeon	ENT service	Psychology service	Anesthesia service	Audiology service	Speech therapy service
Provide perma- nent pros- thesis	If neces- sary remove pre- maxilla					

CHAPTER 6

Physical Examination of Newborns with Cleft Lip and/or Palate

STUART SHELTON STEVENSON

About 20 per cent of children with cleft lip and/or cleft palate have one or more associated anomalies, as compared with about 2 per cent of other children. Comparison of numerous published statistics is difficult or even misleading because the different series cover children of various ages and may or may not include stillborn babies and infants who died in the neonatal period. It is reasonable to estimate, however, that when a lip or palatal defect is present at birth, the child's chances of having one or more other anomalies are increased at least 10-fold. Easily observed lip and palate defects alert the physician to search carefully for less obvious but possibly even more serious anomalies, many of which are fatal if not promptly discovered and successfully corrected. Unhappily, defects in less than 50 per cent of surviving malformed infants are correctly diagnosed in the neonatal period; in fact, defects in 20 per cent of them are not discovered within the first year of life.

The incidence of associated anomalies in children with cleft lip and/or palate is estimated mainly from analyses of patients referred to the plastic surgeon. Since approximately 22 per cent of all infants who die in the neonatal period have congenital malformations, as compared with 2 per cent of infants who survive longer, it is obvious that the plastic surgeon's records will not include statistics on the larger group. Many infants with defects of the central nervous system, the cardiovascular system, and the gastrointestinal tract, and many with multiple anomalies, die soon after birth. Published estimates of the incidence of malformations associated with cleft lip and/or palate undoubtedly err greatly on the low side and show a misleadingly high percentage of musculoskeletal and other nonfatal deformities.

The presence of cleft lip and/or palate in a newborn therefore obligates the physician to search diligently for associated, possibly hidden anomalies that may prove fatal if not promptly corrected.

Family and Maternal Histories

The search for congenital malformations rightly begins with a review of the family history, since many of them are inherited or familial, and a review of the pertinent material from the maternal history. If the mother had rubella in the first trimester of pregnancy, the infant must be carefully examined for signs of microcephaly, hydrocephalus, cataracts, microphthalmus, and cardiac anomalies. Deafness, another possibility, is at present difficult to diagnose in very young infants. Infants born of a mother with hydramnios have almost a 50 per cent chance of being malformed. High intestinal obstruction, the most commonly associated defect, must be diagnosed promptly so that corrective surgery can be performed. Defects of the central nervous system are the next most common, but defects in other organ systems may also occur. Conversely, infants born of a mother with oligohydramnios are likely to have an anomaly preventing urination in utero. Agenesis of the kidneys and polycystic lesions of the kidneys are not presently correctable, but urinary tract obstructions are curable if promptly diagnosed and treated.

Medications taken by the mother during the first trimester must be noted. The tragic effects of thalidomide, which caused phocomelia in numerous infants, is well known. Intestinal atresia, another result of this drug, can be cured with prompt treatment. If the pregnant woman has received tetracycline, the infant may have hand deformities or congenital cataracts. If she has taken androgens or estrogens she may give birth to a masculinized, but chromosomally female, infant. Plastic surgery is required to correct this pseudohermaphroditism. Thiouracil and its derivatives may cause neonatal goiter and temporary cretinism, both of which can be treated. Antifolic acid compounds may create diverse anomalies. Radiation, even in small amounts, during pregnancy may seriously malform the fetus. Lastly, a maternal diet deficient in protein is believed to be teratogenic, although this has not yet been clinically proved.

Umbilical Artery

The umbilical cord stump must be carefully examined for the presence of only one umbilical artery—an anomaly that is often missed. Dipping the cut end of the cord in an alcoholic solution of methylene blue shrinks the Wharton's jelly, differentially staining the blood vessels and facilitating the diagnosis. A single umbilical artery, occurring in approximately 1 per cent of all births, is found in about 50 per cent of infants with severe congenital malformations involving any part of the body or even the chromosomal pattern.

Birth Weight

Low birth weight, especially following a gestation period of 10 lunar months, should alert the physician to possible anomalies. While only about 7 per cent of normal infants weigh less than 2,500 gm. at birth, over 25 per cent of malformed infants have a low birth weight.

SPECIFIC PHYSICAL EXAMINATION

A proper physical examination is obviously the physician's best means of uncovering congenital anomalies in newborns. It is assumed that an adequate general examination will be made. The aspects of the examination discussed below are particularly important. Even the most careful observations will not reveal all possible defects; deafness, which frequently occurs with cleft lip and/or cleft palate, as well as most metabolic and chromosomal defects, are seldom diagnosed at this time.

Central Nervous System

Examination of the central nervous system is difficult, but relatively simple procedures can be revealing. The stigmata of mongolism are usually obvious, as is the presence of meningocele, meningomyelocele, or anencephaly. Bilateral clubfoot may be associated with central nervous system defects. A watery nasal discharge suggests an encephalocele herniating through the cribriform plate. A soft pulsating mass in the midline of the skull is probably an encephalocele. Microcephaly and hydrocephalus can usually be diagnosed by measuring the head circumference. It should be borne in mind, however, that a small skull may indicate premature closure of the sutures. This condition, suggested by ridging along suture lines, is confirmed by skull X-rays and is correctable by surgery. Conversely, a large skull may be merely a familial trait or may indicate macrocephaly, which is usually accompanied by severe mental retardation. It is helpful to remember that in early infancy the head circumference, the chest circumference, and the stem length are roughly equal; a skull measurement considerably out of line with the other two suggests trouble. Hydranencephaly is rarely discovered in newborns unless the skull is transilluminated—a procedure that should be routine.

The eyes should be examined for microphthalmia and cataract. Aniridia, a rare condition, may be associated with a congenital Wilms' tumor.

Gastrointestinal System

Diaphragmatic hernia is usually ruled out if breath sounds can be heard well over the entire chest area. Respiratory distress, however, even with normal breath sounds, demands a chest X-ray. This may reveal a congenital lung cyst that requires surgical removal, or even agenesis of the lung. The latter condition is commonly associated with one or more hemivertebrae.

Esophageal atresia may be ruled out by passing a catheter into the stomach. While the examiner's hand rests gently on the abdomen, a puff of air is blown into the catheter and the air bubble is palpated as it passes through the cardiac sphincter. Usually no more than 5 to 10 ml. of gastric fluid can be aspirated. Recovery of 25 to 50 ml. suggests upper intestinal obstruction.

Imperforate anus is ruled out if a catheter can be passed 4 cm. into the rectum. A lower bowel obstruction should be suspected in an infant who does not defecate within 6 to 12 hours of birth. Vomiting of bile-strained material may point to an upper bowel obstruction.

Genitourinary Tract

Deformed external genitalia are usually obvious, but commonly associated upper urinary tract anomalies are less easily diagnosed. A malformation, such as hypospadias or undescended testicle, is an indication for intravenous pyelography. Although the kidneys are often palpable in newborns, unusual size of these structures suggests hydronephrosis or polycystic kidney—also revealed by intravenous pyelography. An inadequate urinary stream may reflect lower urinary tract obstruction; an infant who does not void at all within 24 hours of birth must be thoroughly and immediately investigated. Absent abdominal musculature and malformed external ears suggest urinary tract malformation, with which a single umbilical artery is frequently associated.

Cardiovascular System

Congenital heart disease is often difficult to diagnose in newborns, but several simple observations may be helpful if cautiously applied. A loud murmur, especially if transmitted, suggests trouble. However, 50 per cent of normal newborns have audible murmurs which later disappear. Constant and generalized cyanosis, more marked when the infant cries, strongly suggests a cardiac anomaly.

Constant cyanosis of the upper half of the body almost always indicates transposition of the great vessels with a patent ductus arteriosus. Coarctation of the aorta proximal to a patent ductus arteriosus causes constant cyanosis of the lower half of the body. Cyanosis involving a lateral half of the body is completely benign. In the neonatal period, cyanosis may also stem fiom central nervous system or respiratory system pathology, or from infection, but it usually varies, abating when the infant cries. A commonly observed slight blueness of the extremities and around the mouth merely reflects the newborn's poor peripheral circulation.

Femoral pulsations, although not always palpable during the first few days, tend to rule out coarctation of the aorta. A seemingly enlarged or overactive heart calls for a chest X-ray, which must be interpreted by an experienced radiologist. Cardiac enlargement is difficult to confirm in small infants; for example, a slide taken during the expiratory phase of respiration may suggest enlargement of a normal heart.

Musculoskeletal System

External musculoskeletal anomalies should be obvious to the careful examiner, but a distressing number of malformations, such as polydactylia or syndactylia, have been discovered by the infant's mother.

Location of the midpoint of the newborn's body above the umbilicus suggests the possibility of achondroplasia, in which case a skeletal X-ray survey should be scheduled.

Atresia of the nasal choanae may be fatal if not discovered and treated promptly. It can be easily ruled out by passing a catheter through each nostril into the oropharynx.

Shakespeare, in *King Lear*, speaks of "the foul fiend Flibbertigibbet" who ". . . squints the eye, and makes the harelip . . . and hurts the poor creature of earth." He may be the product of heredity, environment, or both. In any event, the presence of a harelip and/or cleft palate increases by at least 10 times the infant's chances of having one or more other congenital anomalies. An exhaustive physical examination at birth should reveal these conditions so that treatment can be instituted, leading hopefully to good physiological and cosmetic correction.

CHAPTER 7

Nursing Care

ANN M. RICHARDS

As soon as possible, the attending physician discusses the entire situation with the parents of an infant born with a facial cleft. He tells them that the cause is unknown, and that they should have no feeling of disgrace or self-blame. But the mother—feeling confused, frightened, and perhaps guilty—almost always turns to the nurse for comfort and further reassurance. In addition, she may have forgotten or been too embarrassed to ask the doctor certain questions. To answer these questions accurately and objectively, the nurse should have a thorough understanding of the defect, and of her own feelings in relation to it.

Because our society has placed a high premium on physical perfection, the nurse caring for a child with a surface physical defect sometimes finds it difficult to overcome her own feelings of distress; but only by doing so can she establish a satisfactory relation with the parents and the child. The parents are especially sensitive to the reactions of others; any display of revulsion only compounds their feelings of guilt and inadequacy.

CLEFT LIP

When a child is born with a cleft of the primary palate, the parents usually first want to know how soon he can have surgery to make him look "normal." The suggested time varies with different clinics. Primary cheiloplasty is scheduled within the first few days in many institutions—a policy which the St. Lukes's Cleft Palate Clinic adheres to because it has obvious advantages. For example, the newborn is a good surgical risk, and the parents are relieved to have the surgery performed before they take the baby home. At some centers surgery is scheduled during the first few weeks, provided the infant is in good physical condition and free from a cold or infection. In other clinics, cheiloplasty is deferred several months on grounds that increased lip size facilitates operative precision. In this event, the parents must decide whether the infant should be taken home meanwhile or transferred to the pediatric unit. Although hesitant about taking home a "deformed" infant, many feel guilty about leaving him in the hospital. The nurse may help them to weigh the advantages and disadvantages of the two plans. If they decide to keep the infant with the family, the nurse's responsibility is to instruct them in proper home care.

By the time the infant is discharged, the mother has practiced feeding him, using a soft nipple with extra-large holes (Fig. 7-1). Cradling the child in a near-sitting position and directing the flow of milk against the side of his mouth minimize the danger of aspiration or "snorting" the formula through the nares. A disadvantage of this method of feeding is the child's tendency to swallow air so that he must be "bubbled" often. After the baby is fed, his mouth should be rinsed with a small amount of sterile water and the lip cleaned with an applicator dipped in sterile water. The mother should begin to train the infant to sleep on his side, the position required for some time after surgery.

The parents are cautioned to protect the infant from colds or infections, to which his deformity makes him unusually susceptible. It is important to outline the baby's need for specialized physical care while emphasizing that he is normal in all other respects, including his need for love and attention.

The ideal plan is to have the parents talk with members of the hospital team responsible for the baby's care. Many large hospitals have a cleft palate clinic whose team consists of plastic and dental surgeons, a social worker, a speech therapist, and nurses. The plan for hospitalization and further care, discussed at this time, is modified according to need.

When the parents have had the infant home for a time, their attitudes may undergo a change. They seem to become reconciled to the defect, at least outwardly, but are extraordinarily sensitive to any unfavorable reaction on the part of others. The nurse, usually the first person with whom they are in intimate contact in the hospital setting, should be alert to this possibility. Most parents of children admitted for cleft lip or palate surgery appear aggressive, as if daring the nurse to make an unfavorable comment or gesture. An experienced nurse can accept their attitude matter-of-factly, establishing a smooth and friendly initial contact that is important for good rapport as time goes on.

The infant scheduled for primary cheiloplasty is usually hospitalized a day or two earlier for adequate preoperative preparation: routine laboratory procedures, as well as full-face and profile photographs for the "before-and-after" record. The policy of our hospital is to obtain parental consent for use of these photographs by members of the team for educational purposes. A complete blood count and urinalysis are done routinely. Both are usually normal in this age group. Since blood loss during surgery is minimal, no blood is drawn for typing and cross-matching.

All infants and children admitted for surgery are seen by a pediatrician to check their general state of health and rule out associated anomalies. Any required additional studies, such as a chest

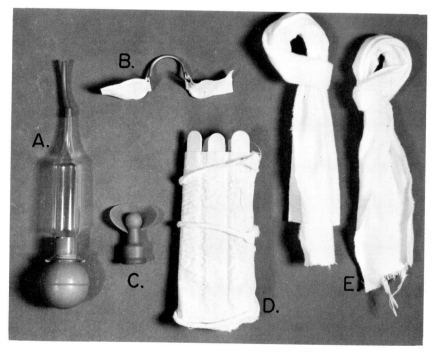

FIG. 7-1 *A. The cleft palate feeder used at St. Luke's Hospital is a Dakin or asepto-bulb syringe to which a small soft rubber tip is attached. B. The Logan bow, a wire wicket devised to relieve tension upon the lip wound, must be tightened daily to remain effective. C. A nipple with a flange is often used to feed the infant before closure of the palatal defect. A soft rubber nipple with large perforations (usually an X cut upon the tip with a razor) will serve as well. D. Elbow restraints (adhesive tape or material into which are inserted wooden tongue blades which parallel the long axis of the arm) are used to prevent the infant from disturbing the recent wound. E. Flannel wristlets may be used to restrain the infant. Also his sleeves may be pinned to his diaper.*

X-ray, are carried out at this time. A visit from the anesthesiologist completes the preoperative work-up.

Before the parents leave the hospital, they must give specific consent for the surgery. The pediatric staff obtains a detailed history, devoting special attention to any problems that may have arisen while the child was at home. A member of the Social Service Department interviews the parents and helps to clarify the future plan of treatment. Also, as part of the research presently under way in our Cleft Palate Clinic, the parents are asked to complete an anomaly questionnaire.

The infant is kept on the same formula in the hospital that he had at home. Experience has shown that if we immediately begin to give the formula with the cleft palate feeder used after surgery, he usually adjusts to it quickly. The feeder consists of a Dakin's bulb syringe fitted with a small rubber tip (Fig. 7-1). The infant (securely wrapped so that flailing hands will not accidentally jar the device) is fed in a near-sitting position on the nurse's lap and is frequently "bubbled," since he swallows a large amount of air. As he attempts to suck, gentle pressure is exerted on the bulb to direct the milk into the side of his mouth. The formula is given at a moderate rate to prevent choking and possible aspiration. If the infant is fed too slowly, he falls asleep. After one or two feedings the correct amount of time needed can usually be determined. Sterile water is used to cleanse the mouth and lip after each feeding, and the infant is returned to his crib and positioned on either side. The nurse must be very patient during the first few feedings in this new manner, which is strange to the infant used to sucking from a nipple.

At our hospital cheiloplasty is performed under sedation and local anesthesia, minimizing the danger of vomiting and aspiration. A feeding is given in the pediatric unit immediately before surgery. No medication is administered preoperatively.

After surgery, the infant is first taken to the recovery room. Maintenance of a patent airway is the nurse's most important responsibility during this period. The baby should be kept on his side and free from mucus. Emergency equipment, such as a laryngoscope, suction machine, airways, endotracheal tubes, etc., should be on hand. If this equipment is needed, it must be used with the utmost care since traumatic handling of the lip could jeopardize the cosmetic success of the surgery. Luckily, most infants with a primary cheiloplasty have little or no distress; however, too vigorous suctioning by an overenthusiastic nurse in one instance resulted in disruption of the wound in unilateral repair.

The infant's hands are restrained to prevent his disturbing the suture line (Fig. 7-1). With small infants, we have found that swaddling adequately restrains the hands and also lends extra security, making them less irritable. With larger infants, we use wrist restraints or pin the shirtsleeves to the diaper. Elbow restraints have proved more effective with older infants. Any type of restraint should be released periodically, when the nurse has time to hold and cuddle the baby.

A Logan bow (Fig. 7-1), placed on the lip in the operating room, relieves tension on the sutured wound. This wire wicket device is attached to both cheeks by adhesive tape. The nurse checks the adhesive frequently, for if it loosens the bow may slip out of alignment. In this event, the surgeon is advised immediately so that the necessary adjustments can be made. The bow should be tightened daily by the surgeon. This is done by cutting the tape attachment at the bow, applying another, and sticking it on top of the old tape, which is left in place. This keeps skin irritation due to tape removal at a minimum.

Since a successful cosmetic outcome depends to a great extent upon keeping the lip completely free of clots and crusts immediately after surgery, continuous saline compresses are applied for the first few days. An ideal dressing that is not too bulky is made by cutting a 2 inch by 2 inch piece of gauze in half. It is held firmly on the lip by tautly applied Scotch tape. We had one incident, fortunately without serious consequences, in which a hungry baby swallowed a loosened piece of gauze. To prevent maceration of the underlying skin, the Scotch tape edges should be affixed to the adhesive tape holding the Logan bow. The dressings are changed frequently to prevent drying and adherence to the sutures.

The parents will undoubtedly wish to visit the infant soon after surgery and should be prepared for his appearance. Regardless of adequate explanations, many parents expect the child's lip to be completely "normal." They should be told, before surgery, that the Logan bow will be in place for several days, and that the baby's hands will be restrained. They are often upset about hand-restraining. The nurse must explain that restraints are necessary to protect the lip but are removed periodically while the child is under careful supervision. If the parents wish to see the completed repair, the dressings may be removed for a few moments. They are told that when the postoperative edema subsides and scar begins to fade, they will be better able to realize the excellent result.

Excessive crying is to be avoided, since it places undue strain on the wound. A bottle of sterile water or glucose water should be on hand for the hungry infant immediately after he returns to his unit from the recovery room. If it is well tolerated, regular formula feeding is resumed with the cleft palate feeder. The child is again held and bubbled in a near-sitting position. Sterile water is given after each feeding to rinse the mouth, and the suture line is cleansed with a gauze square soaked in saline or half-strength peroxide. A cotton swab is not suitable for this purpose, since cotton wisps may adhere to the sutures. When the lip and nostril areas are kept moist with saline, crusts seldom form in the nares. Any crusts can be removed with saline-soaked gauze wrapped around the tip of a small blunt forceps.

One nursing problem may arise following cheiloplasty with the type of anesthesia used in our clinic. Rectal pentothal, which is one type of sedation used with local anesthesia, is sometimes not completely absorbed and often causes skin irritation in the perianal area within a few hours after the first stool. We therefore institute prophylactic "buttocks care" from the moment the child returns to the unit. This consists of removing the diaper and exposing the buttocks to air. The perianal area is carefully cleansed after each bowel movement and a soothing ointment applied. If more vigorous methods are required, the area is exposed to the heat lamp for 15 to 20 minutes after each feeding. We consider the extra time and effort well spent.

The sutures are usually removed by the plastic surgeon on the third to fifth postoperative day, and the saline soaks are supplanted by cold cream applications to help prevent excessive drying that may result in a puckered scar. The Logan bow remains in place until just prior to the infant's discharge. Although the lip is well sealed by this time, direct trauma could spoil the repair. Restraints are still employed and the infant is positioned so that the healing lip is not abraded by rubbing against the sheet.

A child whose lip is healing well and who is gaining weight and free from infection may safely be discharged 7 to 10 days after surgery. Since the mother obviously needs special instructions for home care, we ask her to visit a few days before the infant leaves to practice feeding and handling him. The initial visit is scheduled for a time when the nurse can spend the entire feeding period with them. We have a separate utility room adjacent to the surgical nursery where the mother sits with the baby. To guard against infection, she carefully washes her hands and dons a clean gown. We have dispensed with masks, except in cases of infection. Any indication of infection or illness on the part of the mother is a contraindication to practice feeding.

We have found that it is unwise to expect the mother to remember a great deal of information at a time and therefore generally confine the first session to a demonstration of feeding technique and equipment. If the mother is reluctant to attempt the feeding, the nurse does it, but makes clear that the mother must give the next feeding under careful supervision. Most mothers are eager to try feeding their babies. Their greatest difficulty is learning to exert the correct pressure on the feeder bulb. They usually exert too little, and the infant falls asleep before taking all the formula. This is easily corrected as they become more skilled. When the feeding is over, the cleft palate feeder is briefly explained and taken apart while the mother is still holding and cuddling the baby. Other areas of care are discussed only if she raises specific questions.

In later sessions, as the mother becomes more proficient and less timid, the care is fully discussed. If the formula has been changed, she is given written instructions about the ingredients and preparation. She is told that a 24 hour supply of formula will be sent home with her, along with an asepto-bulb syringe and several rubber tips. Proper sterilization of the feeder is clearly described.

The nurse discusses hand restraints, continued for a few weeks after discharge, and helps the mother work out a plan for their use. The infant may resist swaddling, in which case the easiest method for home care seems to be pinning the shirtsleeves to the diaper. When the restraints are removed during the day, the infant must be watched closely to prevent his injuring the lip by flailing hands. Vitamins, as ordered, may be placed directly on the tongue from a medicine dropper. Solids, given during the first few postoperative weeks only if the baby's hunger cannot be satisfied with formula alone, must be of soupy consistency. They are dropped into his mouth from a spoon.

The Logan bow is generally removed on the day of discharge. The only dressing is a strip of fine-mesh gauze held in place with collodion. The parents are assured that any redness or swelling in the immediate postoperative period is normal and will soon disappear.

Although we are primarily concerned with the mother's role in care of the child following a cleft lip repair, the father is included in the planning if possible. He should witness the proper feeding technique, and some actual practice is most desirable.

The nurse emphasizes that, except for the lip defect, the baby is normal and should be treated like other infants.

If the lip is well healed within 3 to 4 weeks, determined by a follow-up visit to the surgeon, restraints are removed and the child is fed from the bottle. If the infant will require further surgery to correct a flattened nose or revise the scar, the parents are advised of this possibility. Unless he has an associated palate defect, his feeding and care will be essentially the same as for others in his age group.

CLEFT PALATE

A cleft palate defect is usually discovered at birth. An examiner who notes an obvious lip defect will look for a palatal defect; a careful evaluation of the mouth and palate is part of the routine physical examination of newborns. If this is neglected, an observant nurse may be the first to suspect a palatal defect in an infant who has excessive mucus, difficulty in feeding, and regurgitation through the nose. In this event, she reports these signs to the attending pediatrician.

Cleft palate may occur alone or with a lip defect. Although a palatal defect may be more difficult to correct and ultimate rehabilitation may take longer, the parents tend to be more optimistic than those of children with an obvious lip deformity. The nurse, while supporting this feeling, must not minimize the seriousness of a palatal defect.

As soon as cleft palate has been diagnosed, the attending physician should inform the parents. If a plastic surgeon is not available, the attending physician also informs them about the treatment and the prognosis, especially in terms of eventual rehabilitation.

Most surgeons favor early closure of a cleft lip but defer palatal repair for at least a year because the oral cavity is too small for adequate surgical exposure, and the trachea is too small to accommodate an endotracheal tube safely. On the other hand, repair prior to the onset of speech is essential to achieve as near normal anatomy as possible. In our hospital, palatal repairs are scheduled at the end of the first year, unless surgery is contraindicated at that time.

Before the newborn with a cleft palate is discharged from the hospital to await surgery, the mother is instructed in proper feeding methods. If the defect is not extensive, some infants can be fed with a soft, standard nipple with extra-large holes. Others require a commercial cleft palate nipple or the cleft palate feeder described previously. The best method of feeding should be determined before discharge so that the mother can have adequate instruction and practice. Regardless of the feeding method, extreme care is exerted to prevent aspiration, which occurs all too easily. The baby is therefore fed slowly in a near-sitting position. If there is no associated lip defect, he is then placed on the abdomen.

It is often hard to convince present-day parents, guided by child psychologists who teach that too early weaning is harmful, that it is beneficial for these special children to begin taking formula from a cup or spoon at the age of 3 or 4 months. This method facilitates postoperative care, because the infant cannot suck for some time after surgery. Thus, the mother does not have to learn a new method of feeding and the child is less upset by the strange experience of hospitalization and surgery. Admittedly, early weaning is difficult and may require 3 to 4 weeks of diligent effort, but the extra investment of time and patience pays off after surgery.

Solid foods are started at the usual time, but until the child becomes accustomed to swallowing they should be very soft or even soupy. Because solid foods and formula curds tend to cake, the mouth is rinsed with water after each feeding to dislodge all particles. If not done immediately, it may be necessary to remove them with a swab or a gauze-wrapped finger. The latter procedure is not recommended because of the risk of the infant's aspirating food particles.

As soon as the infant can safely tolerate them, various fluids—including juices and soups—are added to the diet. In the immediate postoperative period, when milk is contraindicated, the fluid balance should then be no problem.

Usually the mother of a child with a birth defect tends to be overprotective, insisting upon meeting most of his physical and psychic needs herself. We urge her to delegate some responsibilities so that when the child is admitted to the hospital he is somewhat accustomed to being handled by others. For example, a responsible babysitter can safely feed and care for an older child with a cleft palate.

On admission for primary palatoplasty, the child is examined by a pediatrician. The physicians are especially alert to signs of upper respiratory infection which might make general anesthesia risky, or to associated anomalies that might interdict surgery. Routine laboratory procedures are carried out, and parental consent for surgery is obtained. An anesthesiologist sees the child to determine whether special problems or a surgical risk may be involved. Feedings are withheld for several hours prior to surgery, and the appropriate preoperative medication administered.

Since the fairly recent advent of postanesthesia recovery rooms, most nurses assigned to the pediatric unit are not directly responsible for immediate postoperative care. Obviously, the foremost consideration is maintenance of a patent airway. Any signs of respiratory embarrassment must be immediately reported to the attending surgeon. Luckily, such complications are rare, but tracheostomy has been necessary in a few cases of airway occlusion due to postoperative edema. Because blood loss is minimal, circulatory collapse seldom occurs, and transfusion is rarely needed. When the pulse is stabilized and there is no evidence of respiratory distress, the child is returned to the ward.

Since the new wound could be readily disrupted by the child's placing his fingers or objects into the mouth, he is kept in cuff restraints from the time he leaves the operating room until the repair is well healed—about 3 weeks. Cuff restraints (welcome sleeves) may be made by an ingenious nurse. Several tongue depressors, cut to the same length as the child's arm, are laid side-to-side and covered on both sides with adhesive tape. These restraints are wrapped around the arm from axilla to wrist and tied on with roller gauze. Safety pins attached to the gown or shirt at the shoulders prevent the restraints from slipping if the gauze becomes loosened. The child cannot bend his elbow to put anything into his mouth, but the limited movement permits him to fondle a favorite toy or clutch the blanket for security. Care of the skin of the arms when the restraints are in use must be scrupulous. The restraint's are removed one at a time, and the underlying skin is carefully washed, dried, and soothed with powder or bland ointment. When the mother or a nurse is constantly at hand, both restraints may be removed to permit free movement. Prior to discharge, the mother is reminded to keep the restraints on day and night; otherwise, the infant may suck his fingers or toys, even during sleep.

Feedings for the first few days after surgery consist of water or clear fluids given either by cup, round spoon, or cleft palate feeder. Since milk tends to collect and cake around the suture line, it is usually withheld until the wound has sealed and begun to heal, at about the fourth day. Water is then given after each milk feeding to flush the palate of crusts and detritus.

Crying, which increases tension on the wound, is a problem in the immediate postoperative period. A minimum of crying is easier ordered than accomplished. Liberal visiting hours, with the mother at hand throughout most of the waking hours, diversion by nurses when no family member is present, a favorite toy or blanket—all may be helpful. If all else fails, sedation—usually in the form of phenobarbital —is given to prevent prolonged crying.

Indiscriminate use of antibiotics is to be discouraged. They are prescribed only if there is evidence of infection.

The sutures, of medium silk, are not removed. They are either spit out or swallowed and passed without incident.

If the wound is healing well and there are no complications, the child is discharged in 8 to 10 days.

The mother, who has been given explicit instructions, should have an opportunity to make and apply arm restraints and care for the underlying skin. Liquid and soupy foods are supplanted by a regular diet within about 3 weeks. Hard foods such as dry toast or crackers are avoided for a month after surgery. By this time the palate is well healed, and crying is not dangerous, so the mother need not become overly upset by it.

Rehabilitation problems of the infant with cleft lip or palate have been mentioned only indirectly. Fortunately, the infant born with a cleft lip alone has little or no difficulty in speaking, following repair that has provided a flexible lip of ample length. In our hospital, palatoplasty is accomplished with a primary pharyngeal flap, i.e., the palate is lengthened by adding tissue from the posterior pharynx at the time of closure. An overwhelming majority of these patients learn to speak normally and require no speech therapy. However, recording and evaluation of the child's speech and hearing at the age of 2 years are desirable. If defects are noted, speech therapy is usually started when the child is a little older. There are many things that family members can do in the interim. In fact, the use of the mother teaching under professional guidance has obviated speech therapy in some cases. When needed, speech therapy should be begun at about the age of 4 years. If his development appears slow, he should undergo psychometric testing to determine whether he is sufficiently capable mentally to benefit from such therapy. A secondary palate-lengthening procedure (usually a pharyngeal flap) should be considered for a child who still speaks abnormally after a year of intensive speech therapy.

Dental anomalies are not uncommon in the child with cleft palate, particularly when the alveolar ridge is affected. Such a child will need orthodontia when older. Regular dental visits would be started earlier than usual for prophylaxis against caries. Conscientious tooth brushing, good nutrition, and regular 6-month dental check-ups are essential.

Although the pediatric nurse usually loses contact with patients following primary palatoplasty, problems that may arise in later years will come to the attention of the school nurse. The incidence of ear, nose, and throat disorders is somewhat higher in children with cleft palate than in others. Otitis media, for example, requires conscientious treatment to prevent a chronic condition. If this should occur, the child should have periodic audiometric examinations to detect any hearing loss. In certain centers the nurse may be responsible for scheduling or even administering the tests.

Since it is important for the child to "belong," the nurse may encourage him to gain athletic and social skills, if further cosmetic surgery is contemplated. In any case, nursing care of children with cleft lip or palate is demanding and complex, since rehabilitation often requires many operations over a period of years.

Nursing care of children born with cleft lip and/or palate begins when the diagnosis is made. The nurse should be prepared to give expert care both before and after surgery, and to instruct the parents in proper management in the home. She must therefore be familiar with the specialized equipment and techniques and impart this information clearly and concisely.

By the time the child starts school, most of his initial difficulties will have been corrected or minimized, thanks to vigorous coordinated therapy by specialists of various disciplines.

CHAPTER 8

Anesthesia

ENNIO GALLOZZI

Operative mortality in the surgical repair of cleft lip and palate was 3.8 per cent in 1938 (Veau), and by 1953 it had dropped to 0.2 per cent (Davies and Danks). MacCollum and Richardson in 1957 reported no operative deaths in a series of 2,635 cases. Improved surgical techniques, better knowledge of the anatomy and physiology of infants and children, and modern anesthetic management all share equally in this remarkable accomplishment.

HISTORY

Pierre Franco (1561) and Ambroise Paré (1564) were the first to report on cleft palate in the literature, although cleft lip had been mentioned earlier by several authors, including Celsus and Fabricius d'Acquapendente. Paré was the first to discuss surgical repair of cleft lip and palate. The use of general anesthesia in these operations was not mentioned before 1868. Paré, in his *Introductio Seu Ad Chirurgiam Compendiaria,* indicated that pain was inevitable in such operations: "Quis alia eiusmodi patrare citro dolorem queat." Velpeau in 1839 wrote: "Eviter le doleur dans les opérations est une chimère."

The use of opium for anesthesia in surgical procedures was rooted in antiquity. It became more prevalent after Robert Boyle injected opium into the jugular veins of dogs (1697), often anesthetizing them so deeply that they did not react even to perforation of the tongue. But knowledge of the pharmacology and toxicology of opium was, unfortunately, so rudimentary that many patients died from overdosage.

Chloroform anesthesia in operation for cleft lip and palate was reported by Collins in the *Dublin Quarterly Journal* (1867) and popularized by Thomas Smith during the following year. In 1868 Buszard performed staphylorrhaphy under chloroform.

Chloroform and ether were the most popular anesthetic agents in the latter part of the nineteenth century. Owen's description of the use of chloroform is of interest:

> In my experience there is no operation in which the need of a skilled anesthetist is greater than in that of a closure of a wide palatine cleft in a delicate child. . . . The narcosis should not be deeper than is necessary to keep the child quiet. . . . The chloroformist should not be called to help much in the operative work, still he may be asked to hold the long ends of a suture now and then . . . he may also gently swab the mouth from time to time. . . . The nurse should be instructed to bring the hypodermic syringe filled with ether or brandy. . . .

During the past 60 years anesthesia has been achieved in varying ways—from cyclopropane to hypothermia (Kilduff *et al.*, 1956), and from Avertin (tribromoethanol) to acupuncture (Lu-Ch'ien and Tao-Hsieh, 1960) with varying results. The present good results in anesthesia for cleft lip and palate are due not only to new and safer agents but also to well-trained anesthesiologists, better equipment for pediatric anesthesia, and a broader knowledge of the anatomy and physiology of infants and children.

ANESTHESIA IN THE NEONATAL PERIOD

We now recognize that "the child is not a diminutive adult but an immature organism with anatomical, physiological, and psychological features peculiar to his age" (Anderson, 1959). Most important, from the standpoint of anesthesia, are the child's respiratory and circulatory systems. Still, minute-by-minute functioning of these systems, which are profoundly affected during anesthesia, can be monitored with relatively simple equipment.

Respiratory System

Anatomical differences between the larynx of an infant and of an adult have been well described by Eckenhoff (1951). At birth the tongue is relatively large, the cricoid cartilage is opposite the fourth cervical vertebra, and the hyoid bone is closely related to the thyroid cartilage. The larynx in an infant is therefore more cephalad than in an adult; the large tongue overhangs the epiglottis, which is convex, longer and more "curled" from side to side. The larynx is narrowest at the cricoid ring.

The distance between the vocal cords and the carina is approximately 4 cm. in the newborn infant (Adriani and Griggs, 1954). These authors point out that the right and left bronchi, in a child under 3 years of age, branch from the vertical at an angle of 55°, so that beyond the carina, an endotracheal tube has an equal chance of passing into the left or the right main stem bronchus. Studies by C. Smith (1962) have demonstrated that the division of the trachea in a child is similar to that in an adult, the right bronchus branching at 25° and the left at approximately 70°.

In a newborn the total lung volume in medium expansion is 120 ml. (Engel, 1962). Nonparenchymatous tissue (bronchi, vessels, etc.) accounts for 30 per cent of this volume, as compared with 10 to 15 per cent in an adult. The newborn thus has a relatively larger functional dead space, although this is in part compensated for by tracheal width in relation to total lung volume. In an infant, whose trachea is 6 mm. wide on the average, the ratio of lung volume to trachea is 20:1. In an adult, whose total lung volume in medium expansion in about 3,000 ml. and whose trachea is 15 mm. wide, the ratio is 200:1.

It is generally agreed that the infant's anatomical dead space is equivalent to 1 ml. per pound of body weight, while the tidal volume is equivalent to 3 ml. per pound.

At birth and during the first year of life, the ribs lie horizontally and the intercostal muscles are quite feeble. Respiration is accomplished almost entirely by diaphragmatic movement, which, regardless of muscular force, is limited by the presence of a large liver. Only after the ribs assume an oblique position does the inspiratory volume increase parallel to the increase of the chest's transverse and anteroposterior diameters. Up to that time, an increased demand for oxygen can be met only by increased respiratory rate, the least efficient way of maintaining adequate ventilation. The increased respiratory rate raises the velocity of air flow, which in turn, results in increased resistance.

Minute volume is estimated to be 190 ml. per kilogram of body weight at birth and 220 ml. per kilogram after 1 year of life (Kottgen, 1954). The ratio of minute volume to body surface area changes only slightly from infancy to maturity. Also, the ratio of minute volume to oxygen consumption remains at 0.3 for all ages.

Periodic breathing is a frequent pattern in the neonatal period, especially among premature infants. Their arterial blood has been found to have normal or almost normal oxygen saturation (Graham, 1960). According to Gross (1954), the purpose of periodic breathing is to help the lung expand fully through occasional deep breaths, which are part of the pattern.

Circulatory System

The outstanding characteristic of the newborn's circulation is centralization—i.e., circulation of most of the blood through an inner core at the expense of peripheral flows (Graham, 1960). Narrowness of the peripheral vessels results in increased peripheral resistance. The heart rate is rapid and the stroke volume is small, narrowing the limits of regulation and compensation in the event of hemorrhage.

Investigators agree generally that blood volume in the newborn is 41.3 ml. of plasma per kilogram of body weight and 87.4 ml. of whole blood per kilogram of body weight. The blood hemoglobin level of 17 gm. per 100 ml. at birth decreases gradually to 12 gm. per 100 ml. by the end of the fifth month of life.

Various factors contribute to the newborn's ability to withstand relatively long periods of apnea. Owing to the presence of fetal hemoglobin, the oxygen dissociation curve shifts to the left. The low pH of neonatal tissue, due to the relative anaerobic glycolysis, favors the dissociation of hemoglobin. Infant hemoglobin is 75 per cent saturated at a partial pressure of oxygen of 40 mm. Hg, compared with 50 per cent saturation of adult hemoglobin at the same partial pressure.

Blood pressure in the infant is very labile. Systolic blood pressure is 75 to 80 mm. Hg and diastolic is 40 to 50 mm. Hg on the average. Blood pressure increases only slightly during the first year of life. Sphygmomanometric determinations in newborns and infants are rather difficult. Holland (1954) obtained the most reliable reading with the palpation method using a 2.5-cm. cuff. On the other hand, Kottgen in the same year reported better results with a wide cuff than with a narrow one. Regardless of the method used, subject to individual preferences, it is necessary to stress the importance of monitoring the blood pressure in infants and children because of their tendency to develop shock more readily than adults.

ANESTHESIA FOR CHEILOPLASTY

At St. Luke's Hospital cleft lip is repaired within the first 2 weeks of life, and cleft palate by the end of the first year. The surgical, physiological, and psychological reasons for this timetable are discussed elsewhere. From the anesthesiologist's standpoint it seems the best of many in current use.

Cheiloplasty in experienced hands is performed quickly, with minimal blood loss. Within the first fortnight the infant is best able to withstand the procedure. His anesthesia needs are minimal, and he has not yet developed nutritional deficiencies or infections of the upper respiratory tract or middle ear. Blood chemistry is within normal limits, and short periods of hypoxia, should they occur, are better tolerated than at a later time. Moreover, the plasma's high corticosteroid level provides adequate resistance to stress.

Cheiloplasty is performed under combined sedation and local anesthesia. The operation is usually scheduled for 8 A.M. No preanesthetic medication is used. The infant is fed 2 hours before being taken to the operating room, where thiopental sodium (Pentothal) is administered rectally. The dose, 20 mg. per pound of body weight, was first suggested by Weinstein (1941). A 10% solution of Pentothal in water may be used, although we prefer a prepared suspension in mineral oil packaged in a disposable plastic syringe with a rectal tip. Each syringe contains 10 graduated increments of Pentothal (200 mg. each) with a total dose of 2 gm.*

Administration of rectal Pentothal to an infant requires both patience and exactness. While the nurse holds the infant in her arms, the anesthesiologist lubricates the rectal tip and instills the planned dose, exercising gentleness and caution to avoid trauma. The infant frequently cries and strains, expelling the first dose together with fecal matter. After the infant has become calm, the procedure is repeated. An arbitrary 10 per cent, assumed to have been absorbed, is subtracted from the second dose.

Error is always possible when dealing with an uncooperative patient and with small doses of the agent. We would rather err by giving too light than too heavy a dose. Within 10 to 15 minutes the infant is asleep, though reacting to painful stimuli and with active laryngeal reflexes. We consider this an adequate level of sedation.

An ataractic mixture first described by Laborit (1951) and by C. Smith (1958) may be substituted for rectal Pentothal. The hypodermic administration of this mixture has the advantage of permitting more accurate calculation of the dose. We prefer a combination of Demerol and Phenergan, in a dose of 1 mg. per pound, injected 30 minutes before the operation. Nevertheless, in our experience, when used in a premature infant or an infant of less than 5 pounds, the mixture appears to have a very depressant effect on the respiration.

After the anesthetic has been given, the patient is "mummified" with a drape and placed on a plastic blanket in which circulating water is maintained at 37° C. The head is positioned in extension within a small ring and fixed to the table with a strip of adhesive tape

---

* Abbott Laboratories: Rectal Pentothal.

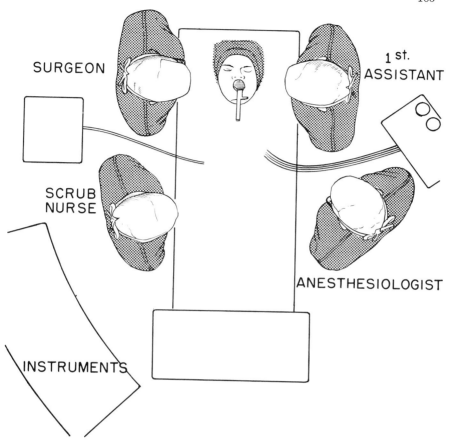

FIG. 8-1   *The anesthesiologist and anesthesia apparatus are on the left side of the patient. The scrub nurse and instrument table are on the right side. The operating surgeon and the first assistant have adequate space and freedom of motion at the head of the table.*

across the forehead. A stethoscope is affixed to the chest and a thermometer is placed in the rectum.

When working in a small surgical field, positioning of the various members of the surgical team is important. We have found that the arrangement shown in Figure 8-1 permits maximum team movement with minimum interference and provides adequate exposure.

After the proposed lip incisions are marked, the surgeon injects a local anesthetic with a vasopressor. Our choice is a solution of 0.5% lidocaine (Xylocaine)* with 1:150,000 of epinephrine. The infant usually reacts to this injection but returns to sleep as soon as the local

* Astra Pharmaceutical Products, Inc.

infiltration has been completed. After allowing 10 minutes for maximum anesthetic and hemostatic effects, surgery is started. The maximum dose of 0.5% lidocaine to be used is calculated according to the formula: Body weight (pounds)/2 = milliliters of 0.5% lidocaine. The anesthesiologist obtains pertinent information about the cardiac and respiratory function by means of the stethoscope throughout the operation. Rectal and water-blanket temperatures are checked at frequent intervals, and necessary adjustments are made to maintain the infant's temperature within physiological limits. Even though the blood loss is very small with almost no risk of aspiration, the first assistant has the suction apparatus at hand and is responsible for seeing that no blood runs into the mouth.

Normally we do not start an infusion, but we would not hesitate to do so or to perform a cut-down should the necessity arise.

Resuscitative equipment, which must be ready for use when anesthesia is started, consists of three sizes of sterile endotracheal tubes, an infant-size non-rebreathing valve, mask, bag, Ayre's T-tube, an infant laryngoscope with straight and curved blades, suction catheters, and a tracheostomy set.

The child should react by the time the operation is completed. The mouth is scrupulously and gently suctioned with a soft rubber catheter to prevent stimulation of the larynx by mucus. With the proper dose of sedation, respiration is satisfactory and the patient retains sufficient muscular tone to prevent drop of the mandible and laryngeal obstruction. In the rare cases of Pierre Robin syndrome, a suture is passed through the tip of the tongue so that it can be pulled forward. We do not use an oral airway because it is not well tolerated by an infant merely sedated and, in addition, may jeopardize the lip repair.

In the recovery room the infant lies prone with the face to one side and is kept under constant surveillance until he is fully reactive. His feeding schedule is then resumed if vital signs are normal.

ANESTHESIA FOR PALATOPLASTY

Surgical repair of the cleft palate is undertaken in St. Luke's Hospital when the child is about 1 year old. Postponement for 1 or 2 months does not affect the surgical result.

A time is chosen when the patient is in "good physical condition"—difficult if not impossible to define. Some anesthesiologists may consider a child's condition to be below the lower limit, while others may find it within normal limits.

The infant's body weight should be within the normal range for his age, and there should be no concomitant disease or infection, particularly of the upper respiratory tract or middle ear. Results of all routine laboratory tests should be within normal limits. Although a "normal" hemoglobin level for a child of this age is controversial, we agree with Salanitre (1962) in considering 10 gr. per 100 ml. of blood as the lower limit of normal. If these criteria are not met the operation should be postponed.

The child is hospitalized in the morning of the day preceding the operation. During preoperative rounds that evening, the physical and laboratory findings are reviewed and operability is assessed. Solid food is withheld for 12 hours and oral fluids for 4 hours prior to surgery.

Atropine sulfate is the only preoperative medication we use for this procedure. The dose for a 1-year-old child averaging 20 lb in weight is 0.3 mg., administered 45 minutes before induction of anesthesia.

We administer the rectal Pentothal (20 mg. per pound of body weight) in the anesthesia room adjacent to the operating room. In rare instances, it may be desirable to administer the rectal Pentothal in the child's room. This procedure should be performed only if resuscitation equipment is available, if the patient can be transferred quickly to the operating suite under the direct supervision of the anesthesiologist, and if there are no other congenital malformations associated with the cleft palate. Once in the operating room the child is positioned on a water-circulating blanket on the operating table; a stethoscope is strapped to the chest wall, and a rectal thermometer is inserted. A 2-inch blood pressure cuff is placed on the right arm. Induction of anesthesia may be completed by the open drop method or by the semiclosed system with one of the infant non-rebreathing valves (Slater, Fink, Frumin) or by the Reese modifications of the Ayre technique. We have no preference regarding the choice of the anesthetic agent suitable for open drop or semiclosed system technique. The choice of the agent should be mostly based on the personal preferences and familiarity of the anesthesiologist.

The anesthesiologist may prefer to omit the rectal Pentothal and induce anesthesia by the open drop, semiclosed, or any other standard technique. With the proper concentration of anesthetic agent, induction is quiet and smooth. All our palatoplasty patients are intubated. Placing an endotracheal tube in a child with a cleft palate is a difficult task, even in experienced hands. The cleft may limit the leverage by the blade of the laryngoscope. It is almost impossible to visualize the larynx in a patient with associated Pierre Robin (micrognathia) or Klippel-Feil (rigid cervical spine) syndrome. Anatomical features of the child's mouth should therefore be evaluated before anesthesia is begun. In cases in which serious difficulties

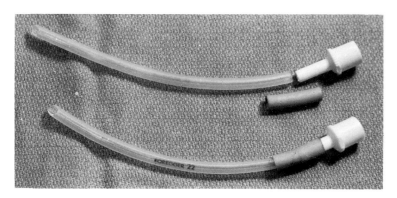

FIG. 8-2   *Connector and endotracheal tube have the same diameter; they are held together by a tight-fitting rubber connection.*

may be anticipated the child should be intubated awake, before in-duction of anesthesia. At any rate, the anesthesia should never be started unless the anesthesiologist is sure that he can control the child's airway at any moment.

When the proper level of anesthesia has been reached, we at-tempt to intubate the child without the aid of relaxant in order to maintain spontaneous respiration. Only if necessary do we administer succinylcholine (1.0 to 2.0 mg. per pound) intramuscularly. A relaxant should be used only by an anesthesiologist very familiar with pediatric anesthesia and, in particular, familiar with cleft palate children.

Oral endotracheal intubation is preferred for surgical and anes-thetic reasons. At St. Luke's Hospital, cleft palate repair involves a primary pharyngeal flap to the uvular area, where a nasal tube would be in the way. We feel that nasal endotracheal intubation in children should be limited to special situations. In routine surgical procedures, the possible trauma to the nasal cavities and the increased resistance to respiration that will result should limit its use.

Anesthesiologists generally agree on the necessity for endo-tracheal intubation in palatoplasty despite the risk of postoperative tracheitis and laryngeal edema, estimated to occur in 1 to 3 per cent of the cases (Morris, 1955). These complications may be prevented by gentle handling and scrupulous attention to myriad essentials during intubation. According to Hollowell (1962), the longer the operation the greater the risk of complication from endotracheal anesthesia. Children 1 to 3 years old are particularly vulnerable in this respect.

Three sizes of sterile endotracheal tubes (Nos. 16, 18, and 20 French) without cuff should be available. The tube is lubricated with a sterile water-soluble emollient cream. It should be long enough so that, when inserted, the tip is no more than 2 cm. below the vocal cords. Aneroid plastic and rubber tubes in the correct size and length all give good results. We prefer plastic transparent tubes because possible foreign bodies inside the tube may be seen. With an aneroid tube a stylet must be used. Despite the most careful handling, soft tissue damage may result if the tip of the stylet accidentally protrudes beyond the tip of the tube.

Insertion of a metal adapter into the endotracheal tube tends to reduce the tube lumen, concomitantly increasing resistance to respiration. Our solution to this problem (shown in Fig. 8-2) is to seal the tube in a wide-bore adapter by means of a tight-fitting rubber connection.

Choice of a laryngoscope blade depends upon the child's anatomical features and the anesthesiologist's familiarity with a particular type. A full set of straight and curved blades should be ready as needed. In our experience, a straight No. 2 blade has proved the most satisfactory.

To facilitate exposure of the larynx, we temporarily plug the palatal cleft with gauze (Leigh, 1960) and use a Dott mouth gag. The proximal end of the tube is anchored by one of the arches of the gag, and the rest of the tube is held between the blade and the tongue, out of the surgeon's line of vision (Figs. 8-3 and 8-4). The pharynx is

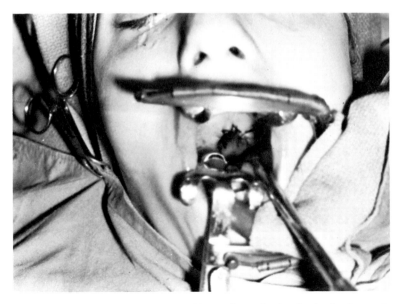

FIG. 8-3 *Dott mouth gag in place. The endotracheal tube is firmly anchored out of the surgeon's line of vision. The pharyngeal flap has been sutured to the soft palate.*

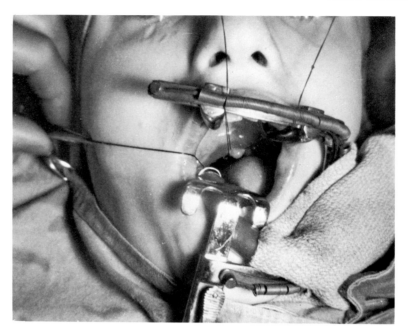

FIG. 8-4 *The Dott mouth gag depresses the endotracheal tube onto the tongue and, at the same time, immoblizies the tube. Thus it affords exposure and safety.*

packed with sterile moist gauze. Anesthesia is then maintained at the lightest level possible, compatible with good operative conditions. We believe that a non-rebreathing technique, utilizing an Ayre T-tube, offers the least resistance to respiration, ensuring an almost physiological level of carbon dioxide in the alveolus.

The T-tube, 1.0 cm. in diameter, has a small inlet tube entering at a right angle. A rubber tube, 1.0 cm. in internal diameter and 0.72 cm.^{2} in internal area, is attached to the open end of the T-tube as a reservoir for anesthetic gases. The tube length is determined by the patient's estimated minute volume. The capacity of a tube with the above dimensions and 2 cm. long is 2 ml. (Ayre, 1956). With this system, concentrations of anesthetic gases and alveolar carbon dioxide depend upon the inflow rate of fresh gas, the patient's carbon dioxide production and minute volume, and the capacity of the T-tube's expiratory limb. Given a flow of gases twice the patient's minute volume, with an expiratory limb capacity equaling one-third of the estimated tidal volume, no rebreathing or anesthetic gas dilution occurs (Inkster, 1956).

If it is necessary to assist or control respiration, this can be accomplished by rhythmic occlusion of the expiratory limb (thumbing) or by connection of a 500-ml rebreathing bag with the tail end open to the expiratory limb (Reese, 1962). Chest movement should be closely observed for signs of excessive pressure in the lungs and for assurance of adequate respiratory exchange. The expiratory limb is always kept in sight to avoid accidental occlusion or compression by drapes.

The desired level of anesthesia can usually be maintained with nitrous oxide and oxygen in a 50% concentration with halothane (0.5 to 1.0%). A total flow of 7 liters per minute is more than twice the estimated minute volume for a 20-lb. baby. Ether and cyclopropane give equally good results, although at present halothane seems to be the preferred agent among anesthesiologists because of the short period of induction and recovery and because it is nonflammable within the range of clinical use.

The surgeon injects a solution of epinephrine and normal saline (1:150,000) in the mucosa of the palate and larynx along the proposed line of incision—a technique that has reduced bleeding from palatoplasty-pharyngeal flap procedure to about 60 ml. Even though ill effects from clinical use of halothane anesthesia and hypodermic use of epinephrine have been reported, a continuous ECG has revealed no cardiovascular changes in our patients given the two drugs in the prescribed doses and concentrations. Papper and coworkers (1962) demonstrated the safety of this combination experimentally.

We use no mechanical devices over the child for protection, feeling that they give a false sense of security. Constant attention to all essential details related to the patient's welfare is still the best safety measure available to the anesthesiologist. He should never permit himself to be distracted by happenings in or out of the operating room.

An infusion of 5% dextrose and water is started percutaneously by microdrip, with the infusion bottle holding only one-third of the patient's estimated 24-hour fluid requirement.

Gentle removal of the endotracheal tube is essential to good repair. When the operation is completed and the patient is still in a surgical plane of anesthesia, any pharyngeal packing is removed and the larynx and pharynx are carefully aspirated. Anesthesia is then discontinued and the patient is allowed to breathe pure oxygen for several minutes. When respirations are regular, the tube is removed at the end of an inspiratory act. Aspiration through the tube is avoided unless necessary, but if necessary, it is done as rapidly as possible. No such attempt should be made while the tube is being removed. A rubber oropharyngeal airway is inserted, and the patient is placed prone with the head to one side. He should remain in the operating room until the pharyngeal reflexes are present and regular and adequate respiration is established.

In the recovery room the child is kept under constant surveillance. A tracheostomy set must always be available. At first signs of laryngeal edema, treatment consisting of steroid infusion and administration of antihistaminics and high humidity oxygen is instituted (Deming and Dech, 1961).

Repair of cleft lip and cleft palate has been carried out during the past 9 years at St. Luke's Hospital with no operative deaths. The surgeon's and anesthesiologist's understanding of each others' problems is believed to be a basic factor in our rewarding experience. To obtain the best possible results, the anesthesiologist should be aware of the patient's anatomical and physiological problems and should be unwilling to compromise in the matter of proper equipment for pediatric anesthesia. When choosing anesthetic agents, he should realize that while no one agent, at present, has been proved definitely superior, nevertheless there is a superior way of using any agent. Familiarity with the technique for optimal use of the anesthetic agent may represent the difference between success and failure of any given procedure.

CHAPTER 9

Initial
Repair of
Cleft Lip

CLAYTON R. DEHAAN

Repair of the congenitally cleft lip has challenged the operator's ingenuity for almost four centuries. Although techniques are constantly being improved, most plastic surgeons are not satisfied with the over-all results and continue their unrelenting search for methods offering better functional and cosmetic effects.

A few basic methods have endured, and the others are simply variations. The myriad innovations in cleft lip surgery are reviewed elsewhere in this volume. Only the techniques found most useful in our experience at St. Luke's will be discussed in detail here.

The degree of involvement of the lip, nose, and alveolus (primary palate) varies greatly and largely determines the method of repair employed in each case. Our team has always considered it illogical to adhere strictly to a single technique, no matter how satisfactory the reported results. Rather, our policy has been to select the type of repair which appears best suited to the patient at hand.

OBJECTIVES AND CONSIDERATIONS

The principal objective in cleft lip surgery is to form the lip and other involved structures into a state as near normal as possible, both functionally and anatomically (Fig. 9-1). The essentials are: (1) a symmetrical lip with a natural appearing cupid's bow, (2) a full vermilion with preservation of the mucocutaneous (white) line, (3) a natural appearing philtral ridge and dimple, (4) a symmetrical nose with restoration of the nostril floor and sill and elongation of the columella, and (5) negligible scarring.

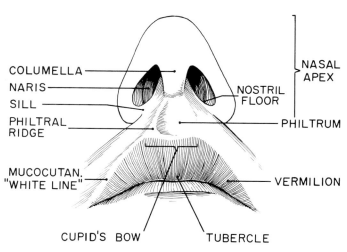

FIG. 9-1 *The anatomical features of the normal nose and lip.*

With some minimal clefts, all the above aims may be achieved at the time of primary surgery. But with many severe clefts, especially if bilateral, the repair leaves much to be desired, and secondary surgery is mandatory.

It is commonly believed that cleft lip surgery is made difficult by inadequate tissue, but actually the only significant deficit is in the prolabial region of the bilateral cleft—a conviction strengthened after reviewing a series of incomplete unilateral and bilateral clefts of widely dissimilar degrees. There seems to be little doubt that the basic problem is tissue displacement rather than deficit. This in no way contradicts the theory that cleft lip and palate result from mesodermal deficiency, which has been well demonstrated by embryological studies. The mesodermal deficiency may be a factor of time, i.e., the tissue is delivered to the lip area but not at the critical period of development.

It is fortunate that certain landmarks on which the repair should be based are invariably preserved in unilateral cleft lip; a careful inspection reveals the midpoint of the lip and also the peak of the cupid's bow on the uncleft side. Regrettably, these points are seldom identifiable in bilateral cleft lip and therefore must be arbitrarily selected.

The cleft margins are drawn upward into the gap toward the nostril floor, shortening both sides. Any design for repair must correct this shortening, so that the lip will be the same length as on the normal side. Creation of a symmetrical and natural appearing lip with a well-defined cupid's bow, a distinct mucocutaneous (white) line, and a full vermilion with midline tubercle is essential. Involvement of the nose increases the magnitude of the problem immeasurably.

In unilateral cleft lip, the columella is short on the cleft side, with its base rotated downward and toward the normal side. The non-rolled ala nasi is rotated downward and laterally, with flattening and depression of the entire alar cartilage on the involved side. The nostril floor, which may be intact, is invariably broadened and flattened, having lost the sill so noticeable in the normal nostril floor. Such marked distortion can be corrected only by a relatively radical approach.

The situation in bilateral cleft lip is somewhat different. Symmetry is easier to achieve, but this advantage is outweighed by the necessity of correcting the protruding premaxilla and broad prolabium, which lacks a philtrum, the markedly shortened columella, the absent alveolabial sulcus, and the flattened, depressed nasal tip. Alveolar involvement may be negligible, but in most cases ranges from definite notching to a total fissure with a prominent premaxillary element leading to early posteromedial collapse of the maxillary segments on the cleft side. Maximal deformity with a complete bilateral cleft may include a premaxilla pushed far forward and upward or even rotated toward one side. Repositioning and stabilizing the maxillary segments and retropositioning the premaxilla are important considerations, and the surgeon must decide whether the steps should be included in the primary operation or postponed. In any event, the anterior palate (alveolar cleft) must be repaired, if possible, in cases of complete cleft lip to prevent persistent oronasal fistulae and to facilitate later closure of the cleft secondary palate.

SURGICAL PROCEDURES

Timing

What is the optimal time for initial cleft lip repair? Although fully cognizant of the controversy on this point, we elect to perform the surgery during the first week of life. (We avoid operating the first 24 hours of life, when the perinatal mortality is so high.) The very young infant who still has immunity from the mother and high resistance to infection tolerates surgery well and requires minimal anesthesia. Blood loss, a serious factor in newborns, can be limited to 3.0 to 5.0 ml. by using local anesthesia with a dilute epinephrine solution (1:150,000). If growth and weight gain are to progress at a normal rate, adequate nutrition is essential. For an infant who finds it difficult if not impossible to suck effectively, this presents a sizable problem which can, however, be solved by early surgical intervention.

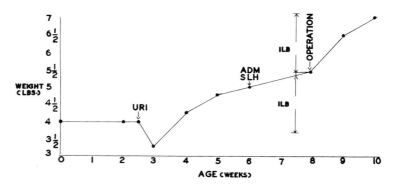

FIG. 9-2 *Weight chart of infant born with bilateral cleft of primary and secondary palates. Cheiloplasty was delayed because of prematurity. Marked weight loss occurred, associated with upper respiratory infection (URI) contracted at age 2½ weeks. No significant weight gain took place until following admission to St. Luke's Hospital (ADM SLH), the lip was repaired at the age of 7½ weeks.*

A moist, healthy nasopharyngeal mucosa—a great deterrent to respiratory tract infections—is assured by early surgery, which effectively blocks the drying column of cool air entering the wide cleft.

Early repair of the nonunited orbicularis oris musculature will provide a biological orthodontic band augmented by the buccinator muscles, which exert a powerful molding action upon the cleft maxillary segments. The greatest narrowing of the cleft occurs anteriorly, although the cleft narrows throughout its length.

One of our patients dramatically demonstrates some of the difficulties that can be encountered with an unrepaired cleft (Fig. 9-2). Since this infant was born prematurely with a bilateral cleft of the primary palate and weighed only 4 lb., it was decided to delay surgery until he reached a normal birth weight. He not only failed to gain weight but also developed an upper respiratory infection at the age of 2½ weeks which reduced his weight by 8 oz., one-eighth of the total body weight at birth. Part of this loss was certainly due to dehydration, but, whatever the cause, it was impressive and serious. Corrective surgery performed at 7½ weeks was followed by a prompt and steady weight gain. In retrospect, deferring surgery because of prematurity was a mistake, as our pediatric colleagues agreed.

Proponents of later repair argue that the size of the lip in the newborn makes accurate repair difficult. We have not found this to be true and, in fact, feel that the slightly longer (1.0 to 2.0 mm.) lip at the age of 3 months is no easier to correct.

Another reason for early definitive surgery is the psychological effect on the parents and siblings. Few parents are prepared for the shock of seeing a cleft lip in their own child. Returning home with a relatively normal looking infant can therefore be extremely important to their morale. Certainly, siblings tend to be confused and frightened by the appearance of a new baby with an unrepaired cleft.

Repair of Unilateral Cleft Lip

Linear

LINEAR CLOSURE

Paring and coaptation of the lip margins was the earliest type of repair of a unilateral cleft lip (Paré, 1510–1590). This simple means of closure has the distinct disadvantage of being useful only for the most minimal clefts—usually with very slight distortion of the nose, slight or no shortening of the lip, and possibly no notching of the alveolus. No attempt is made to correct any nasal distortion at the primary operation, and the lateral elements do not have to be undermined. The cleft margins are trimmed, using a gently curving incision which, when closed, lengthens the lip slightly (Figs. 9-3 and 9-4). The closure line falls along the philtral ridge and crosses the vermilion at the peak of the cupid's bow on the cleft side. Since the orbicularis oris muscle is intact and well developed, a through-and-through incision is unnecessary and inadvisable.

ROTATION FLAP

Rotation

The majority of incomplete clefts present much more complicated problems then described above and call for a more sophisticated approach. Millard has described a repair which we consider excellent for an incomplete cleft. A triangular flap is shifted from one lip mar-

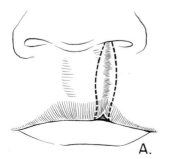
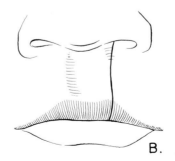

FIG. 9-3 *A gently curved incision to lengthen the lip is used in cases of incomplete minimal clefts. When the orbicularis oris muscle is intact, the incision is carried only through the skin.*

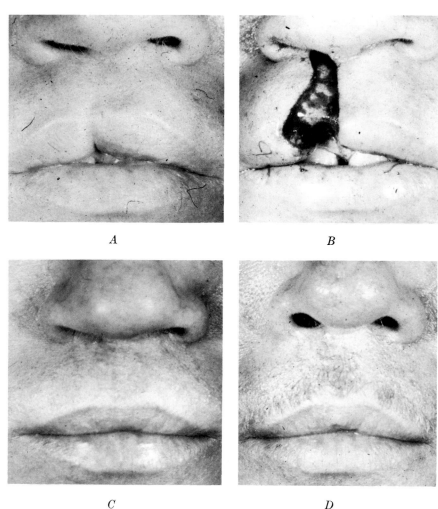

A

B

C

D

FIG. 9-4 *Adult patient with minimal cleft of lip. Simple notching of vermilion is associated with a shallow fissure extending to the nostril floor and deformity of the nose (A). Straight-line repair along philtral ridge (B) results 6 weeks after operation in improved appearance (C and D).*

gin to the other, but, in contrast to other techniques, the tissue is shifted at and below the nostril floor so that a minimal amount of lip tissue is discarded. Advancing the flap beneath the columella gives adequate length to the lip, and the wound is closed along a line closely simulating the normal philtral ridge. At the same time, the columellar base is rotated upward and the flaring ala nasi is drawn medially, thus creating a longer columella and a natural appearing nostril floor and sill (Figs. 9-5 through 9-7). This repair, which has yielded excellent results, is relatively simple technically and does not rely on a set of predetermined points; any adjustments required in the length of the flap can be readily made. An additional advantage is that secondary repair can be accomplished by simple reduplication with extension of the original incisions.

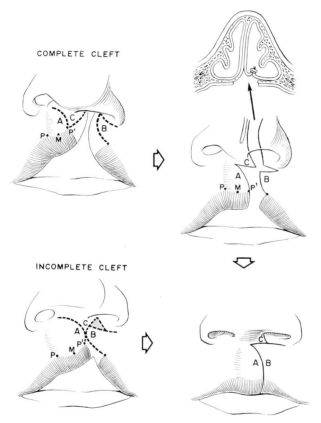

FIG. 9-5 *Rotation flap for repair of incomplete and complete unilateral clefts of lip (primary palate). Point P′ represents peak of cupid's bow on cleft side, easily calculated by measuring distance from midpoint to peak of cupid's bow on normal side, and then measuring equal distance from midpoint of cleft side. Incision carried upward from point P′ just inside vermilion curves inward beneath base of columella. Flap C is created by trimming mucous membrane in complete cleft or excising wedge from nostril floor in incomplete cleft. From point lateral to cleft where the mucous membrane begins to thin out, triangular flap B is outlined. In incomplete cleft flap is carried onto persistent Simonart's bridge. Medial incision in alveolabial sulcus allows mobilization of flap C. Ala nasi is freed from maxilla by similar incision laterally. Wound is closed in layers using fine chromic catgut and fine silk or monofilament nylon.*

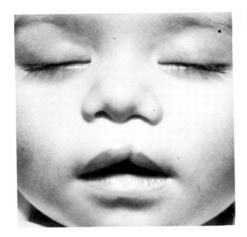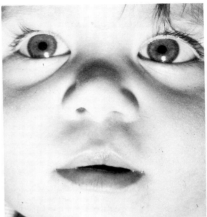

FIG. 9-6   *Incomplete unilateral cleft of primary palate with minimal distortion of nose and alveolus, repaired by rotation and advancement principle of Millard.*

The majority of infants undergo surgery with rectal thiopental sodium or parenteral barbital for basal sedation plus approximately 5.0 ml. of 0.5% lidocaine for local infiltration combined with epinephrine in a 1:150,000 concentration to aid in hemostasis. These agents afford good anesthesia for a period of 2 hours (Chapter 8). Blood loss does not exceed 5.0 ml. (Roth *et al.*, 1963).

After calculating the distance between the midpoint of the lip and the peak of the cupid's bow on the uncleft side, the surgeon measures an equal distance along the vermilion away from the midpoint toward the cleft to establish where the peak of the cupid's bow should be located on that side. A through-and-through incision carried superiorly from this fixed point, just inside the vermilion, to the base of the columella, then across and beneath this structure allows the cupid's bow to drop into its normal horizontal position. In most instances, the incision must be extended across the midline toward the uncleft side to achieve adequate downward rotation. After judging the distance visually, the surgeon can extend the incision if required. A slight overcorrection is advisable.

The rotation incision creates a small triangular flap (*C* in Fig. 9-5) at the columellar base on the uncleft side from which mucous membrane must be trimmed in cases of complete or high incomplete cleft. In most incomplete clefts this flap is created only after a small wedge of skin has been excised from the nostril floor for appropriate narrowing of this area.

The next step is to select a point lateral to the cleft where the vermilion begins to thin, to start a through-and-through incision which is carried upward just inside the vermilion and then laterally beneath the alar rim. A broad Simonart's band, usually present in incomplete clefts, can be used advantageously in forming the triangular flap, obviating a long lateral extension of the incision beneath the ala. In complete clefts, the apex of the triangle is carried high onto the nostril floor and extended farther laterally beneath the alar rim.

Incising the mucous membrane along the alveolabial sulcus medially and laterally frees the small triangular flap (*C* in Fig. 9-5) on the medial side so it can be rotated upward with the columellar base. The ala, freed from its maxillary attachment through the lateral alveolabial incision, can be rotated upward and inward to correct the flare and permit medial advancement of the lip.

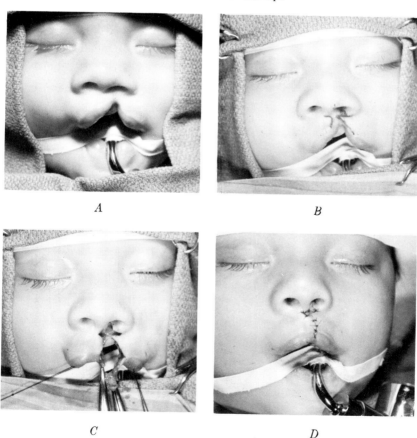

A

B

C

D

FIG. 9-7 *Rotation flap repairing incomplete unilateral cleft lip. Triangular flap formed from Simonart's band is placed beneath columella to rotate the lip downward.*

The complete cleft presents greater problems, since less tissue is available and more radical advancement of the lateral elements is required. Furthermore, an opening in the forepart of the palate (alveolar cleft) should be closed posterior to the incisive foramen as part of the primary repair. An incision is carried posteriorly from the base of the columella along the vomer, and mucoperiosteum is elevated superiorly. Similarly, an incision is carried posteriorly from the vestibule along the lateral nasal wall, and a mucoperiosteal flap is elevated.

The forepart of the palate is first closed by approximating the medial and lateral mucoperiosteal flaps with interrupted 5-0 chromic catgut sutures. The lip is closed in layers with 5-0 and 4-0 chromic catgut for the mucous membrane and muscle, respectively, and fine silk or monofilament nylon for the subcutaneous tissues and skin. The lateral triangular flap (*B* in Fig. 9-5) is advanced beneath the columella and any necessary adjustments are made. The flap (*C*) is sutured beneath the ala, followed by approximation of the vermilion margins at the peak of the cupid's bow. The vermilion is trimmed appropriately and closed with 5-0 chromic catgut. No vermilion is sacrificed before this stage, since it may be needed for deficient areas evident medially, laterally, or on both sides of the cleft.

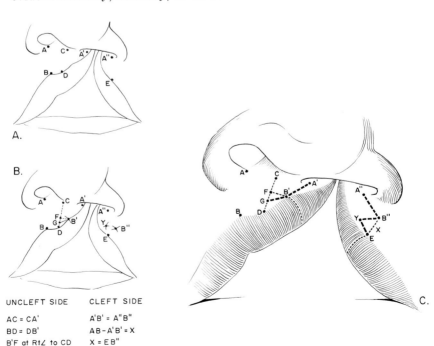

A.

B.

UNCLEFT SIDE	CLEFT SIDE
AC = CA'	A'B' = A"B"
BD = DB'	AB − A'B' = X
B'F at Rt∠ to CD	X = E B"
G = ½ FD	B'G = EY = YB"

C.

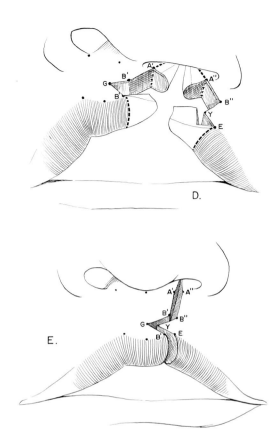

FIG. 9-8   *Triangular flap for repair of complete cleft of lip.*
Drawing A

    A, floor of uncleft nostril at superior end of philtral ridge.

    B, peak of cupid's bow on uncleft side.

    C, midpoint of base of columella.

    D, midpoint of cupid's bow.

    A′ and A″, floor of nostril on medial and lateral side of cleft, respectively.

    E, point at which vermilion begins to narrow on cleft side.

    $AC = CA'$.

Drawings B, C, D, and E

    $BD = DB'$.

    AB minus $A'B' = X$ or required drop from peak of cupid's bow on cleft side to achieve symmetry.

    B′F is drawn perpendicular to CD (midline of philtrum).

    G, point midway between FD on line CD.

    Arc with radius X is inscribed from point E.

    Arc with radius A′B′ is inscribed from point A″.

    Intersection of two arcs establishes point B″.

    Arc with radius B′G is inscribed from points E and B″.

    Intersection of arcs establishes point Y.

    $GB' = EY = YB''$.

The major nasal distortion is corrected by the basic lip repair; no further refinements are attempted at this time. Millard attributes the generally good results to lengthening the columella by upward and inward rotation of its base and repositioning the alar base at the time of advancement. The nostril floor and sill created by upward rotation of the columellar flap (*C* in Fig. 9-5) appears more natural than with other repairs used by the St. Luke's group.

TRIANGULAR FLAP

Results in complete clefts of the lip have been consistently good with an inferiorly placed triangular flap advanced just above the vermilion line (Figs. 9-8 through 9-11). We have had somewhat more

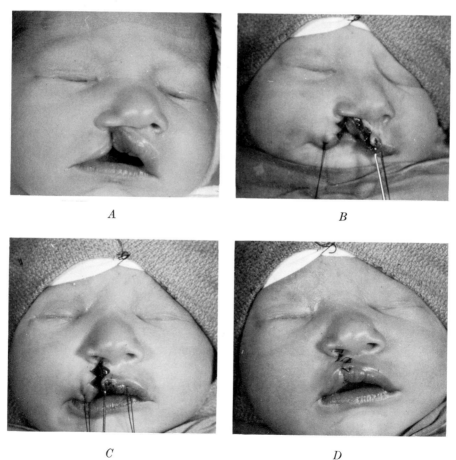

A

B

C

D

FIG. 9-9 *Triangular flap used in complete unilateral cleft lip with Simonart's band.*

success with this method than with Millard's superiorly placed flap, which is sometimes difficult to advance adequately.

Numerous variations of the triangular flap have been advocated. Our clinic relies mainly on a variation of the Tennison "stencil" method described by Brauer (1953), Randall (1959), Marcks (1953), Hagerty (1958), and others, in which all points are predetermined rather than arbitrarily selected.

The columellar base is freed through an incision in the alveolabial sulcus medially. A similar incision laterally frees attachments of the alar base and lip to the maxilla and pyriform sinus.

The palate anterior to the incisive foramen (alveolar cleft) is repaired by carrying incisions posteriorly from points A' and A'' (Fig. 9-8) and developing superiorly based mucoperiosteal flaps along the vomer and lateral nasal walls.

Once the alar base is completely freed, dissection superficial to the alar cartilage on the involved side frees this structure from the skin anterior to the lateral crux so that the ala nasi can be turned inward with less difficulty and the deformed nasal tip can be partially corrected. We do not attempt the more radical repositioning of the alar cartilage advocated by Berkeley and others, preferring to correct any residual deformity when the child is older.

Coaptation of the prepared cleft margins is begun by closing the anterior palate and nostril floor with interrupted sutures of 5-0 chromic catgut. The mucous membrane and orbicularis oris muscle are approximated with similar or slightly stronger material. Fine silk or 5-0 monofilament nylon is used to close the skin after key points such as the vermilion margin have been approximated. We have found a straight vertical incision at the vermilion superior, but occasionally must resort to an onlay flap or interdigitation of tissue from the thicker to the thinner side to produce full and even vermilion at the closure line.

A single through-and-through mattress suture retains the position of the alar cartilage without buckling. Tied over a small ointment-treated gauze bolus to prevent scarring, the suture is removed about 1 week postoperatively.

QUADRILATERAL FLAP

The quadrilateral flap (Figs. 9-12 and 9-13), advocated by LeMesurier, is an excellent repair method, but we feel that certain drawbacks make it less acceptable for general use than the triangular rotation flap. An operator experienced in cleft lip repair by LeMesurier's technique probably has learned to adjust for various deficiencies, but a novice is unlikely to achieve as satisfactory results as with the other procedures described.

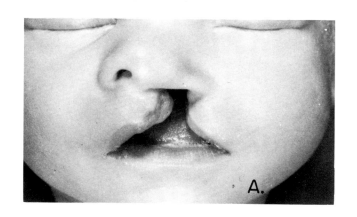

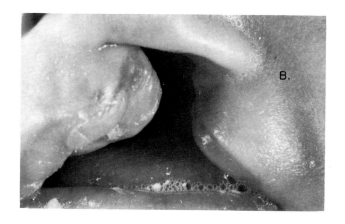

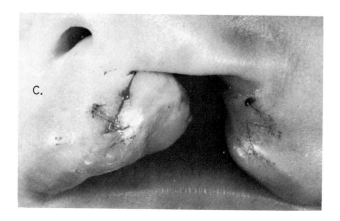

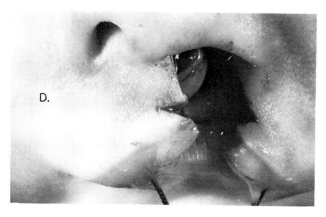

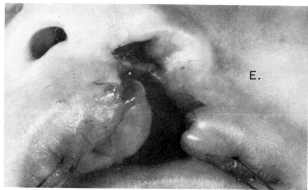

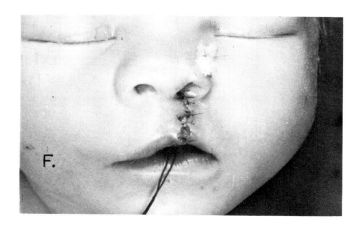

FIG. 9-10 *A and B. Complete unilateral cleft lip. C. Markings made for repair by triangular flap. D. Incisions made. E. Nostril floor formed. F. Repair completed. Through-and-through suture in ala nasi is tied over bolus to minimize "warping" of alar cartilage.*

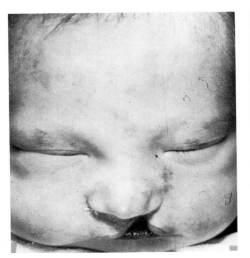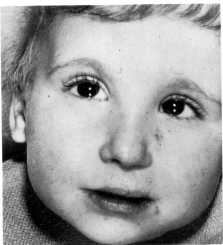

FIG. 9-11 *Complete cleft of primary and secondary palates; lip repaired by triangular flap.*

Measurements made from the cleft side are arbitrary and are designed to construct a cupid's bow that is already present, albeit distorted. An asymmetrical lip with the cupid's bow pulled toward the cleft frequently results. Even a slight miscalculation in the size of the quadrilateral flap can make the lip too long or too short on the cleft side. Although there is adequate tissue to effect repair, no excess can be discarded with impunity; yet we know of no other repair in which a greater amount of tissue is sacrificed. Finally, what appears to be a good primary repair may later be disappointing since unequal growth on the two sides may cause the lip on the cleft side to be too long vertically. For these reasons, we believe the quadrilateral flap should be reserved for secondary lip repair; if the lip already has most of its growth, the results are often better than with other methods.

Repair of Bilateral Cleft Lip

A bilateral cleft of the lip is considerably more complex than a unilateral cleft. Surgical correction is likely to be less satisfactory, since the cleft may be characterized by poorly defined physiological landmarks, a small prolabium with deficient vermilion carried far forward by a protruding and rotated premaxilla, a nasal tip flattened by an unduly short columella, and absence of the alveolabial sulcus.

Good surgical repair rests on two basic concepts: (1) the prolabium, which constitutes the entire soft tissue of the central portion

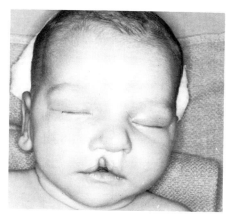
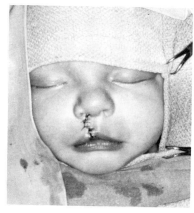

A   B

FIG. 9-12   *Quadrilateral flap inserted into the inferior lip above the vermilion.*

of the lip, must be preserved; and (2) the lateral lip elements should not be used to lengthen the prolabium regardless of its size, since the lip as it develops will become too long vertically.

There is a good deal of controversy over whether lip repair should be done in one or two stages. The two-stage operation is less satisfactory, in our opinion, for several reasons. Two operations are required, each with attendant risk and expenses. When one side only is corrected, the premaxilla rotates toward it, widening the cleft on the other side and twisting the prolabium; thus, the second side is technically more difficult to correct, greater tension is placed on the secondary repair line, and symmetry is not easily achieved. Surgeons also

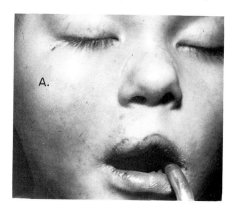
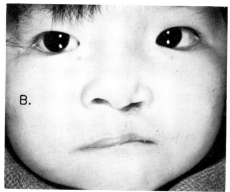

FIG. 9-13   *A. Lip that is too long upon the repaired side (right) following use of quadrilateral flap. B. Lip that is too short upon the repaired side (left) following use of rotation flap.*

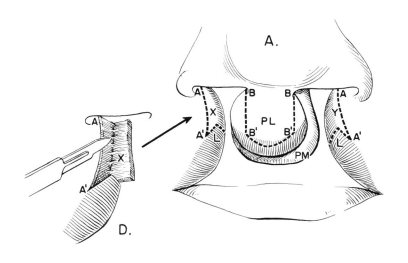

A.

PL

PM

D.

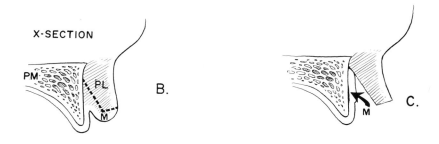

X-SECTION

PM

PL

M

B.

M

C.

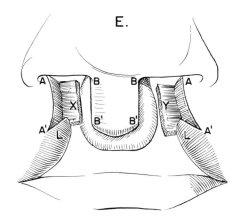

E.

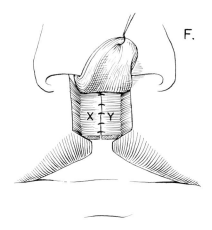

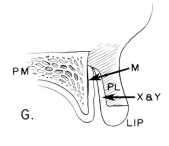

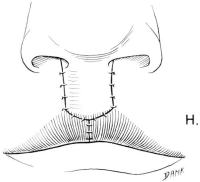

FIG. 9-14 *Operation for bilateral cleft lip.*

Drawing A

   B, point located at base of columella on skin side of mucocutaneous line.

   B′, arbitrarily chosen point at peak of cupid's bow on mucous membrane side of mucocutaneous line.

   A, point at inferior edge of ala on skin side of mucocutaneous line.

   A′, point on mucous membrane side of mucocutaneous line.

   AA′ = BB′.

   Skin lateral to BB′ is discarded. Mucous membrane is incised between B′B′, preserving mucocutaneous white line.

Drawings B and C

   Prolabium is dissected from premaxilla. Mucous membrane flap is formed to surface premaxillary side of alveolabial sulcus.

Drawing D

   AA′ is incised; vermilion and mucous membrane flaps (X and Y) are unfolded.

Drawings E, F, and G

   Mucous membrane (X and Y) is advanced beneath prolabium to surface labial side of sulcus.

Drawing H

   Flaps (L) are advanced inferior to prolabium to form central portion of lip vermilion.

131

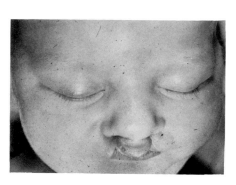
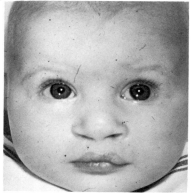

A   B

FIG. 9-15   A. Bilateral cleft lip with protruding premaxilla. B. Postoperative view following closure of both sides at initial operation.

disagree on whether the premaxilla should be recessed at the primary operation. We have not found the prominent premaxilla a serious problem; once the lip is closed, it usually exerts sufficient pressure for the desired retrodisplacement. We feel that operative recession of the premaxilla may well interfere with growth of the central third of the face.

We prefer a straight linear repair of both sides of the lip in a single stage (Figs. 9-14 through 9-16). Prolabial vermilion surfaces the premaxillary side of a deepened alveolabial sulcus, while vermilion from the lateral lip elements is advanced to the midline beneath the prolabium. This repair is strong and assures a deep alveolabial sulcus and a full prolabial vermilion; the esthetic results are consistently good.

Millard has applied his advancement-rotation principle to repair of the bilateral cleft lip. We have not tried the technique, but feel that it warrants consideration, especially for repair of incomplete clefts.

The preoperative preparation, sedation, and anesthesia for infants with bilateral cleft lip are the same as for those with a unilateral cleft. Approximately 5.0 ml. of 0.5% lidocaine containing epinephrine hydrochloride affords good anesthesia and is an aid to hemostasis.

As the definite landmarks facilitating repair of unilateral clefts are not discernible, all points on which the repair is based depend upon the surgeon's judgment and experience. A small prolabium makes the correction relatively more difficult, but it may still form the entire central lip element since under tension the growth potential of this tissue is phenomenal.

The prolabial segment is often too wide following repair and lacks the desired normal appearing philtral ridge with dimple. No attempt should be made to narrow it at this time, as this segment will later furnish ample tissue for lengthening the columella.

We attribute the greater strength of this repair than of most others to two main factors: approximation of mucous membrane flaps from the lateral lip elements in the midline, and wound closure in two planes so that one suture line does not immediately overlie another.

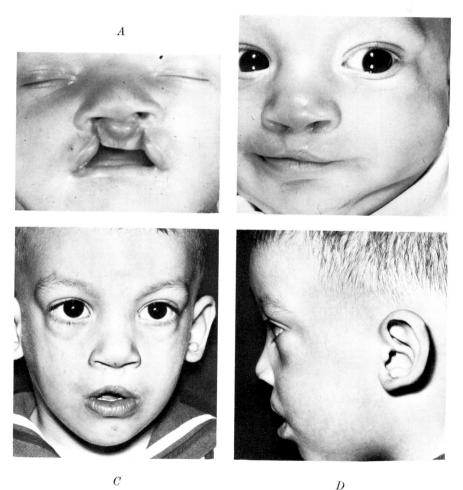

FIG. 9-16 *A. Bilateral incomplete cleft of lip. B. Postoperative view following closure of both sides at initial operation. C. At age of 3 years. D. Profile view shows lax lip with normal "pout."*

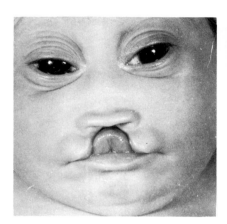
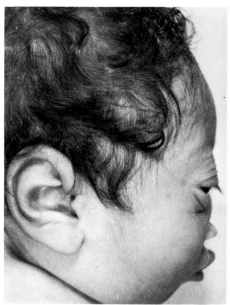

FIG. 9-17 *Median cleft of lip with arhinencephalia, orbital hypotelorism, and absence of nasal septum, columella, prolabium and premaxilla.*

Repair of Median Cleft

Fortunately true median clefts of the lip are rare. They are almost invariably associated with a central nervous system defect (e.g., arhinencephalia; Fig. 9-17) which is incompatible with life, and with hypoplasia of the central third of the face.

We have treated four such infants, all with a typical appearance: microcephaly; ocular hypotelorism associated with bilateral exophthalmos; absence of the entire central portion of the lip, including the premaxilla, anterior to the incisive foramen, but with a normal secondary palate; and a single central ostium (nasal pit) leading into a nasal cavity devoid of vomer, septum, and ethmoid plate. The clefts were repaired by a simplified straight-line technique during the first week of life to facilitate feeding. The infants tolerated the surgery well, but none survived longer than 5 weeks.

Repair of Atypical Clefts

A few clefts of the lip vary anatomically from the commonly encountered unilateral and bilateral types, lying farther laterally and extending upward toward the alar base rather than the nostril floor (Fig. 9-18). All those observed by our clinic have been associated

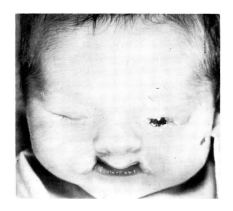

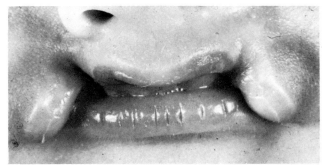

FIG. 9-18 *Bilateral atypical clefts associated with coloboma of the left lower eyelid.*

with defects of the eyes and eyelids. The cleft sometimes crossed the medial cheek adjacent to the nose, connecting the lip to the eyelid (oblique facial cleft). Such rare cases are thought to result from faulty embryonic fusion of the nasolacrimal duct. They have been repaired by the methods described above.

POSTOPERATIVE WOUND CARE

Immediately following surgery a Logan bow is placed across the lip. Although we are not convinced that the device significantly reduces tension, it affords some protection and anchors the moist saline compresses that help keep the wound clean for the next 3 to 5 days. Alternate skin sutures and the alar suture are removed on the third day, and all sutures as well as the Logan bow by the fifth day. A strip of collodion-saturated gauze or Micropore tape across the lip gives external support for another 5 to 7 days.

CHAPTER 10

Secondary Repair of Cleft Lip

RICHARD B. STARK

Secondary repair of the cleft lip, at varying intervals after the initial surgery, is performed to correct elements of the primary palate or to improve the relation between maxilla and mandible. A single imperfection is rare in these cases. Indeed, in bilateral total cleft of the primary palate, many defects may require later correction. A number of imperfections that may remain after the first repair will be discussed, along with appropriate methods of correction.

UPPER LIP VERMILION

Irregular Inferior Margin

The inferior margin of the upper lip may be irregular, overly full, or notched, owing to mismatching at the time of primary correction. In bilateral cleft lip, the lateral lip segments may be too full in comparison with the skimpy prolabial vermilion, or the tubercle may be absent.

The affected vermilion may be removed as a wedge, with accurate approximation. Occasionally, the wedge must be continued into the skin with thorough coaptation of the lip layers and vermilion. When possible, it is well to avoid transecting the mucocutaneous or white line; reflected light makes this ridge between vermilion and lip skin appear white. A surgically interrupted white line never looks normal after resuture.

A minor notch can be corrected by a Z plasty (Fig. 10-1). The central limb of the Z is the excised notch, with one of the Z's end limbs placed along the inferiormost margin of the vermilion. By switching the two triangular flaps, the notch is obliterated.

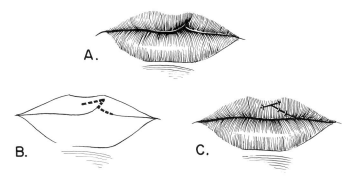

FIG. 10-1 *A minor notch of the lip may be corrected by Z plasty. The central limb of the Z corresponds to the notch, while one of the elective end limbs corresponds to the lower vermilion border. By switching the two triangular pedicles, the notch is obliterated.*

In bilateral cleft lip, the lateral vermilion segments are often excessively full in relation to the prolabial vermilion. The excess vermilion is thinned by removing wedges in the vermilion's axis (transverse or coronal plane), and the suture line is placed at the inferiormost portion of the vermilion (Fig. 10-2). Placing many inter-

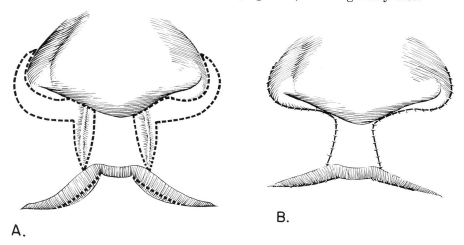

FIG. 10-2 *In bilateral cleft lip, the problems left for secondary surgery consist of excessively wide prolabium, obvious scars, relatively long lateral lip elements, and overly wide lateral lip vermilion as compared with the vermilion of the prolabium. The prolabium is narrowed as the scars are resected. The height of the lateral lip elements is diminished at the nostril base by removal of a perialar crescent. The wide vermilion on the lateral elements is removed at its inferiormost margin and the defect is sutured with multiple fine interrupted catgut sutures placed near the wound margins so as to avoid serration.*

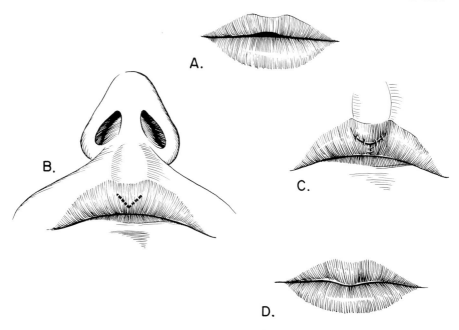

FIG. 10-3 *The median tubercle of the upper lip, which often is missing, especially in bilateral clefts of the lip, may be produced by V-Y advancement. The flap is placed so that its base is at the inferiormost vermilion. As the flap, or V, is advanced from the posterior lip inferiorly, a prominence or tubercle is formed. The V is sutured as a Y.*

rupted sutures of fine chromic catgut close to the wound margins prevents serration of the margin.

The median tubercle of the upper lip, missing in such cases, may be produced by a V–Y advancement flap elevated from the inner or posterior mucosal surface of the lip and based at the lowermost vermilion (Fig. 10-3). This flap is advanced downward, forming a small protrusion. Sutures of fine chromic catgut close the V-shaped donor wound as a Y.

Irregular Superior Margin

Irregularities of the superior margin range from a slight mismatching of the vermilion, forming a stairstep, to gross asymmetry or absence of the cupid's bow.

A stairstep defect is corrected by removing a small triangle of skin, advancing the vermilion, and placing fine chromic catgut sutures (Fig. 10-4). These are placed as horizontal half-buried mattress sutures in the vermilion, picking up only the dermis on the skin side of the wound.

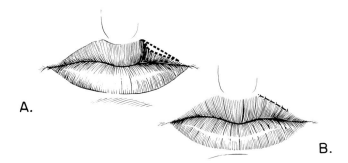

FIG. 10-4 *A stairstep defect of the vermilion at the mucocutaneous line is corrected by removing a triangle of skin and advancing the vermilion upward. To preserve the precise color division between vermilion and skin, it is well to use a half-buried mattress suture, which is placed from the vermilion side and which picks up only the dermis of the skin. (See also Fig. 10-5.)*

When repair involves the mucocutaneous or white line, the points to be coapted should be marked preoperatively, with the patient upright. Accurate location of this line in the supine patient is difficult since most of the blood pools dependently on the dorsal aspect of the torso.

It is occasionally necessary to construct the entire cupid's bow, which in the male child should not be exaggerated. A cupid's bow is carved in the skin; vermilion is undermined and advanced outward and upward and sutured to the "pattern" in the skin (Gillies). Half-buried mattress sutures, catching dermis only on the skin side but tied on the vermilion side, leave virtually unnoticeable scarring (Fig. 10-5). This technique avoids cross-hatch suture marks that obliterate the white line.

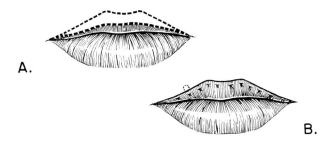

FIG. 10-5 *Occasionally it is necessary to construct the upper vermilion configuration or cupid's bow. This is done by carving or incising the desired bow in the lowermost skin of the upper lip and advancing the vermilion upward. Half-buried dermal mattress sutures are placed from the vermilion so as to preserve the precise color division between vermilion and skin.*

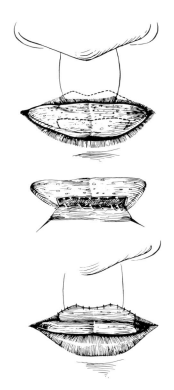

Fig. 10-6 *Another way of providing vermilion in the cupid's bow operation is to use a flap of mucosa from the tip of the tongue. Similarly a flap of mucosa from the lower lip may be used. In either case, the flap must remain attached to tongue or lower lip for 2 weeks or more before it can be transected safely.*

A flap of mucosa and submucosa from the lower lip (cross-lip flap) may be substituted for the vermilion (Lexer). Another method is to suture a flap of mucosa from the tongue tip to the denuded upper lip after carving a facsimile of the cupid's bow (Fig. 10-6). In both instances, the flap remains in situ about 2 weeks, then is freed and inset. Guerrero-Santos (1963) reported no case of wound disruption with the tongue flap.

UPPER LIP SKIN

Notch

Excision of the notch through some of its layers, with straight-line closure, may suffice to correct this defect. In most instances, however, the lip must be incised through-and-through to obtain maximum coaptation of the muscle.

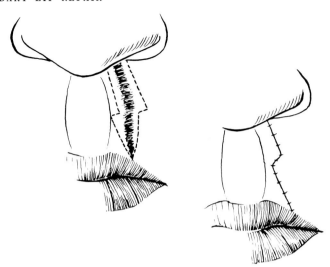

FIG. 10-7 *A notch and/or a furrow of the upper lip may represent a minimal form of cleft lip or the sequel of previous surgery. It may be necessary to lengthen the lip as well as to correct the defect. A through-and-through three-limb correction, a modification of the triangular flap procedure, accomplishes both purposes.*

We feel that correction of an incomplete cleft of the lip, which may be little more than a notched furrow, may require lengthening as well as through-and-through incision of the lip (Fig. 10-7). A three-limbed closure, marked according to Brauer's modification (1953) of Tennison's procedure (1952), postoperatively suggests a traumatic wound rather than a congenital defect. The lip is closed in layers with fine chromic catgut sutures for the mucosa, medium sutures of the same material for the muscularis, and fine interrupted silk sutures for the skin.

Following lip closure, a furrow may occasionally develop owing to incomplete approximation of the deeper structures. It is excised and the muscle is closed as a discrete layer with buried knots. The skin is closed with fine interrupted silk sutures on the surface. A small Z plasty in the central part of the skin closure may be necessary to create a better result.

Obvious Scar

The scar from previous surgery may have widened and become unsightly. If total excision with careful coaptation is not indicated, the appearance may be improved by dermabrasion of the scar and adjacent epithelium. In effect, the scar is made less obvious by blanketing it under the same new cells that epithelialize the surrounding area. As with all other secondary corrections of the lip, this is performed preferably before the child enters school where he may be subjected to cruel taunts from his schoolmates.

Unequal Wound Margins

Unequal wound margins usually result from incorrect measurement of the lip segments in bilateral clefts where the prolabial wound is shorter than the margins of the lateral elements. If closure has been effected without equalizing the length of the wound margins, the longer lateral sides must be shortened secondarily. The least obvious correction results from removal of a perialar crescent of skin and subcutaneous tissue down to the muscularis (Webster) on one or both sides. The crescent must be sufficiently wide to reduce the lateral segment of the same length as the opposite wound margin. Occasionally the shortening must be accomplished at the white line, with skin removed immediately above the vermilion.

Tight Upper Lip

The upper lip frequently becomes tight, lacking a rounded profile and natural pout. Factors causing this condition are erroneous removal of the intermaxillary segment (prolabium and premaxilla), lip closure under tension, and traumatic and widespread undermining over the maxillae. Subperiosteal undermining over the middle third of the face may deprive the developing maxillary bones of blood supply needed for appositional (subperiosteal) bone growth; membranous bones of the face grow in this way up to approximately the fifth year of life (Sarnat and Gans, 1952).

Tight upper lip may be corrected in several ways. When the premaxilla is absent, the alveolar gap may be spanned by a tooth-bearing bridge with a plumping device. The widely flanged "gum" in the labial sulcus pushes the lip forward in the midline, allowing it to fall in a more relaxed position. Fullness can also be added to the tight upper lip by rotating tissue from the nasolabial area; with the removal of perialar crescents, lip tissue may be brought toward the midline without occluding the nares.

When the prolabium is absent, or when it is small and tight, a full-thickness pedicle flap from the protruding lower lip is turned up and hinged on a blood-bearing vermilion pedicle. Abbe (1894) first suggested this technique in the secondary repair of bilateral cleft lip (Fig. 10-8). Since the lips must be locked for over 2 weeks, the Abbe procedure is best performed under local anesthesia to circumvent problems of maintaining a patent airway during and after surgery. No epinephrine should be added to the local anesthesia, to avoid embarrassing the circulation to and from the pedicle. Scar tissue is dissected from the upper lip, which is opened through-and-through. The defect is then measured. The proposed lower lip pedicle flap is located slightly lateral to or below either margin of the upper lip wound. A rectangular flap usually suffices, although it may require a triangle at the inferior aspect to facilitate closure of the donor defect. As the blood-bearing vermilion pedicle is swung upward, the triangle may be split into an M and inset to embrace the columella. The Abbe flap should be no wider than the simulated philtrum. The inferior labial artery and vein, which constitute its vascular supply and which lie between muscle and mucosa, must be preserved to ensure viability. A sound precautionary measure is to incise the lower lip several millimeters below the mucocutaneous juncture with a pointed scalpel. If the nourishing vessels are intact, the flap is developed; if the vessels are transected, the flap may be nourished by the same vessels coming from the opposite side of the flap.

The lips must be immobilized for over 2 weeks. Insertion of a 1.0-cm. piece of rubber tubing through the large apertures on each side of the vermilion pedicle facilitates breathing in the immediate postoperative period. The patient is given semisolids and fluids by straw through one of the openings. The vermilion pedicle is divided and inset at a second operation under local anesthesia.

PHILTRUM

The philtrum, absent from the prolabial segment in bilateral total cleft of the primary palate, may be reconstructed using subcutaneous implantation of palmaris longus tendon (Pickrell) or a U-shaped piece of auricular cartilage (Schmid).

ALVEOLABIAL SULCUS

Part or all of the upper sulcus may be absent. It is always absent in bilateral total cleft of the primary palate. The sulcus is best repaired at the time of the original cheiloplasty (see Chapter 9).

Usually, a partially occluded sulcus can be corrected by a Z plasty of the obliterating mucosal web, or by excising the obliterating band or scar and closing the defect with an advancement flap from the neighboring mucosa and submucosa of the sulcus lateral to the new defect.

When the sulcus is absent, as is often the case in bilateral cleft lip, the structure can be dissected. A mold of the defect is made with wax dental compound softened in hot water; it hardens as it cools.

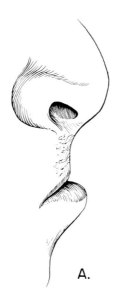

A.

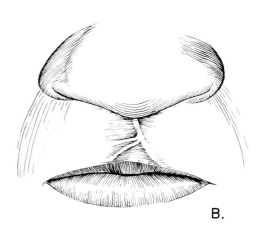

B.

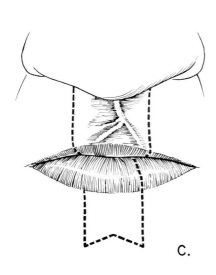

C.

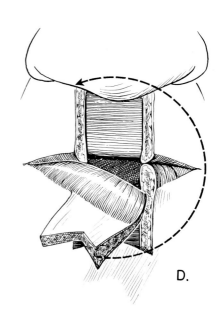

D.

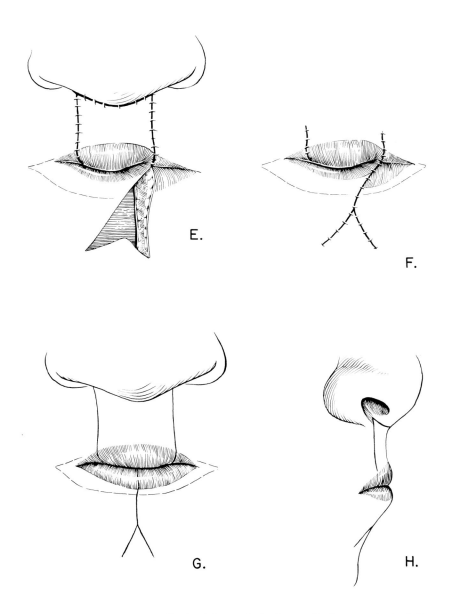

E.

F.

G.

H.

FIG. 10-8 *When the upper lip is tight and the lower lip is excessively full, the Abbe flap will equalize the disparity as seen in the profile view. The scarred section of the upper lip is removed, usually the size of the philtrum; a through-and-through flap from the lower lip is formed lateral to the defect above. The vermilion alone is preserved to provide blood supply to the pedicle flap until the time of vermilion division, a period usually of from 2 to 3 weeks.*

Two such castings are made. The first is wrapped with either buccal or, in the case of girls, vaginal mucosa or with skin taken from a hairless donor site, e.g., the upper inner arm. The graft is glued to the mold with Dermatome cement. The mold is maintained in situ either by sutures of medium silk or by affixing it to a dental appliance with a metal outrigger. A plastic duplicate fabricated from the second mold is attached to a dental appliance and worn after the first dressing for at least 3 months, to prevent creeping obliteration of the sulcus by graft contracture.

Oral-Nasal Fistula

In total cleft of the primary palate there is discontinuity of the alveolus, and teeth are missing. When the cleft is wide, it is difficult to close the alveolar gap at the first operation. Some narrow the gap by maxillary orthopedics; then use an autogenous graft of bone. An oral-nasal fistula develops however, in many cases of complete cleft of the primary palate even after successful lip closure.

Ideally, the operation to close the oral-nasal fistula is performed in the preschool period, and preferably is combined with secondary repair of the lip (correction of vermilion irregularities and/or abrasion of the scar of the skin of the lip). The procedure, under general anesthesia, is facilitated by the use of epinephrine and saline solution (1:150,000) as a vasoconstrictor. The fistula is repaired by a two-layered closure (Fig. 10-9). A semicircular turnover flap from adjacent tissue provides epithelium for the nasal side; an advancement flap of mucosa and submucosa from the sulcus opposite the turnover flap provides oral epithelium.

MOBILE PREMAXILLA

In the newborn, bilateral total cleft of the primary palate with protrusion or 90° forward rotation of the premaxilla (intermaxillary segment) attached to the septum may make its oral surface horizontal. No method for complete correction of this hideous anomaly has yet been perfected. In the past, the premaxilla was brought into normal relation with the alveolar ridge either gradually, by having the mother push it backward manually, or by union of the orbicularis oris musculature through early closure of the two clefts, creating a biological orthodontic band to retrodisplace the segment slowly. Once the premaxilla is properly aligned with the two maxillary segments, they can be joined by fibrous union via adjacent mucoperiosteal flaps across the clefts.

Fibrous union of the bony margins of the cleft may also be achieved by a lateral nasal flap and a small mucoperichondrial flap

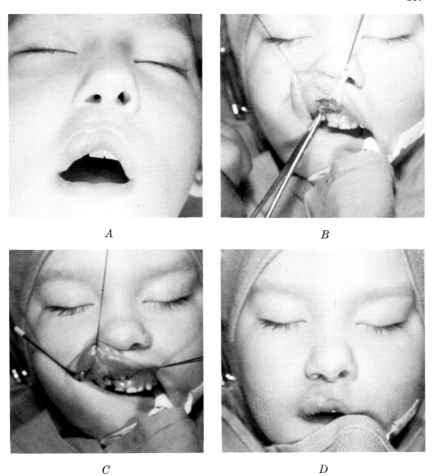

A B

C D

FIG. 10-9 *Correction of nostril asymmetry, dermabrasion of lip scar, correction of disparity of vermilion width, and closure of oraonasal fistula in the preschool period.*

from the nasal septum. If the nasal floor is closed with the cheiloplasty, the surgeon avails himself of the good exposure afforded by the cleft. The septal flap, based superiorly is gently raised from below, then swung lateralward from the midline and sutured to a mucoperiosteal flap on the lateral nasal wall of the cleft. The resulting triangular dead space will close by secondary fibrous union.

If the premaxilla remains mobile instead of fusing with the maxillary segments, the few incisors that erupt are generally of poor quality and must be replaced. The premaxilla is removed, but not before it is no longer needed to plump out the upper lip so that it (and the prolabium as well) may reach its full growth potential. The usual practice is to remove the mobile premaxilla and insert a tooth-bearing prosthesis for lip propulsion and cosmetic effect. Some clinics are removing the premaxilla, then replacing it in a more advantageous position as a free graft of bone.

Recently, in bilateral total cleft of the primary palate, an attempt has been made to unite the three distinct maxillary segments during the first year of life (see Chapter 9). Once they are in close proximity, following maxillary orthopedics, the lip is repaired and the discontinuous alveolus is simultaneously solidified by autogenous bone grafts (Schmid, 1955; Johanson, 1955; Schuchardt, 1958). The cleft's alveolar segments are united by raising mucosal flaps from the alveolabial sulcus as a covering for segments of cancellous bone used to fill the bony gaps.

NASAL DEFECTS

Unilateral Distortion of Nostril and Nasal Apex

In a complete unilateral cleft of the primary palate, almost invariably the affected side shows a widened nostril, with the axis of the naris lateral rather than medial, a widened nostril floor, a flattened nasal apex, and a buckled ala.

The operation to correct the nose definitively should not be performed before adolescence. The nostril floor is narrowed by removing a wedge of excess tissue, the incision involving only the sill and stopping short of the lip. The flattened nasal apex is corrected by the following steps: exposure of the alar cartilages through bilateral intercartilaginous incisions, transection at the medial crus of the normal ala but lateral to the medial crus on the cleft side; free dissection of the two crura and rounding of their sharp margins; joining of the crura with a single medium chromic catgut suture and repositioning them beneath the nasal apex. The twisted cleft ala is corrected by dissecting out and discarding the involved twisted lateral crus. A through-and-through horizontal mattress suture placed in the alar skin furrow counteracts any postoperative buckle. It is tied outside over a small ointment-gauze bolus to prevent skin scarring.

A recent innovation by Reynolds and Horton (1965) sutures the medial crus of the transected alar cartilage on the cleft side to the lateral cartilage of the normal side.

Bilateral Flaring Nostrils

This defect is occasionally found in bilateral total cleft of the primary palate with a normal columella (Fig. 10-10). An excessively wide nasal floor, rather than a snub apex, becomes the problem. The

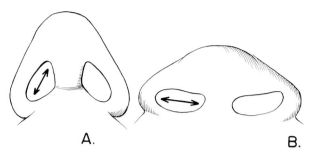

FIG. 10-10 *A. Axis of the naris in the normal nose. B. Axis of the naris commonly found after repair of the bilateral cleft lip.*

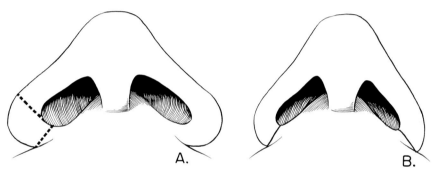

FIG. 10-11 *The excessive ogee curve at the nostril base may be corrected by the Weir excision.*

nares' axes are lateral and the alar cartilages are buckled. Vestibular skin is exposed and the vibrissae are prominent. Correction involves narrowing the nostril floor by wedge incisions and removing the excessive ogee curves of the lateral crura by Weir excisions (Fig. 10-11).

Snub Nasal Apex and Short Columella

In the classic defect following cheiloplasty for bilateral total cleft of the primary palate, mesodermal deficiency of the intermaxillary process results in a short columella and nasal septum and a snub nasal apex. In most instances, use of the entire prolabium to form the central lip has left wide-set and bowed vertical scars. In the ideal correction, the prolabium is narrowed so that the vertical scars more nearly simulate the philtrum; the columella is lengthened; the nasal apex is sharpened; and the nostril floors are narrowed (Fig. 10-12).

After removal of the vertical lip scars, a forked flap (Burian, Pešková, and Fára, 1943; Millard, 1958; Stark, De Haan, and Washio, 1963) is raised from each side of the prolabium with the bifurcation

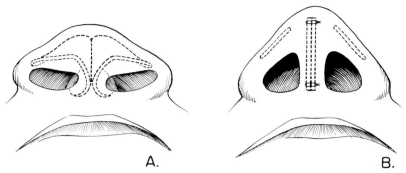

FIG. 10-12 *The snub nasal apex may be corrected in some instances by transection of the lateral alar crura so as to include the domes, by straightening the curved domes, and by suturing the two medial crura together.*

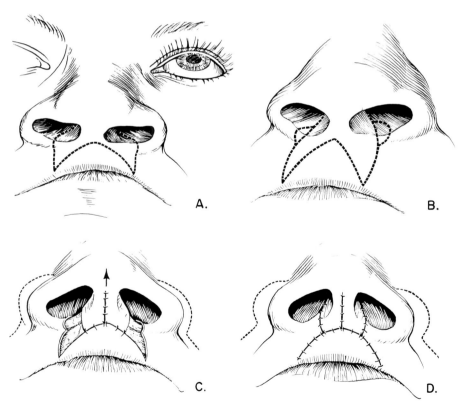

FIG. 10-13 *The classic postoperative defect in bilateral cleft of the lip is the overly wide prolabium, the snub nasal apex with short columella and wide nostril floors. The forked-flap columellar advance operation of Millard is ideal to correct all the defects simultaneously.*

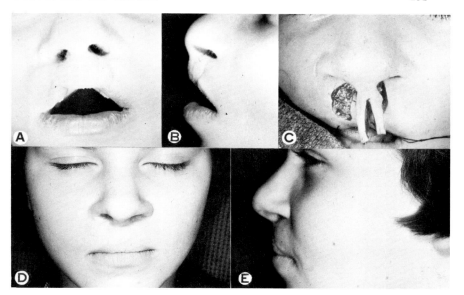

FIG. 10-14 *Forked-flap columellar advance in patient with wide prolabium (A), snub nasal apex, and short columella with obtuse columellar-labial angle (B). A bifid forked flap is raised from prolabial skin and subcutaneous tissue (C). The two flaps are advanced upward and sewn together to form additional columella. The nasal apex is released through intercartilaginous incisions. The postoperative result (D and E) shows increased height of the nasal apex and lessening of the columellar-labial angle. (Courtesy of Cleft Palate Journal 1:116, 1964.)*

at the columellar base (Figs. 10-13 and 10-14). The two prongs of the fork are advanced upward as the columella is separated from the septum. Bilateral intercartilaginous incisions are made by continuing this incision upward. The prolabium is narrowed by removing this pronged flap of skin and subcutaneous tissue, mobilizing the lateral lip skin medially, and suturing it to the prolabial wounds. The two resulting vertical wounds now simulate the philtrum. The columella is lenghtened by advancing the fork prongs upward toward the nasal apex and suturing them together in the midline. The degree of upward advancement of the blunt nasal tip, which has been freed by intercartilaginous incisions, will determine its ultimate sharpness and narrowness. The nostril floors are narrowed by wedge incisions.

Deviated Nasal Septum and Nasal Deformity

Because the nasal septum tends to be deformed and deviated in bilateral total cleft of the primary palate, patent nasal airways depend on a thorough submucous resection including elements of the vomer. The nasal apex can be raised and its shape improved or the entire nose can be reshaped, but these procedures should be undertaken only by surgeons thoroughly familiar with rhinoplastic technique. Kazanjian's method of elevating the snub apex is recommended. Here the alar cartilages, transected lateral to the medial crura, are dissected from the soft tissues of the tip and their sharp margins are rounded. The angles of the two crura are straightened in the midline and joined with a single medium chromic catgut suture. They are then repositioned beneath the nasal apex, which is raised and reinforced by joining of the two alar cartilages together as a supporting post.

The snub nasal tip may be elevated by an autogenous bone or cartilage graft, but this usually elevates the dorsum as well. The graft should be united to the nasal bones at the nasion by subperiosteal transplantation to ensure solid support without movement.

THE MAXILLA

Flattening of the maxillary and zygomatic bony promontories may occur in general hypoplasia of the adjacent facial bones or the skull base. It may be due also to interference with normal bony growth, usually from excessive undermining of soft tissues over the cheeks during the initial operation to close the lip cleft. The flat profile (dish-face) on viewing the face obliquely may be improved by onlay grafts of structural tissue such as cartilage or, preferably, bone. Cartilage grafts may be in the form of blocks, and bone grafts either in blocks or chips (Mowlem, 1952). The chips are introduced via an incision in the alar crease (Ragnell, 1952) or combined with a Weir excision. For dish-face, Gillies and Harrison (1950) advocated osteotomy of all maxillary suture lines and forward repositioning of the midfacial complex, with intermaxillary fixation.

CHAPTER **11**

Initial
Repair of
Cleft Palate

RICHARD B. STARK

A cleft of the secondary palate is a considerable handicap because an incompetent velopharyngeal valve results in defective speech
and deglutition and, in some cases, defective hearing. A cleft that tra-
verses the alveolus as well (cleft of the primary and secondary
palates) affects dentition, both functionally and cosmetically, and
articulation may be faulty. Because of these inherent problems, initial
cleft palate surgery has many goals.

The foremost goal is to construct a competent, functioning, air-
and watertight valve at the junction of soft palate and pharynx, permitting the air stream necessary for speech to be directed not through
the nose but through the oral cavity, and fluids, semisolids, and solids
to be directed not through the nose but into the esophagus. This surgery should be performed early enough to enable the child to begin
speech with a functioning velopharyngeal valve, free of edema. Faulty
surgical closure may lead to fistula formation, compromising the effectiveness of the valve, and to a short velum due to scarring.

The velopharyngeal valve is a complex one, unlike any other
of the bodily petcocks. The soft palate or velum is elevated backward
and upward in a flap-like motion to the level of the atlas mainly by
the paired levator veli palatini muscles. Complementing the flap is the
forward and medianward gripping movement of the superior constrictor hemisphincteric muscle. Both are innervated by the vagus nerve;
both contribute about equally to the effectiveness of the valve.

Among secondary goals are the preservation of normal hearing
by early closure of the palatal cleft, normal development of bony
growth of the central face, and functional and attractive dentition.

Although there is no general agreement on the optimum time

153

for surgery of the secondary palate (and, if needed, the primary) at our center, the palate is closed atraumatically at the age of 1 year to achieve the best speech and to preserve hearing.

Supporting data for palatal closure at various times appear to be somewhat contradictory. On the one hand, dental colleagues indicate that up to about the fifth year of life growth of membranous bones of the central face is appositional or subperiosteal. Growth later than the age of 5 years is largely at the suture lines of the facial bones. These data have been construed as interdicting or limiting early surgery, on the theory that wide undermining of the periosteum of the palatal shelves and anterior surface of the maxillae presumably could inhibit bony growth of the central face. Some centers, mostly European, therefore prefer to delay surgery until the child is of school age.

We do not consider bony growth as our primary goal in cleft palate surgery. Also, when the palatal cleft is left open for several years, air-drying of the mucous surfaces of the palate and pharynx deprives these areas of their valuable defense against upper respiratory infection (the continuous mucous bath). Such children seem to have a continuous cold, which often precludes surgery at the appointed time.

Closure of the palatal cleft when the child is more than 18 months old means that speech in phrases must begin with an abnormal and incompetent velopharyngeal valve. Such speech of necessity is faulty. Whatever the method of closure used, a large percentage of these patients require speech reversal by means of speech therapy and possibly require secondary surgery to lengthen the palate.

OPERATIVE PROCEDURES

Closure

Early velar closures or staphylorrhaphies were accomplished mainly by sutures only slightly less strong than the tissues they were binding together; yet, many staphylorrhaphies were successful, as witness Jonathan Mason Warren's success in 88 of 100 cases in 1867.

However, when the cleft extended into the hard palate, either up front to the incisive foramen or through the alveolus, the task became formidable. Often the soft tissues dissected from the bony shelves of the hard palate were too thin and the sutures cut out. It was von Langenbeck in 1861 who divined that closure would succeed only if mucous membrane were dissected with periosteum as a single layer from the underlying bone. Thus the mucoperiosteal flap came into being.

But this dense layer could not be closed by elevation alone, since it is completely inelastic and incapable of being stretched to

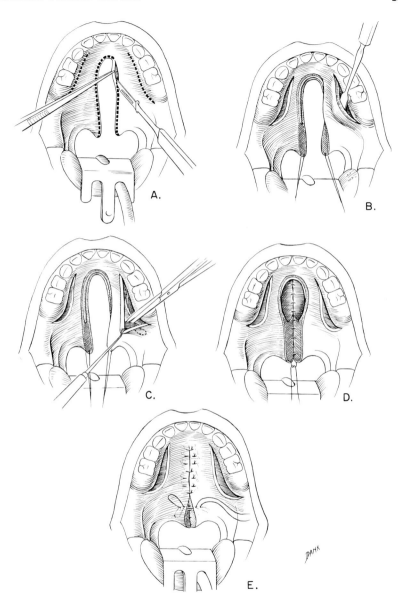

FIG. 11-1 *The commonly performed Dieffenbach-Warren-von Langenbeck procedure consists of paring a strip of mucosa from the palatal cleft, formation of bilateral relaxing incisions, elevation of two bipedicle flaps of mucoperiosteum, fracture of the hamular process, incision of the aponeurosis between hard and soft palates, closure of the nasal side of the flaps, and suture of the oral side, which consists of the placement of vertical mattress sutures through muscle and mucosa.*

cover the open cleft. To effect closure, something else had to be done. That something was a contribution of Dieffenbach in 1826: the relaxing incision was made immediately inside the alveolus, extending backward from the canine tooth around the maxillary tubercle in the region of the last molar; occasionally it was carried along the lateral margin of the velum as well.

Sir William Fergusson of England elucidated the cleft palate problem from an anatomical point of view in 1844, placing the onus for postoperative wound disruption upon contraction of the tensor veli palatini muscles during swallowing.

There followed operations that were designed to reduce tension upon the suture lines by myotomy and fracture of the hamular process (Billroth).

In modern times closure of the cleft secondary palate is most commonly accomplished by paring (rather than incising) a strip of epithelium from the cleft margins, mobilizing the soft tissue surface from the hard palate as a single layer (mucoperiosteum), advancing this layer bilaterally toward the cleft after making a relaxing incision (around the maxillary tubercle and inside the alveolar ridge), fracturing the hamular process, freeing and/or transecting the aponeurotic connection between hard and soft palate, and suturing the cleft margins (Fig. 11-1). These basic steps of the Dieffenbach-Warren-von Langenbeck procedure are essential to close a palatal cleft without tension and with a good chance of surgical success. If done gently and skillfully, this closure method meets all the above goals except that the speech results fall short of the desired standards.

As patients were followed in the dimension of time, success in closure was not tantamount to success in speech. Indeed, a startlingly high proportion (40 per cent) of patients whose palates had been closed uneventfully went on to develop characteristic cleft palate speech typified by nasality and denasality. Dorrance termed this "congenital insufficiency of the palate." Unsuccessful speech, the phenomenon of successful surgery, was dubbed "velopharyngeal incompetence" by Calnan.

Closure Plus Propositioning of the Pharynx

A movement developed to not only close the palatal cleft but also to position the velum closer to pharynx. A number of ingenious attempts were made, many of which have not stood the test of time. Those still viable are procedures to project forward the posterior pharyngeal wall, procedures to move the velum backward, and procedures to tether velum to pharynx.

In 1878, Passavant elevated a pharyngeal flap which he doubled upon itself so that, in essence, he built a pharyngeal shelf. A biological approach to the problem was made by Hynes (1950) who elevated two superiorly based lateral salpingopharyngeal muscle flaps which he interpolated 90° and set horizontally into the posterior pharyngeal wall above Passavant's ridge. By closing the donor defects, the pharynx was narrowed, thus reducing nasal air escape. Others have and are implanting autogenous grafts or inert implants into the pharynx. The list of these inert implants is long: paraffin (Gersuny, 1900; Eckstein, 1902); cartilage (Perthe, 1902; Peet, 1959; Hagerty, 1960); fascia (Halle, 1925); fat and fascia (von Gaza, 1926); and silicone rubber (Blocksma, 1963). When enticed by a "new inert substance," it is well to remember the usually dismal fate of the long line of its predecessors, inserted because no donor wound was required. Also the effect of gravity on these implants, causing migration, must still be appraised.

Closure Plus Retropositioning of the Palate

The attempts to move the velum backward have been more than moderately successful, but even in the best hands they permit normal speech in only about 75 per cent of patients. The best known procedure for palatal retroposition, the V-Y advancement, is that devised by Ganzer (1920) and adopted by Veau and Ruppe (1922) (Fig. 11-2). Other proponents of what is truly a W-V flap were Ernst (1925), Moorhead (1928), Wardill (1928), and the late great Professor T. Pomfret Kilner (1937). Operating very effectively at the United

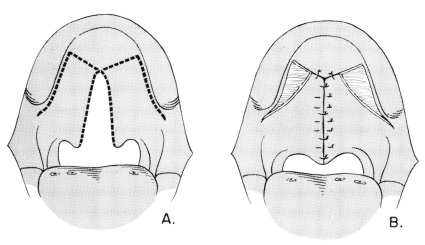

FIG. 11-2 *The push-back palatoplasty based upon the V-Y advancement principle of plastic surgery closed the palatal cleft as well as lengthened the palate.*

Oxford Hospitals in the 1940's and 1950's, Professor Kilner perfected the W-V flap procedure and passed it on with his own exquisite craftsmanship to his immediate disciples—Peet, Osborne, and Reidy—who perform this operation with consummate skill.

With this push-back procedure, the palate was closed and lengthened at the same time. If there were also a cleft of the primary palate (alveolus), bilateral bipedicle flaps were raised, as in the Dieffenbach-Warren-von Langenbeck procedure, and transected obliquely to form four single-pedicle flaps. These were mobilized to the midline to close the alveolar as well as the palatal cleft (four-flap procedure of Wardill and of Kilner).

The crux of the permanent retropositioning lies in the avoidance of raw surfaces upon the nasal side which will granulate and heal by cicatrization. If this occurs, the retroposition achieved at operation will be short-lived, since the contracting scar inexorably pulls the velum forward again.

To avoid open granulating nasal surfaces, many ingenious operative steps have been added to the parent procedure. The Oxford group dissects the pterygoid and vomerine mucosa. The vomerine mucosa then is sutured to the mucosa of the lateral nasal wall, thus lining the nostril floor (Figs. 11-3 through 11-5). In clefts of the

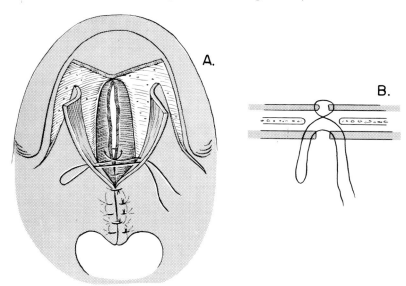

FIG. 11-3 *Closure of the nasal mucoperisteum and mucoperichondrium was considered of primary importance by Veau and those who followed him in the use of the push-back procedure. The potential dead space at the junction of hard and soft palates was closed by use of a figure-of-eight suture placed as a vertical mattress upon the oral side.*

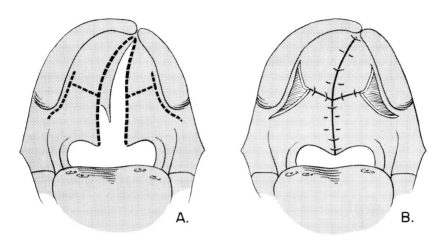

FIG. 11-4 *In complete cleft of the primary palate (cleft alveolus), a four-flap procedure is carried out to close as much of the hard palate as possible.*

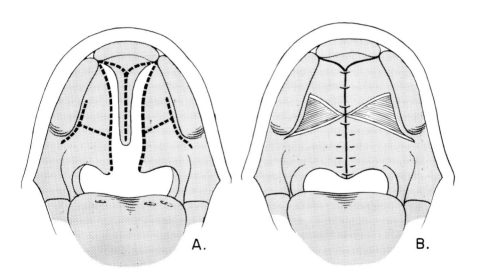

FIG. 11-5 *In bilateral cleft of the hard palate (with vomer exposed), muco-periosteal and mucoperichondrial flaps are elevated and sutured to close the nasal side. A four-flap procedure is used to close as much of the bilateral alveolar clefts as possible.*

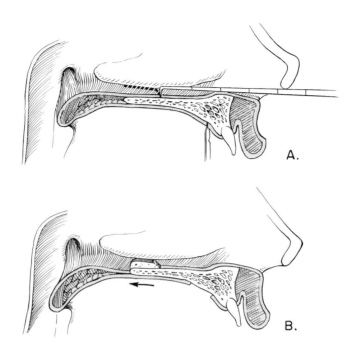

FIG. 11-6 *In incomplete clefts of the secondary palate, Cronin (1957) lined the raw nasal side of the flaps of his push-back operation with nasal mucous membrane. Using a right-angle knife, he transected, dissected, and retro-displaced the mucous membrane of the posterior nasal floor which he used for nasal lining. The resultant raw donor defect was upon the stable bony floor of the nose and did not pull the palatal flaps forward as it spontaneously epithelialized.*

velum, the raw surface produced on the nasal side by pushing the velum backward has been lined by transecting, dissecting, and retro-displacing the posterior portion of the nasal mucous membrane to cover the defect (Cronin, 1957) (Fig. 11-6). The raw surface of the nostril floors thus produced plays no role in the dynamics of wound healing of the velum. As a preliminary step, Dorrance (1943) lined the raw surface with a free skin graft before palatal setback (Fig. 11-7). Millard proposed that a forward area of mucoperiosteum be sacrificed to provide an island flap for the nasal defect (Fig. 11-8).

To obtain additional retroposition, some surgeons chipped the greater palatine neurovascular bundle out of its bony canal to remove its tethering effect (Limberg, 1927; Brown, 1940; Marino, 1944; Conway, 1947) (Fig. 11-9), while Edgerton dissected it away from the soft tissues of the velum.

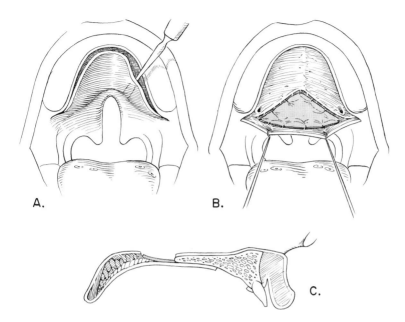

FIG. 11-7 *Before he retrodisplaced the palate, Dorrance (1943) lined the nasal side with a preliminary skin graft. The sagittal view depicts the graft upon the nasal side, immediately posterior to the hard palate.*

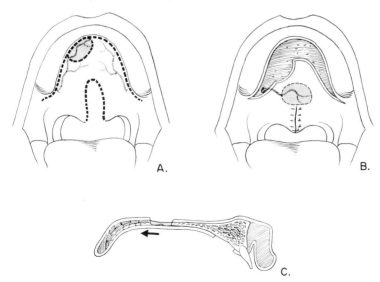

FIG. 11-8 *Millard sacrificed anterior mucoperiosteum to form an island flap, nourished by the greater palatine vascular pedicle, which he turned over and transplanted to line the raw nasal side.*

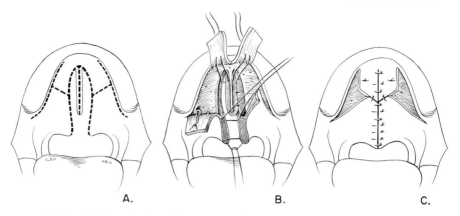

A.   B.   C.

FIG. 11-9 *Besides closing the mucoperiosteum and mucoperichondrium of the nasal side, some surgeons released the tethering effect upon the flaps of the greater palatine vessels. Limberg, Brown, Marino, and Conway removed the posterior bony wall of the greater palatine canal, while Edgerton partially dissected the vascular bundle from the flaps.*

Closure Plus Tethering of Pharynx to Velum

Another approach to the problem was one which added length to the velum by a pedicle flap from the posterior pharyngeal wall. Since the donor wound was closed to promote healing, the pharyngeal diameter was narrowed and the nasal escape of the air column diminished. Schoenborn (1875) described the first truly successful pharyngeal flap:

> I cut at the posterior pharyngeal wall an oblong flap, longitudinal axis medianly, its base down, about 2 cm. wide and 4 to 5 cm. long. . . . The flap has to start as high up as possible at the posterior pharyngeal wall, so that it reaches, after separation, comfortably and without the slightest tension, at least as far as the posterior margin of the hard palate. The incision cut through the mucosa and the muscles underlying it. . . . Then, the mucoperiosteal cover of the palate is separated sufficiently in the usual manner, and it and the soft palate are sufficiently mobilized. Then I . . . sutured it between the two halves of the soft palate. . . . When the patient woke from chloroform anesthesia her speech was tested immediately and was found to be very much clearer than before the operation.

In 1924, Rosenthal of Germany began to use an inferiorly based pharyngeal flap, occasionally combining it with a closure of the Dieffenbach-Warren-von Langenbeck type. The use of the pharyngeal flap as a secondary operation of the "failed cleft palate" increased apace. Padgett (1946), Moran (1951), Conway (1951), Dunn (1951), and

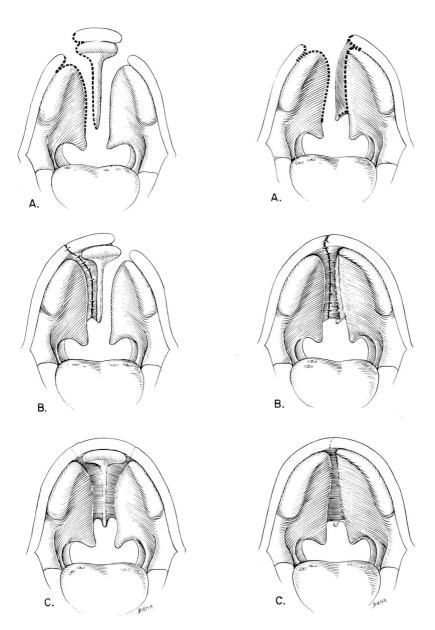

FIG. 11-10 *Some surgeons convert a complete cleft of the primary and secondary palates into an incomplete cleft of the secondary palate at the time of the cheiloplasty. They avail themselves of the unparalleled exposure afforded by the open lip cleft to close the anteriormost part of the cleft of the hard palate. This is done following the principle of Lannelongue (1872), elevating a mucoperichondrial flap from one or both sides of the vomer and suturing it to a mucoperiosteal flap of the lateral nasal wall.*

others were gratified with the high percentage of salvage that the procedure afforded.

The use of the pharyngeal flap as a primary operation has had less attention. Freund (1927) used it upon one occasion. In 1954, the author performed his first primary pharyngeal flap at the time of palatal closure on a 1-year-old child, prior to the onset of speech. Today, at St. Luke's Hospital, we have performed over 60 such operations before speech has begun. We have performed roughly an equal number of primary pharyngeal flaps *after* the onset of speech. The number of secondary flaps performed is now into the second hundred. Webster *et al.* (1958), Cox and Silverstein (1961), and Pool (1966) have reported upon the use of the primary pharyngeal flap as well.

At St. Luke's Hospital we have performed palatoplasty and primary pharyngeal flap at about 1 year of age so as to construct the roof of the mouth which will be free of edema by the time the infant begins to speak. Anticipating that there will be a quartile (25 per cent) of poor speakers by palatoplasty alone using any of the standard operations and lacking methods by divining which children will fall into this group, we have elected to lengthen as well as close the palate. Certainly, the pharyngoplasty (pharyngeal flap procedure) can be performed with ease due to maximum exposure afforded by the open palate.

From our studies, we feel that the primary pharyngeal flap functions in several ways. First, by tethering the velum posteriorward it appears to increase the length of the soft palate as the infant grows in a manner akin to the rapid growth of the minuscule prolabium in bilateral cleft lip, once the prolabium has been attached to the lateral lip elements and put, thereby, upon stretch. Second, although the velar flap does not rise as high as normal in speech, as demonstrated by cineradiography, there is increased and compensating coaptation of velum and pharyngeal flap to the posterior pharyngeal wall. Third, the role of the superior constrictor hemisphincter is augmented as it squeezes against the pharyngeal flap in a side-to-side motion.

Two pharyngeal apertures are left open lateral to the midline pharyngeal flap through which secretions from the nose and paranasal sinuses flow. The pharyngeal flap does not act as a trap to "puddle" secretions. If adenoids must be removed later, skill and a small adenotome are all that are required.

The operation for cleft palate as performed at St. Luke's Hospital is done under general endotracheal anesthesia, with the patient in the supine position. The head is secured in a doughnut and slightly extended by adding two or three folded towels under the shoulders. The entire face is prepared and draped into the field. The Dott mouth gag with the Kilner suture-holder is carefully positioned. The gag must depress the endotracheal tube as well as the tongue, thereby keeping the tube completely out of the surgeon's field. One must be careful not to compress the tube between the blade of the gag and the lower incisor teeth. Once the mouth gag is in situ, however, the operation can proceed with great security. With this unparalleled visibility, the posterior pharyngeal mucosa and musculature are infiltrated as are the velum and the mucoperiosteum of the hard palate, using a saline and epinephrine solution (1:150,000). Approximately 5 to 10 minutes are allowed to pass before the operation is begun so as to obtain maximum vasoconstriction.

Traction stitches of 3-0 black silk are placed into each half of the uvula, and the bifid velum is retracted lateralward, thereby affording unparalled exposure to the posterior pharynx (Fig. 11-11). After the eustachian orifices have been identified, two parallel incisions are made medial to the fossae of Rosenmüller, but so placed to provide the widest possible pharyngeal flap, yet without directly impinging upon the orifices of the eustachian tubes. The incisions are carried down to the prevertebral fascia; a hook is used for retraction, and the superior constrictor muscle is dissected from the fascia using right-angle scissors. By gently spreading the scissors, the muscle dissects from the fascia with ease. The end of the flap is then transected using the same scissors.

Which end is transected (i.e., superior or inferior) depends upon which direction one is basing the flap. The decision is often dictated by whether or not an adenoid pad is present at the superior end of the flap. If so, we feel it is better to transect the inferior end (which is free of adenoid tissue), thereby constructing a superiorly based flap. We do not feel that there is any special intrinsic merit to either an inferiorly or a superiorly based flap.

Traction stitches are placed in the end of the pharyngeal flap so as to keep it out of the field. The lateral margins of the flap's donor site are undermined, using scissors to spread, and three or four 3-0 black silk sutures close, the donor defect in the midline. A small triangular area necessarily is left at either end of the wound to granulate.

Attention is now paid to the cleft palate. (In this description, we are dealing with a complete cleft of the secondary palate.) We prefer to pare away the mucosal margins of the cleft so as to expose the muscle, using a pointed knife blade (No. 11). We try to do this as one continuous rim of mucous membrane; we are certain thereby that no epithelium has been left behind which will produce a fistula.

Bilateral relaxing incisions are made. These are carried from the anteriormost extension of the cleft palate at about the canine tooth, inside the teeth, around the posterior molar and the maxillary tubercle, and then for about a centimeter along the lateral cheek wall

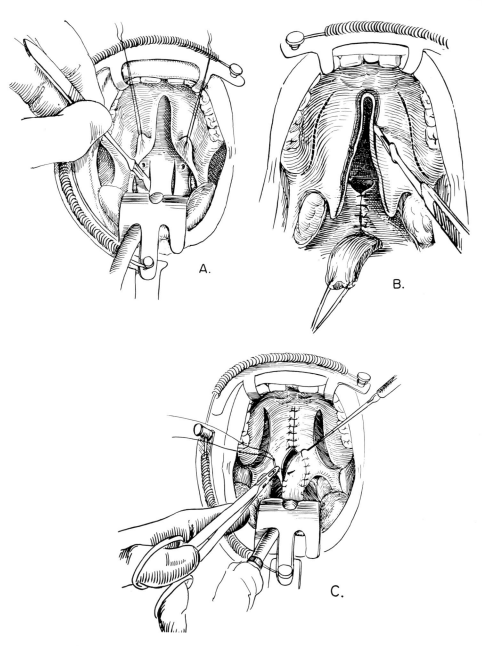

FIG. 11-11   *A. The superb exposure provided by the open palatal cleft permits elevation of the primary pharyngeal flap under direct vision, a safeguard to the fossae of Rosenmüller. The flap is made as wide as possible without encroaching upon these fossae. Incision is carried down to the prevertebral fascia, and the flap is elevated. It appears not to matter which direction (superiorly or inferiorly) the flap is based. B. The palatal cleft is closed in the manner of the Dieffenbach-Warren-von Langenbeck procedure. C. A small trapdoor of mucosa and muscle is turned back to line partially the pharyngeal flap which is sutured into the resultant defect.*

anterior to the tonsillar pillar. Using scissors, these incisions are spread slightly and packed with 1-inch nasal packing which has been soaked in saline and epinephrine. In this manner blood loss will be minimized. The mucoperiosteum is dissected from the hard palate in gentle fashion as a single layer, using a freer periosteal elevator. It is well to elevate this tough layer using a side-to-side movement of the elevator rather than pushing the instrument forward with a motion that is apt to tear the tissues. As one gets posteriorward, using dissecting scissors, one then can spread the incision in the velum, defining thereby the position of the hamular process, which is transected by scissors.

The median advancement of the two flaps that have been formed is impaired by the attachment of the aponeurosis between the hard and soft palates; this is transected using scissors. A raw nasal surface is left, but the attachment of the pharyngeal flap will exert backward traction so the raw surface does not become a factor in shortening the velum.

The bipedicled flaps are brought easily to the midline without tension. Closure is started anteriorward with 3-0 black silk interrupted sutures in the mucoperiosteum. One can place approximately three or four 4-0 chromic catgut sutures in the nasal mucosa and approximately three or four of the same sutures in the musculature of the velum. Following this, using 3-0 black silk, several vertical mattress stitches are placed in the velum, including muscle in the deep bite and mucosa in the shallow bite.

At this point, the pharyngeal flap is brought forward. A small amount of mucosa in the posterior aspect of the velum is trimmed away and the flap is inserted on the muscularis of the velum, again using approximately six or seven 3-0 black silk interrupted sutures. No packing is used. The lateral apertures produced by the relaxing incision rapidly epithelialize and pose no problem in the postoperative management.

All infants undergoing this operation are sent to the recovery room until they have reacted fully. We have not had to transfuse a single one of these patients. Sutures are left to come out spontaneously.

We have been charged with unnecessary surgery by using the pharyngeal flap upon the 75 per cent of patients who would have spoken well by other surgical means. If we could diagnose at 1 year those patients who are endowed with adynamic and insufficient soft palates, of course we would add the pharyngeal flap only in those cases. Unfortunately, we cannot as yet make this diagnosis. We have been charged, in the same vein, with performing prophylactic surgery. In response, we can only say that although only a small number of us in the United States will be exposed to smallpox, few would eschew

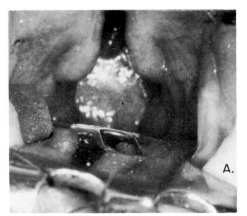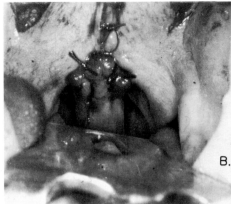

FIG. 11-12 *A. Open palatal cleft. The two tags of the bifid uvula are stuck to their respective tonsillar pillars. B. Palatoplasty and primary pharyngeal flap for a cleft of the secondary palate in a 1-year-old infant.*

prophylactic vaccination against this devastating disease. Since the addition of the pharyngeal flap to primary palatoplasty adds little to the operating time (average total time for the combined procedure is 95 minutes) and virtually nothing to blood loss (average blood loss is 60 ml.), we do not find ourselves in agreement with these disclaimers.

The author feels strongly that in areas of the world where the cleft palate patient may never return to the hospital and where there is no follow-up, the combined palatoplasty and pharyngeal flap procedure offers this patient the best hope for the development of normal speech.

It is obvious to those of us using this approach that the procedure has great merit. It is equally obvious that we shall not convert any of our colleagues by enthusiasm alone. We are studying these patients carefully. Unfortunately, one must wait until the patient is about 5 years old before an accurate appraisal of speech can be made, hence the final opinion of this combined palatopharyngoplasty will not be forthcoming for another decade.

CHAPTER 12

Secondary Repair of Cleft Palate

RICHARD B. STARK

Secondary surgery becomes necessary when primary palato-plasty has resulted in poor or unintelligible speech, but is rarely resorted to in cases of faulty deglutition with nasal regurgitation. Some of the procedures used as primary operation are used as well for secondary surgery: palatal retroposition (W-Y) and pharyngeal flap. Hynes operation to produce a shelf on the posterior pharyngeal wall; Moore's and Sullivan's bilateral palatopharyngeous flaps; Kiehn's sling to put the velum in ready position; Gillies' tubed pedicles from a distant site inserted through a cheek defect; and transplants and "inert" implants into the posterior pharyngeal wall, all are reserved by their advocates largely for correction of the failed palatoplasty.

The usual procedure in most cleft palate centers (and this pertains in our own) is to allow the patient who has had an initial palatoplasty to develop his or her speech until the time that it can be accurately appraised. Because there is a delay in language development in many patients with cleft palate, owing to social forces (timidity, fear of ridicule, excessive efforts of the parents to understand, etc.), often it is difficult to assay speech accurately until about school age (about 4 to 5 years in the United States). If it is determined that speech is not "normal," speech training is begun and continued for approximately a year; then, if "normal" speech has not been achieved, reassessment should be made by the center, and it is highly likely that a secondary operation must be undertaken.

DIAGNOSIS

First, the skull should be inspected. Is it excessively wide (oxycephalic)? The palate should be inspected. Are there fistulae along the line of palate closure? Is the velum short, more than 1.5 cm. from the posterior pharyngeal wall? Does the palate rise upward and backward? Does the pharyngeal hemisphincter contract when the patient says "Ah"? Does the pharyngeal papilla appear to approximate the posterior pharyngeal wall? Is the transverse diameter of the pharynx excessive?

What is the condition of the tonsils and adenoids? Palpation should be undertaken to determine whether the velum is excessively scarred and whether a notch replaces the posterior nasal spine at the back of the hard palate; the latter is pathognomonic of a submucous cleft. Is the tongue of normal size and mobility? Is there a cleft of the alveolus (complete cleft of the primary palate)? Is there a dental gap? Is there an oral-nasal fistula? How mobile or how tight is the upper lip?

Speech evaluation should include assessment of language development and voice production as well as rate and rhythm of speech. Speech problems such as deficits of articulation must be noted. These would include omissions, substitutions, and distortions of plosive; fricative, lateral, and nasal consonants; vowel sounds involving lingual-dental, lingual-alveolar, lingual-palatal, and lingual-velar movements; as well as labial-dental, bilabial, and labial rounding movements of speech production.

Audiography is needed to rule out deafness as the cause of poor speech.

The child's standing in school should be ascertained. Is he or she doing poorly? Do the parents complain of the child's slowness? If so, psychometric evaluation should be obtained.

If a fistula is present and regurgitation is a problem, it must be corrected surgically. In general, fistulae in the soft palate are detrimental because they produce scarring and shortening of the velum.

Neuromuscular paralyses resulting from such diseases as poliomyelitis, meningitis, and diphtheria may present formidable problems to speech improvement.

Hypertrophic tonsils usually can be controlled medically and rarely must be removed in the patient with cleft palate. Adenoids may have to be removed for serous otitis media (which may cause loss of hearing in high frequencies).

The most frequent cause of poor speech in the patient with cleft palate who has been operated upon previously is a short and/or scarred velum. Usually the superior constrictor hemisphincter is active. Such a patient can be aided in several ways.

Addition of Superior Constrictor Muscle to the Velum; Secondary Pharyngeal Flap

The addition of a pharyngeal flap to the velum for the velopharyngeal insufficiency was attempted first by Schoenborn in 1875. Although it was performed in 1889 by Schede, it was championed by Rosenthal in 1924 and Sanvenero-Rosselli and Padgett in the early 1940's. Later Conway (1951), Moran (1951), and Dunn (1951) gave impetus to the procedure, leading to its widespread use.

The pharyngeal flap is raised with its base (point of attachment) either superior or inferior. It is felt by many that the superiorly based flap is more physiological, since it allows the levator papilla to approximate the posterior pharynx at a more normal height, i.e., near the atlas. Its disadvantage is that the flap retracts, often out of sight, making it difficult to assay whether or not it remains attached.

Technically, the inferiorly based flap is easier to attach to the velum, and it can be observed through the open mouth (Fig. 12-1). This flap is not recommended if there are adenoids present, since if they are located at the tip end of the inferiorly based flap, their friability will weaken the tip attachment. Contrary to the opinion of some, the inferiorly based flap is as physiological as the superiorly based flap, since the mechanism of action of this altered velopharyngeal valve is one of hemisphincteric muscle (superior constrictor) hugging the midsagittal flap.

The velum that is tethered to the pharynx by a flap does not rise to the level of the atlas, and hence its flap-like function is somewhat vitiated. This is more than compensated for by the increased role that the hypertrophied superior constrictor musculature plays as a hemisphincter to achieve valvular closure. In cineradiographic studies it is actually hard to tell which way the pharyngeal flap has been based, since after a time, the base migrates to a point midway between the superior and inferior sites of origin.

The pharyngeal flap should be raised so as not to impinge upon the fossae of Rosenmüller, else hearing may become impaired. When this precaution has been observed, however, the flap should be as wide as possible for most effective valving, since in time, the flap will become narrowed as it becomes tubulated.

The donor site for the flap should be closed. By so doing, the pharynx is narrowed, producing an adjuvant pharyngoplasty.

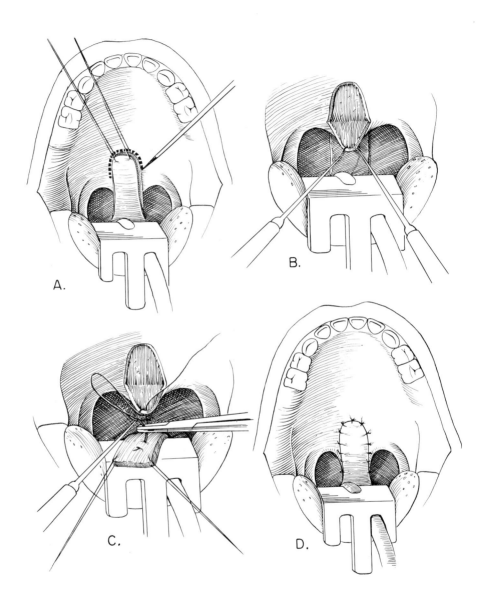

FIG. 12-1 *The velum is retracted and an inferiorly based pharyngeal flap is elevated. The site of inset into the velum is estimated. A trapdoor turnover flap of mucosa and muscularis is fashioned. The flap is inset.*

Occasionally, the velum may be so scarred that it cannot be retracted out of the way and may have to be split to form effectively the pharyngeal flap and close the donor site. The velum is resutured as the flap is attached.

Addition of Superior Constrictor Muscle to Levator Papilla

F. T. Moore of England and D. E. Sullivan of the United States, have devised bilateral, superiorly-based vertical flaps of superior constrictor muscle from the posterior pharyngeal wall. Because the flaps are raised 90° over normal tissue, they resemble those of the Hynes operation, but are set into the nasal side of the velum (Fig. 12-2). They come to lie in the coronal plane at the level of the levator papilla. The velum is split, then resutured, to perform this operation. A certain amount of denervation necessarily follows this procedure for a time.

Palatal Lengthening by Retroposition

A palate that is too short for velopharyngeal closure (usually a velum that is 2 cm. or more from the posterior pharynx at rest, physically cannot perform the function of valving) may be retrodisplaced by a push-back procedure. It is not important whether the previous repair was by the Dieffenbach-Warren-von Langenbeck method or by the V-Y principle of Ganzer-Veau-Wardill-Kilner. The rationale in performing a second V-Y pushback in the face of one that has failed previously is that additional efforts are made to line entirely the nasal side of the velum with epithelium. This has been achieved in a number of ways: wide undermining and mobilization of epithelium from the medial pterygoid lamina; undermining and retrodisplacement of mucosa from the nasal floor to line the nasal surface (Cronin, 1957); using an anterior island flap based upon the greater palatine vessels from one side (Millard, 1962); using an inlay graft of skin performed at an earlier operation (Dorrance and Bransfield, 1946; Baxter and Cardosa, 1947). In shape, the push-back may be of the W-V type or of the U-shaped type described by Dorrance and Bransfield (1946).

Forward Extension of the Pharynx

A number of attempts have been made to move the pharyngeal wall forward so that a mobile, though short, velum may meet it. The best effort of this type to date has been that of Hynes (1950) (Fig. 12-3). He has raised bilateral vertical mucomuscular pedicles from either lateral pharyngeal wall. Each flap incorporated its respective

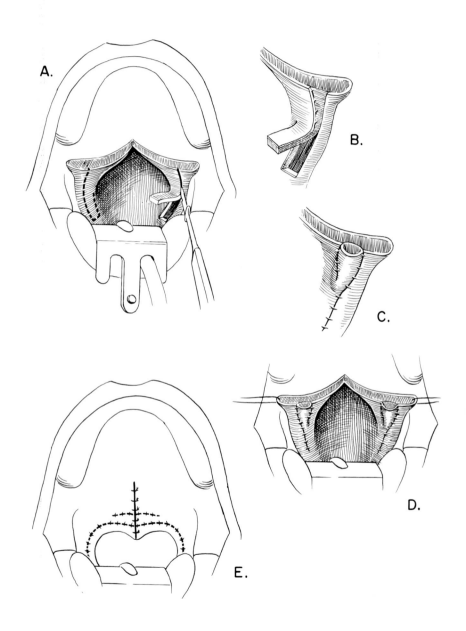

FIG. 12-2 *To obtain more levatory power for the inert velum, Moore and Sullivan have raised flaps that are similar to those of Hynes, but have set them into the nasal side of the soft palate.*

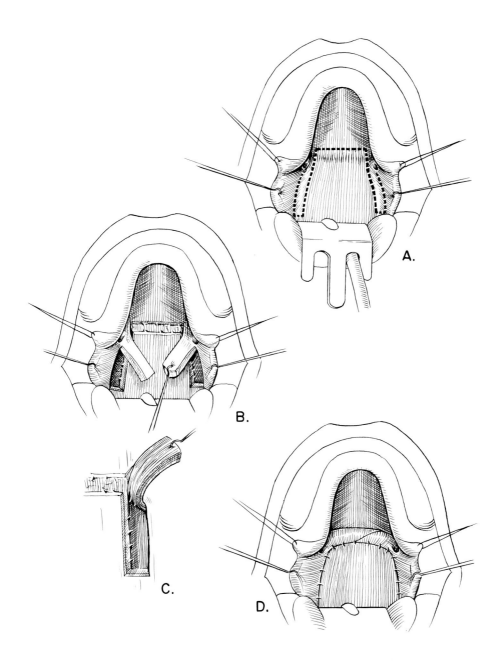

FIG. 12-3 *Hynes (1950) has permanently extended the posterior wall of the pharynx forward to meet a short soft palate by raising two superiorly based mucomuscular pedicles (using salpingopharyngeus muscle), turning each 90° medianward, and inseting them side-by-side in the horizontal plane.*

salpingopharyngeus muscle, and each was based superiorly. Hynes then turned the pedicles toward the midline and set them side-by-side into a horizontal defect created in the posterior pharynx. A prominent, permanent, and often contractile shelf is produced above Passavant's ridge. By closing the donor defects, the transverse pharyngeal diameter is reduced. Hynes performed this pharyngoplasty a month or more before he retrodisplaced the palate by either a V-Y procedure or a Gillies-Fry operation (1921). To gain exposure, Hynes split the velum. The horizontal ridge lies just below the fossae of Rosenmüller. Hynes rightly pointed out that if the velum is immobile, augmenting the posterior pharynx will be of no avail.

Attempts to extend the pharynx forward by the use of free grafts and inert implants have largely been disappointing.

Addition of Dynamic Power to the Velum

Kiehn and his coworkers have attempted to increase the levitation of the velum in patients with an adynamic soft palate by using as motors the bilateral temporal or masseter muscles which are innervated by the motor branch of the trigeminal nerves. Removing the attachment of the temporalis muscle from the coronoid process of the mandible, Kiehn then attaches this muscular insertion to its twin upon the opposite side by means of a free graft of fascia lata (taken from the tensor fascia lata of the thigh) after passing the graft through the velum in the neighborhood of the levator papilla. Kiehn feels that the best results have been obtained in cases of velar paralysis.

CHAPTER 13

Repair of
Cleft Alveolus

RICHARD B. STARK

MAXILLARY ORTHOPEDICS

With so much attention paid to the lip and velum, it was inevitable that interest would switch to the cleft alveolus, so lightly regarded in the past.

The early report from Glasgow by McNeil (1954) and the careful work thereafter by Burston in Liverpool have made amply clear that in complete clefts of the primary and secondary palates (with cleft alveolus) the two maxillary segments involved may be moved rapidly into good alignment by artificial means which have come to be called maxillary orthopedics. This consists of plastic splints which fit the palatal segments and are held in situ by suction. The splints are split in the midline and realigned periodically so as to move the separate elements into near-normal anatomical relation. A variation of this type of splint is one which is split and which incorporates a jack-screw in the midline for arch expansion. The parents are taught to expand the splint periodically by means of a key.

A variation in the molding force is the use of an extraoral elastic band, employed historically by Desaut in 1791 and advocated in modern times by Collito (1966) and by Griswold (1966).

A preliminary lip adhesion has been used by many (Millard, 1964; Spina, 1964; Randall, 1965; Johanson and Ohlsson, 1960; and Walker *et al.,*) (1966) to bring the maxillary elements into satisfactory alignment before the lip is closed definitively; when it is closed one does not have to resort to undermining the lip.

Despite all the effort expended upon preliminary maxillary orthopedics, however, Burston (1964) has reported recently that only about one-third of those treated have maintained good results while another one-third were frankly "disappointing."

BONE GRAFTING OF THE CLEFT ALVEOLUS

Surgeons treating facial clefts have long realized that it is desirable to stabilize the maxillary elements in complete unilateral clefts and to solidify the premaxilla in bilateral clefts. Until recently, these measures have been achieved by fibrous union, by orthodontia with retainers, and by prosthodontia. Within the past decade attempts were made, largely in Sweden and Germany, to stabilize the disparate elements by bone grafting. The first successful attempts were by Johanson and Nordin in Sweden and by Schmid in Germany, both reporting in 1955. They were followed by Schrudde and Stellmach (1955) and by Schuchardt and Pfeiffer (1958), then by a host of others.

Two divergent goals were pursued. One was to solidify the alveolar arch primarily, then to align it properly using maxillary orthopedics (primary bone grafting). The other goal was the reverse: to align the alveolar segments first, then to solidify the arch by bone grafting the alveolar cleft (secondary bone grafting).

It has been abundantly shown that bone grafting of the alveolar cleft in infancy and childhood may be carried out without infection or extrusion and with a high percentage of surgical success. Homografts (allogenic grafts) of bone were found, not surprisingly, to be largely unsuccessful; autogenous donor areas of rib, ilium, and tibia were used.

The right fifth, sixth, or seventh rib is used, taken from the lateral chest. To conserve operative time, two teams were used by Lynch, one team preparing the alveolar bed while the other obtained the graft. The instruments for the two operative areas are kept separate. No infections have occurred in the chest donor area in Lynch's 92 cases (1966). Some surgeons have used the lateral face of the ilium below the crest to obtain cancellous bone. Others, Johanson (1960) among them, have used the tibia as the donor area, using a vertical incision, medial to the tibial crest, which is curved upward and lateral below the tibial plateau. This donor area is not a good one in girls because of the obvious scar. Johanson has reported that the donor leg has grown from 1 to 4 mm. more than the opposite normal leg in 3 to 4 years.

The bone used has been mostly cancellous, although cortical pieces are used for onlay grafts and combined cortical-cancellous grafts are used for large-piece grafts. The latter are often H-shaped, X-shaped, or rib-struts put in the crevasse in the axis of the alveolus.

Cancellous bone chips are packed about solid pieces. Some surgeons use only cancellous chips.

Closure of the alveolar cleft must be in two layers so as to protect the bone. The nasal side of the cleft has been closed variously: by a lateral nasal flap of mucosa, by a vomerine flap, or by a lateral nasal plus a vomerine flap. Closure of the oral side has seen greater variation used. Schuchardt and Pfeiffer (1960) have used an interposition mucosal and submucosal flap taken from either the cleft side or the premaxillary side of the alveolabial sulcus. Burian (1932) (and later Muir) has closed the oral side using a throw-away flap of vermilion at the time of the cheiloplasty. Stellmach (1955) uses an elaborate anteriorly based flap from the vomer that is wrapped around the bone graft from behind. Schuchardt has used this flap when needed.

Johanson (1960) has an ingenious approach to the problem. In a preliminary (the terms primary and secondary have become particularly muddied in surgery of the alveolar cleft) operation at 1 month of age, he has closed the alveolar cleft with a vomerine flap and has sutured the lip by straight-line closure. Following healing, maxillary orthopedics using a screw-plate is resorted to until maxillary alignment is achieved. The lip is reopened at about 6 months of age and with the oral closure left inviolate, a pocket is formed superiorly. For exposure, the hyperplastic inferior nasal turbinate is resected. Bone chips are packed into the pocket; then a lateral nasal flap forms the nasal floor. The lip is closed definitively in this 2-hour operation.

Finally, closure of the entire cleft of the hard palate by bone graft has found advocates. Baeckdahl and Nordin (1961) bring the maxillary elements into occlusion. At about 6 months, they reopen the lip, resect the inferior turbinate, and then close the nasal side with a lateral nasal flap and the oral side with an inferiorly based vomerine flap. Between the two they place their bone graft. There is no elevation of mucoperiosteal flaps to close the cleft hard palate. Longacre (1964) has done this as well, finding that the grafts are incorporated by fibrous union which does not preclude growth.

The union by bone of the cleft maxillary elements must still be considered experimental. Only a few clinics can report upon patients followed for a sufficiently long time to provide meaningful data, since the dimension of growth is all-important in the treatment of congenital anomalies. At St. Luke's we have had only limited experience with bone grafting, using this modality of treatment to solidify the premaxilla after it had been aligned by orthodontia. We have preferred to close the cleft of the lip early and to allow the united orbicularis oris muscle with the now effective buccinator muscles to act as a biological orthodontic device.

The claims and counterclaims of the various proponents and the antagonists, however, may be summed up as follows: The proponents point out that bone grafting completes the alveolar arch, allowing it to develop normally and perhaps obviating the need for early orthodontia. With this is stabilization of the premaxilla in cases of bilateral cleft lip. Some believe that by uniting the lateral element to the central vomerine growth stem, the lateral element will be pulled along with it. Others point out that the well-aligned elements may be stabilized after orthodontia in the periods of mixed or permanent dentition. The ability of tooth buds to migrate into bone grafts is useful to the orthodontist. It is claimed that the bone graft will provide the lip with greater symmetry, will "shore up" the sagging ala nasi, and will improve the nasal airway.

The opponents to bone grafting of the alveolar cleft point out that the procedure does not prevent malocclusion and that it does not prevent collapse, as noted by Johanson, who has had 10 years' experience with the procedure. The fact that autogenous grafts of bone either do not grow or do not grow with the same increment as the surrounding facial bones would make collapse a logical sequel. Also the double suture lines in the two soft tissue layers inevitably contract and this militates against the expansion desired.

The bone grafting procedure requires an additional operation or operations and with them additional anesthesia. All this means more postoperative visits and more expense, with the possibility of overhospitalizing or overtreating the patient.

The procedure itself is not innocuous. It may involve a prolonged operation in infancy, sometimes requiring transfusion. Morbidity may result from the donor wound: perforation of the pleura, hematoma of the iliac area, scarring of the leg, and the possibility that the donor leg may grow longer than normal. In addition, the bone graft may fail due to extrusion.

Maxillary orthopedics and even bone grafting are not yet established as needful procedures to the patient with complete cleft palate. It now seems that if bone grafting of the alveolar cleft is left until the maxillary elements have been aligned by orthodontia during the period of mixed or permanent dentition, better results may be expected.

Certainly bone grafting is the frosting on the cake. Treatment of the cleft alveolus by bone grafting has a priority below the surgery for speech and appearance, below the preservation of hearing and dentition. What it proposes to achieve can be accomplished conservatively by our orthodontic and prosthodontic colleagues without the danger of overhospitalization or overtreating the patient.

EDWARD STROH, JR.

CHAPTER **14**

Oral

Surgery

The participation of the oral surgeon in the treatment of the patient with cleft palate is varied with many interesting aspects. In addition to those areas of the mouth which might be considered normal, but which develop abnormalities requiring the intervention of the oral surgeon, the patient with cleft palate presents numerous specific problems requiring his skill. These problems include teeth impacted in the cleft, a mobile premaxilla, a shallow alveolabial sulcus, an enlarged frenum, a prognathic mandible, and ankyloglossia.

The immediate goal is to restore the child to a functional state in regard to speech, mastication, appearance, and psychological attitude, thus permitting him to take his place in society unabashed. It must be stressed that such oral surgery as may be required should be conservative, with preservation of as much tissue as possible, since the patient has a lifetime ahead of him and may well, in later life, desperately need all tissues that can be retained for him.

Decision to perform oral surgery and the extent of such surgery should be arrived at by the cleft palate team, especially the prosthodontist, orthodontist, and speech therapist, in consultation with the oral surgeon.

ROUTINE EXTRACTION OF TEETH

Every effort is made to retain all normally erupted and positioned teeth. Often for orthodontic or prosthodontic reasons, or because of uncontrollable disease, it may be necessary to extract teeth or to remove cysts or neoplasms. This is done in the usual manner, under either local or general anesthesia as each particular case indicates. Many times multiple extractions are required under general anesthesia. In all cases particular attention is paid to the preservation and suitable preparation of the alveolar ridge for the possible placement later of a dental prosthesis.

REMOVAL OF IMPACTED TEETH

It is not uncommon in a patient with complete cleft of the alveolus to find after extensive radiographic studies impacted teeth and/or supernumerary teeth in unusual positions. All such teeth should be removed. Their removal requires maximum dexterity, as the bone surrounding such teeth frequently is very thin; thus, in removing the teeth, any undue or misdirected pressure may result in loss of the tooth into the soft tissues or confines of the cleft.

Under local or general anesthesia an appropriately large flap is made and reflected to assure good exposure. Bone is carefully removed with a hand chisel. The tooth should be sufficiently well exposed so that it can literally be picked from its socket. The alveolar process is smoothed and shaped and the flap sutured back into position with medium black silk.

CORRECTION OF SHALLOW SULCUS

Heavy fibrous bands and low muscle attachments in the area of the alveolar cleft not infrequently create a shallow alveolabial sulcus. This shallow sulcus presents a restoration problem for the prosthodontist, since if uncorrected, it will not accommodate an extended flange or any restoration that must be inserted.

Surgical intervention is necessary to create an epithelium-lined sulcus that will accommodate the extended flange. Of the many known techniques, the Clark labial technique is the simplest and most applicable (Fig. 14-1). Incision is made over the crest of the alveolar ridge. By supraperiosteal sharp and blunt dissection, the desired sulcus depth is obtained. The lip mucosa is then undermined from the free edge of the incision to the vermilion border. A black silk suture is placed through the free edge of the mucosal flap, carried down through the depth of the wound or sulcus and out through the skin. The needle is removed and the other arm of the suture is threaded onto it and passed through the mucosa and skin 2 mm. away from the first suture and parallel to it. The two suture ends are then tied on the outside of the face over a cotton roll. Several such sutures are placed, depending upon the width of the sulcus extension. Thus the raw surface of the lip is covered, leaving the periosteum-covered raw surface

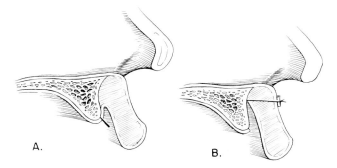

FIG. 14-1 *Clark technique for deepening the shallow alveolabial sulcus. The mucoperiosteum is incised at the alveolar crest and dissected supraperiosteally upward to the desired depth of the new sulcus. The mucoperiosteum is sutured so as to surface the posterior lip. The raw surface of the anterior alveolus spontaneously epithelializes.*

over the bone to epithelize, a process that takes about 10 days. Postoperative care should emphasize mouth hygiene.

FRENECTOMY (FRENOPLASTY)

The abnormal insertion of the labial frenum at such a point as to cause a diastema of the maxillary incisor teeth or to prevent the proper insertion of a prosthetic appliance may be encountered. To assist the orthodontist or the prosthodontist in achieving a desirable esthetic result, the frenum must be removed.

Usually the base of such a frenum is a hard fibrous band of varying thickness, well attached to the alveolar process and sometimes growing to it. This band must be completely dissected free from the bone, some of it removed, and the remainder replaced at a higher, more natural level in the labial sulcus. This procedure might be called frenoplasty as well as frenectomy.

Many methods of frenectomy or frenoplasty are in common use; virtually all are simple and effective. However, some procedures produce more scarring than is desirable and eliminate any semblance of a frenum, thus occasionally resulting in an unnatural control of the upper lip.

A satisfactory technique, which avoids the undesirable sequelae, is accomplished by using a V incision in what is essentially a V-Y procedure (Fig. 14-2). Under local anesthesia the frenum is put in tension by raising the upper lip. The incision is started along the outer edges of the frenum at that point on the labial surface of the alveolus where the replaced frenum is to be based. The incision is

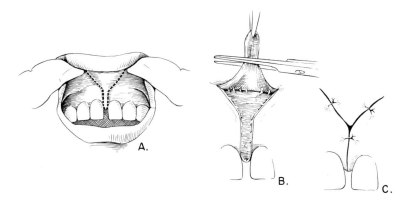

FIG. 14-2 *Frenoplasty and partial frenectomy performed as a V-Y procedure.*

carried down on each side of the fibrous band to the point where it is attached to the nasopalatine pad. The incisions forming the arms of the V are started at the top of the original vertical incisions and carried laterally and upward several millimeters. The frenum and fibrous attachment are dissected free from the bone, from the nasopalatine pad to the ends of the arms of the V. The base of the V is then excised. The flap resulting is sutured into position with one suture in each arm; a tension suture is placed in what was the base of the V but which is now a Y. Postoperative care is routine.

CORRECTION OF TONGUE-TIE

Ankyloglossia, or tongue-tie, is caused by a short lingual frenum firmly attached to the mandible. Operation is indicated in some cases of tongue-tie if, in the infant, it interferes with nursing, or in the older child or adult, it interferes with mastication and speech. If teeth are lost it may interefere with proper fitting and retention of a denture. Difficulties with dentures may be encountered due to the pull exerted by the thick broad cord or multiple fibrous strands which are attached to the lingual aspects of the alveolar process of the mandible.

Frequently, speech defects cause the patient to seek advice. However, other more plausible causes for abnormal speech should be investigated, such as mental and neurological disturbances, submucous cleft palate, hearing deficits, etc.

Operation is indicated in all cases of symptomatic tongue-tie. In the newborn the condition is corrected simply by cutting the frenum with scissors. In the older child and adult a more careful procedure is

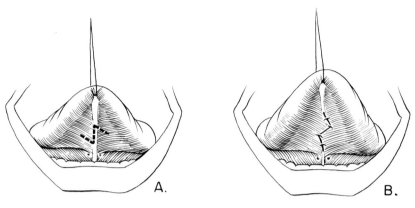

FIG. 14-3   *Ankyloglossia (tongue-tie) is corrected by Z plasty.*

indicated. Anesthesia can be local or general. If local anesthesia is used, a bilateral block of the lingual nerve is the method of choice, since local infiltration distorts the tissues and thus may prevent an accurate incision. The mouth is propped open and a suture is passed through the tip of the tongue for retraction during the operation. The fibrous lingual frenum is put on stretch by upward traction on the tongue. A Z plasty will also turn the offending vertical band into the horizontal plane where it will no longer tether the tongue (Fig. 14-3). This correction not only gives the desired freedom to the tip of the tongue, but also results in an increase in length.

Following ankylotomy many older patients are benefited by speech therapy to correct the faulty diction which may have developed.

REMOVAL OF PREMAXILLA

The premaxilla may not become retrodisplaced or it may remain mobile. In some instances it may be wise to solve the problem by removing the premaxilla, forming an alveolabial sulcus, and utilizing a fixed prosthesis. Circumstances of time, expense, overhospitalization of the patient, etc. may dictate this solution.

The premaxilla is chiseled off the vomer, while three flaps are preserved or fashioned (Fig. 14-4). One mucoperiosteal flap is dissected from the anterior surface of the premaxilla, while two alveolabial flaps are fashioned. One of these is turned over to line the nasal side of the defect; the other is advanced to surface the oral side. The premaxillary flap is turned 180° to line the labial side of the new sulcus (Clark technique).

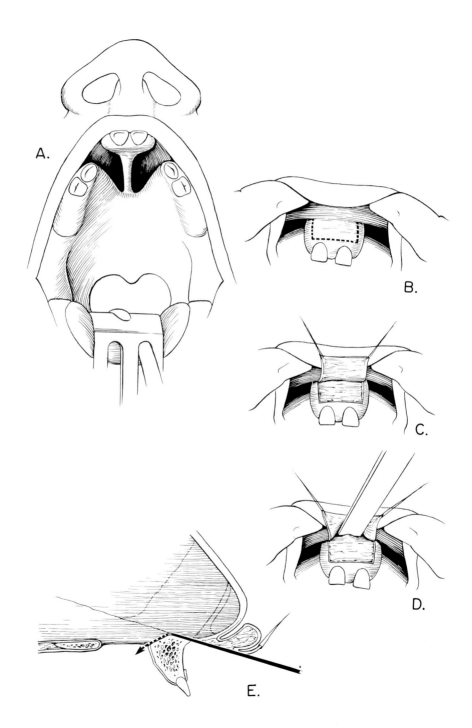

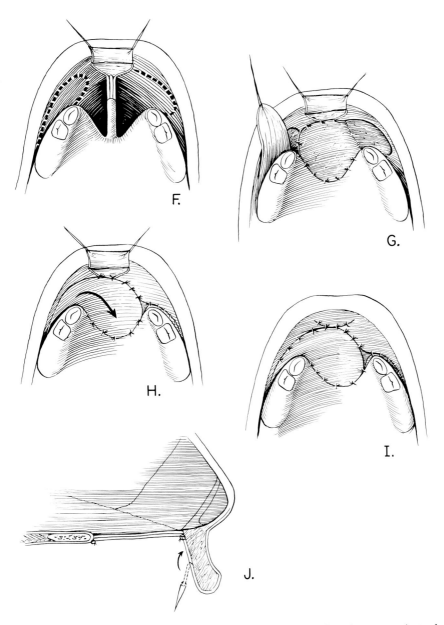

F.

G.

H.

I.

J.

FIG. 14-4 *In removal of the premaxilla, a superiorly based mucoperiosteal flap is dissected from the premaxilla, which is chiseled off the vomer. Two alveolabial sulcus flaps are elevated. One is turned over to line the nasal side, while the other is advanced to surface the oral side. The premaxillary flap is turned 180° to surface the posterior side of the lip, thereby forming a deep sulcus (Clark technique).*

CORRECTION OF MANDIBULAR PROGNATHISM

The disharmony of facial bones known as mandibular prognathism usually has a genetic basis; however, it may be intensified or repressed to varying degrees depending upon environmental factors. Thus, in the patient with cleft palate, the prominence of the mandible may be true prognathism or merely relative prognathism due to lack of maxillary development.

A deformity of this nature is frequently associated with other problems: psychic disturbance (introverted personality, mental anguish), interference with employment, lack of social success. There may be functional difficulties as well, such as speech difficulties and improper occlusion and mastication. Such a skeletal deformity generally is irrevesible except by surgical intervention. Surgical intervention is undertaken for a threefold purpose: (1) to correct occlusion, (2) to enhance the esthetic appearance of the face, and (3) to improve the function of the mandible.

The method used to establish a new maxillomandibular relation is either osteotomy or ostectomy. The anatomical site of the surgery may be either the ascending vertical ramus or the horizontal body (Fig. 14-5). The choice of site is dependent upon the degree of prognathism and the status of osseous structures and of existing dentition.

In all instances, the treatment plan is of paramount importance. The plan entails: (1) determination of degree of prognathism, (2) determination of postoperative occlusal position, (3) choosing the best surgical approach for the existing situation, and (4) determining the type and manner of postoperative fixation. Although each method has its proponents, superior results are achieved when the plastic surgeon avails himself of the services of a skilled dental colleague.

Advantages of cross-sectioning the ascending ramus are (1) simplicity of the operative procedure, (2) lack of interference with the inferior alveolar nerve, and (3) the fact that no teeth are sacrificed. It is safer to section the ramus under direct vision than to do it blindly. A 3-cm. incision is made below the angle and parallel to the mandibular body via the Risdon approach. Through this incision, the masseter muscle is raised from the ramus by a periosteal elevator as far up as the sigmoid notch. It is retracted using a finger-shaped retractor. With a power saw, osteotome, or chisel, the ramus is sectioned.

Ramusotomy may be performed horizontally or vertically. In either instance, the inferior dental nerve (mandibular branch of the trigeminal nerve) must be preserved. If a horizontal ramus section is

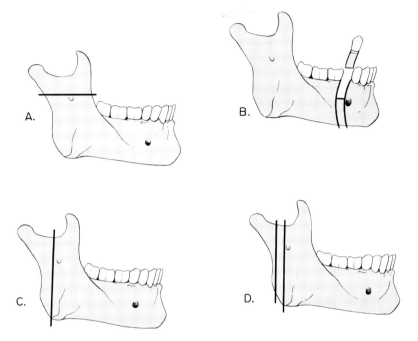

FIG. 14-5   *The prognathic jaw may be set back by operations upon the ramus (horizontal or vertical ramusotomy) or by one- or two-stage operations upon the body.*

being made, the cut must be above the mandibular foramen into which the nerve enters; therefore, it should be made no lower than $\frac{9}{16}$ inch below the sigmoid notch. The plane of section should be horizontal along the face of the ramus, but when viewed from its anterior edge it should run obliquely downward and laterally, thus preventing the external pterygoid muscle from pulling the proximal fragment medially.

If the ramus is being sectioned vertically, the nerve is spared by making the line of section posterior to the mandibular canal. The cut is beveled here as well, so that the body glides backward medial to the ramus. With the beveled surface, bare bone rests against bare bone. By using a dental burr, a wider beveled surface of cancellous bone can be afforded. If the mandible is being retrodisplaced more than 1.5 cm., the temporal muscle tether is released by removing the coronoid process.

Ostectomy of the horizontal body of the mandible can be completed in one operation, although most surgeons advocate the two-stage procedure (Dingman, 1948). This approach is used more frequently in the pseudoprognathic patient or in the patient who has missing molar teeth.

The mandibular body may be sectioned under inferior dental nerve block with local infiltration of the skin overlying the section line. An incision is made below and parallel to the mandibular body, through which two vertical cuts are made in the mandible with a power saw, from below up to the inferior dental nerve. A horizontal cut is made parallel to the nerve canal. Entering the mouth, two vertical cuts are made downward through the upper half of the body and the mandible. These are not continuous with the cuts made below. The distance between the cuts above and below the nerve canal is equal and the same as the desired setback, as judged from study models. Intervening bone between the two cuts is removed above and below. The bony incision now simulates a stair step. The area around the nerve canal is scooped out to house the lax nerve without pinching it. The alveolar mucosa is sutured. The jaws are immobilized by interdental wiring, using an arch bar if there is an imperfect complement of teeth. The lowermost portion of the mandible may be wired directly if insufficient teeth are available and the skin is closed.

CHAPTER 15

Orthodontics

E. CLINTON VOLLMER

In recent years a revolution has been taking place not only in the orthodontic approach to cleft palate treatment, but in the over-all handling of palatal clefts. Previously, treatment was administered often in a haphazard and disjointed manner, with little or no cooperation among the various disciplines, and with understandably poor results. The team approach to these complex problems has proved a savior to today's more fortunate patients and, in one form or another, has been adapted throughout the United States.

So, too, have the orthodontist's skills been recognized as an integral part of the problem and are no longer relegated exclusively to the art and science of treating malocculsion for a large part of the population. The orthodontist is well aware of the important role that the lower half of the face plays in facial esthetics, and through his skills of manipulation he is able to influence this vital area beneficially. The widespread use of cephalometrics has been helpful not only in research but also as a tool in appraising treatment. By means of cephalometry one can see what changes have resulted from orthodontic intervention as well as from the normal growth and development potential of the individual.

TIMING OF TREATMENT

For many years, orthodontists felt generally that the optimum age for treatment was approximately 12 years, an age when most of the permanent teeth have erupted; by then, it used to be said, malocclusion was well established. Today, however, owing to closer cooperation by specialists through the team approach, there is an increased awareness of the advantages to be gained by earlier recognition and treatment of orthodontic problems. We feel that cephalometrics has been an underlying force in this philosophy of treatment. Cephalometrics has enabled the orthodontist to define facial esthetics in positive terms instead of relying on visual methods and individual appraisals, with their necessarily subjective and variable interpretations. He has tried to understand and forecast growth and development by cephalometric means, and although admittedly there is still much to be learned in this respect, progress is being made toward this end. Thus more orthodontists now begin treatment at 8, 9, or 10 years of age so that they may take advantage of the facial growth that occurs in these years instead of waiting until the damage has already been done.

The dilemma of early vs. late treatment was pointed up in the early 1950's when McNeil of Scotland advocated intervention soon after birth. This was a radical departure, for it suggested the performance of orthodontics without the presence of even deciduous teeth. The very derivation of the word orthdontist appeared to give the lie to this approach. We feel, however, that McNeil's work did much to demonstrate that the field of orthodontics was overemphasizing teeth themselves and not recognizing that the main deformity to be dealt with was the collapse of the dental arch, which was followed by deviations of tooth position. It was suggested that perhaps early correction of the maxillary segments would permit more normal development of this area and less deterioration in the subsequent dental pattern. It was shown that such molding of the palate was more easily and quickly accomplished than by conventional methods at the conventional time. Then scar tissue, dense calcification, and well-developed musculature limited orthodontia, which thus became more time consuming and was more prone to relapse. There is an inherent psychological value as well for the patient, for he is no longer subjected to interminable treatment in later life when he is occupied with the trials of adolescence.

This is not to say, however, that we consider early treatment a great panacea. We have encountered problems with this early approach: for example, the difficulty of retention of orthodontic appliances, often coupled with poor cooperation from the young patient. In addition, the length of the treatment, which must be continued until the second stage can be completed following the eruption of the permanent teeth, strains the patient's enthusiasm. It has been our experience that the orthodontic patient, regardless of the nature of the deformity, generally begins treatment enthusiastically; but before long his interest lags and the inevitable question arises, "When are the braces coming off?"

TREATMENT PROGRAM

Our program is modified to fit our particular circumstances at St. Luke's, where orthodontic therapy is initiated at approximately 4 years of age. Prior to this, the patient is followed by the General Dental Service, and all caries are treated. We find that a 4-year-old is more cooperative and manageable than a younger patient, and still young enough to benefit from the advantages of early treatment. By the time of orthodontic treatment, X-ray examination has been completed and other diagnostic aids have been employed, including evaluation by the cleft palate team at its regular monthly conference.

During the first stage of treatment, we generally employ a recurved lingual arch for expansion, in both unilateral and bilateral complete clefts. Rather than banding the second deciduous molars, we have found the use of Rocky Mountain preformed stainless steel crowns to be superior. They are stiffer than most other makes and hence exhibit greater retentive properties. Copper band compound impressions are taken, and amalgam or copper plated dies are formed of these teeth. The correct size crowns are selected, festooned, and swagged on the die for very close adaptation. These are then inserted in the proper position in a full compound impression of the arch, and a stone model is produced.

Half-round tubes (DL-10) are soldered on the lingual aspect of each crown, and the recurved lingual arch is constructed of .038 gold wires. These are inserted and adjusted approximately every 3 weeks.

We feel that there are advantages inherent in this design. As opposed to the acrylic jack-screw appliances, the need for the patient's cooperation is minimal as the arch is not removable by the patient. A great variety of adjustments is possible: notably, the anterior portion of the segment can be rotated laterally while relative stability of the maxillary tuberosity is maintained. There have been objections raised to early expansion techniques, namely, that widening the tuberosity region may result in a broader pharynx and impaired velopharyngeal valving, thus producing further speech defects. We feel that with proper manipulation of the appliance, this can be held to a minimum.

Proper alignment of the segments is usually attained within 6 months. The result may be retained with a removable appliance or more often by the lingual arch mechanism itself.

Missing or extracted teeth in the line of cleft may be replaced by fusing acrylic teeth on the arch itself or in the usual manner on an acrylic retainer. The patient is observed periodically until the time of the second stage or final positioning.

Cleft of Primary Palate (Unilateral, Bilateral, or Median)

The deformity is generally mild, with no or very little segment collapse. Teeth adjacent to the cleft are usually rotated, lateral incisors are sometimes missing, and there may be supernumerary teeth, which are usually removed. The treatment described above can be accomplished quite readily in either the mixed or the permanent dentition, and followed by the fitting of a fixed or removable prosthesis in the affected area. This presupposes that there is no malocclusion present which is unassociated with the cleft itself.

Cleft of Secondary Palate Only (Complete, Incomplete, or Submucous)

The severity of the malocclusion is largely dependent upon the extent of the cleft and the accompanying repair. There is occasionally some lateral collapse, although not nearly as severe as in other cases. The malocclusion should be treated early, just as any crossbite, and the orthodontic appliance should be retained until good interdigitation is obtained in the permanent dentition.

Complete Cleft of the Primary and Secondary Palates (Unilateral, Bilateral, or Median)

The patient with unilateral cleft is best treated early to permit unlocking of crossbite and the more normal development of the maxilla and mandibular position, as there is often an accommodating mandibular shift. We employ a recurved lingual arch as described earlier and often obtain good alignment within 6 months.

In the patient with bilateral cleft early treatment is also necessary. These patients differ from those with unilateral cleft in that the premaxilla presents a major problem. There are various means available to manage this aspect. If there is not too much anterior displacement, frequently the rotation of the palatal shelves is sufficient to permit physiological positioning. Some clinics advocate setback procedures for the premaxilla, with varying results. We prefer to let the orbicularis oris muscle, united at the time of cheiloplasty, serve as a biological orthodontic device. If necessary the premaxilla can be removed surgically. Some elect to remove the premaxilla and to replace it in a more advantageous position as a free bone graft. For all bilateral clefts in which the right and left segments are to be rotated, the recurved lingual arch is the appliance of choice. Appliance manipulation does not vary significantly from that employed in unilateral clefts.

The final decision about the disposition of the premaxillary segment usually is left until the permanent dentition has erupted. Retention is accomplished by removable prosthesis because nasal patency may be present. We feel that management of the premaxilla is one area that needs more intensive investigation. This may prove to be the major indication for early orthodontia and retention by means of autogenous bone graft.

We employ the edgewise arch mechanism for the second phase, although excellent results are certainly obtainable by other means. We work in close conjunction with the prosthodontic staff, as their services are indispensable for successful completion of treatment. Our hopes are to attain the most physiologic results by utilizing a fixed prosthesis to allow optimum dental function and appearance together with normal speech through the use of palatoplasty and pharyngeal flap.

We feel that in this manner the patient may be restored to a responsible position in society with a minimum of artificial contrivances. We realize that this is a long and hard therapeutic road, but we have been heartened by the progress which has been made through our concerted team efforts. We eagerly await greater break-throughs which will benefit mankind so afflicted.

CHAPTER 16

Prosthodontics

ANTHONY S. CARUSO

The prosthodontist's objectives are to restore as well as possible the functions of mastication, deglutition, and speech, and to achieve an esthetic result, thus improving the patient's psychological and physiological outlook. Once the corrections have been instituted, they must be maintained.

In approaching the patient with cleft palate, the prosthodontist should be aware of the importance of good rapport and a high degree of proficiency. Thanks to cleft palate centers throughout the country, these essentials are being more and more fully realized.

The prosthodontist is concerned with separating the pharynx from the nasal cavity and, according to Spriesterbach, "with those oral deviations which prevent the speaker from making the proper impetus of the breath stream as it passes through the oral cavity."

The patient's hypo- or hypernasal speech results from insufficient velopharyngeal closure. Such closure is effected by a hemisphincter and a flap valve. The hemisphincter is produced by simultaneous contraction of the pterygopharyngeal portion of the superior constrictor muscle, the palatopharyngeus muscle, and the salpingopharyngeus muscle. The flap valve raises and pulls the soft palate backward by contracting the levator veli palatini muscles. However, the palate takes a different position in producing nasal sounds such as "em," "en," and "ing." Contraction of the palatopharyngeus muscles aided by the tensor veli palatini forces the soft palate downward against the tongue. The palatoglossus muscles contract simultaneously in sphincter fashion, completely closing off the oral cavity from the pharynx and the nasal cavity.

Deviation of the teeth and dental arches is often treated by the orthodontist, but in some cases he cannot close a severe open bite or fully expand an underdeveloped maxilla. The prosthodontist is then consulted. These specialists should cooperate closely in the hope of achieving optimal occlusion.

The prosthodontist consults with the speech therapist before making an appliance for correction of open bite in patients who cannot pronounce sibilants ("s" and "z") well, those with disharmony of the jaws and poor speech articulation, and those requiring a speech aid and/or obturator.

The oral surgeon is consulted with reference to deepening of a sulcus, a low and closely attached frenulum, a prognathic mandible, bulbar tuberosities, an extremely low alveolar process, flabby alveolar tissue, severe undercuts on alveolar ridges, as well as extraction of malaligned and impacted teeth.

The plastic surgeon is called upon to close an oronasal fistula and redivide a short and scarred soft palate so that a speech aid may be conveniently fitted. A pediatrician and/or internist is needed when a cleft palate patient with a systemic disease or a cardiovascular lesion requires prophylactic antibiotics during treatment. The social service department works closely with clinicians to see that appointments are kept. Occasionally we feel that a psychological (psychometric) or psychiatric consultation would be helpful.

During the examination, diagnosis, and treatment phases, and in arriving at the prognosis, the prosthodontist seeks the opinion and assistance of team members from other disciplines who are similarly eager to develop the best possible treatment plan for each patient.

Whenever surgery is feasible, it is considered more economical than long-term use of an appliance. But when there is insufficient local tissue (Fig. 16-1) or when the patient is a poor surgical risk, an appliance may be the primary treatment of choice (Fig. 16-2). The patient whose surgery is delayed until the proper stage of development often needs a transitional appliance. With a prosthesis making speech training feasible, available functional tissue may become hypertrophied so that in later velopharyngeal closure no appliance will be needed.

Occasionally it is difficult to foretell whether a pharyngeal flap will improve the patient's speech. A prosthetic appliance may aid in evaluating the effect of this surgery (Fig. 16-3). A prosthesis is needed when teeth or missing segments of alveolus must be replaced (Fig. 16-4). A speech aid is useful in treating the patient with a short, immobile, or otherwise inadequate soft palate resulting in nasal speech. A complementary appliance is useful when a pharyngeal flap is too narrow or the pharynx too wide.

The prosthodontist treating cleft palate patients must also be

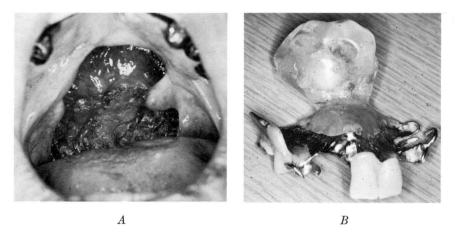

A   B

FIG. 16-1   *A. Cleft of soft palate with tissue insufficiency. B. Frontal view of appliance.*

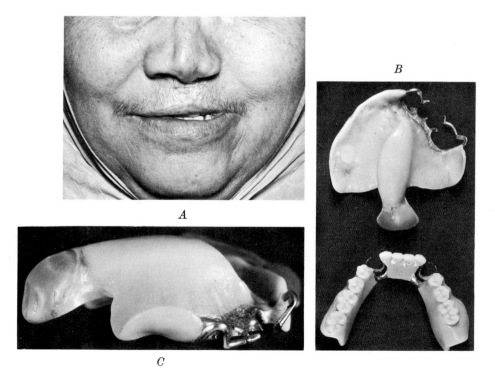

B

A

C

FIG. 16-2   *A. Patient with cleft palate who, because she was a poor surgical risk, was fitted with a maxillary appliance. Patient is shown here wearing appliance. B. Superior view of maxillary appliance and lower denture. C. Lateral view of appliance.*

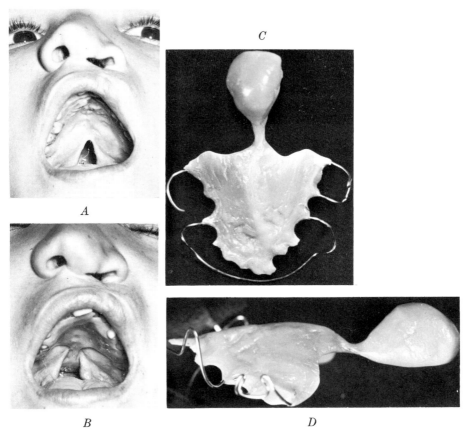

FIG. 16-3   A. Cleft of the soft palate. B. Diagnostic speech aid appliance in place. C. Superior view of appliance. D. Lateral view of appliance.

skilled in areas such as the construction of a speech appliance for an insufficient palate, the use of chrome cobalt alloy to cover the palate when there is a low vault with a small space of Donders (this alloy can be used thinly as it is very strong), and the design of a prosthetic configuration with the superior part sloped laterally to avoid "puddling" of secretions. Also, he must have a working knowledge of the mechanics of speech.

Of the three principal designs of speech appliances, the *fixed,* *meatus,* and *hinged* types, the fixed type is the most commonly used in our clinic and elsewhere. The palatal and velar sections follow a straight horizontal plane anteroposteriorly. The pharyngeal section is directed superiorly so that the appliance lies immediately above Passavant's ridge. The meatus type requires no muscle trimming and is efficient for edentulous patients with clefts of the soft palate at least

A

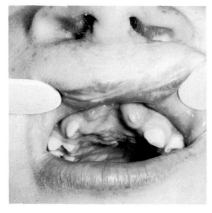

C

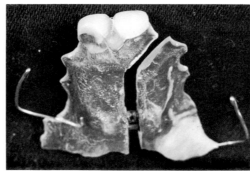

B

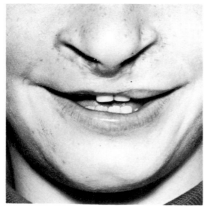

FIG. 16-4

A. Edentulous cleft.
B. Orthoprosthetic appliance.
C. Patient with appliance inserted.

2.0 cm. in width. The hinge type, the most difficult to construct, is generally reserved for cooperative patients who have teeth and an active velum. On films, a well-made hinge appliance closely resembles a normal velum.

In making a prosthodontic moulage, the palate and face are measured prior to intubation for anesthesia. The wax trays for the facial and maxillary areas are then formed (Fig. 16-5) to reduce anesthesia time. With the patient unconscious and intubated, the space around the endotracheal tube in the oropharynx is packed with gauze treated with petroleum jelly to prevent entrapment of the alginate hydrocolloid impression material. The tray for the maxillary area, filled but not overpacked, is inserted without undue force to obtain as extensive a negative mold of the velum and pharynx as possible without depositing any impression material (Technique of Shatkin).

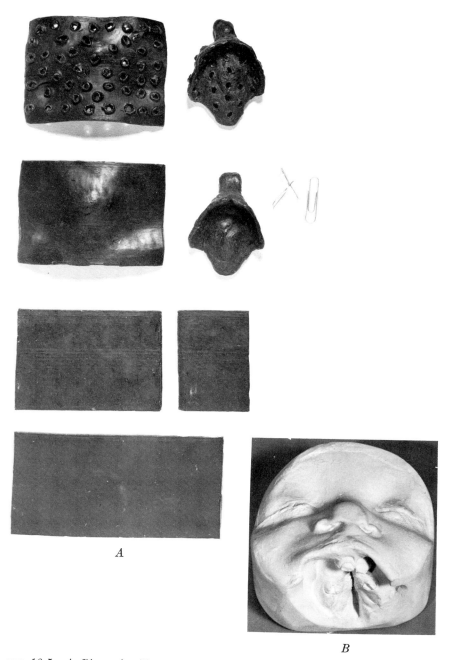

A

B

FIG. 16-5   *A. Piece of utility wax (145 by 72 by 5 mm.) cut into two sections. The smaller piece is shaped into a tray for the maxillary area and is perforated. The larger piece is shaped into a tray for the middle third of the face and is perforated. B. A stone model is made of the negative mold (Technique of Shatkin).*

The following is a prosthodontic summary of J. S. (St. Luke's No. 48-78-80), whose bilateral complete cleft of the primary and secondary palates had been repaired at another institution. She was referred to our clinic for plastic surgery, speech therapy, and dental care.

On examination, the maxilla was hypoplastic, the premaxilla and lateral dental arches were badly collapsed, and the patient had a marked overbite with relative prognathism. Because of rheumatic fever contracted at age 8, she was given standard antiobiotic treatment 2 days before and 2 days after each session of prophylactic dental work.

She first had a transitional appliance of plastic which could be readily adjusted with 0.030-gauge orthodontic wire. The prosthesis was constructed with several factors in mind: a plan for the occlusion to be employed, means of inserting and retaining the removable partial appliance, as well as extending it later onto the oral mucosa in the vestibule and the hard palate. The appliance meanwhile has been a diagnostic aid.

The patient received cast gold crowns to cover the nine remaining maxillary teeth and a cast chrome cobalt partial denture, supported by the crowned teeth, utilizing the guidelines for occlusion and esthetics arrived at by means of the diagnostic appliance.

CHAPTER **17**

Tonsillectomy
and
Adenoidectomy

NORMAN N. OSTROV

A child with an unrepaired palatal cleft or a cleft repaired by a pharyngeal flap should undergo tonsillectomy only if absolutely necessary. The posterior pillar of the tonsillar fossa is composed of the palatopharyngeus muscle, and the anterior pillar is composed of the palatoglossus muscle, both of which are integral components of the soft palate. Since a considerable number of tonsillectomies result in slight to extensive injury of one or both tonsil pillars, e.g., total avulsion or excision, plastic repair of the cleft palate may be partially destroyed. Since tonsillar disease can be controlled indefinitely by medical treatment, as rheumatic fever can by prophylactic administration of antibiotics, tonsillectomy can usually be avoided in the patient with cleft palate.

Indications for adenoidectomy are not nearly as rigidly defined. Diseased hypertrophic adenoids, responsible for numerous cases of respiratory and/or middle ear infections as well as eustachian salpingitis with hearing impairment, can be easily removed without danger to any tissues involved in palatal reconstruction. It is not necessary to free a pharyngeal flap; at least with flaps constructed in our clinic at St. Luke's, there is always adequate space on each side for the required maneuvering. A skilled surgeon who handles the tissues gently and selects adenotomes, curettes, and basket punches of the proper size and type should be able to perform adenoidectomy without injuring the palatal repair in any way.

The otolaryngologist, closely associated with the plastic surgeon and respecting his reconstructive work, should intervene to the minimum degree consistent with the child's health and safety.

CHAPTER **18**

Hearing
Evaluation

STANLEY WHITFIELD

Every youngster with a cleft palate requires a complete ear, nose, and throat examination and a hearing evaluation because of the high incidence of hearing problems reported in this group. Each center may estimate hearing loss somewhat differently, depending on the testing system, competence of the technicians, and their criteria for significant hearing loss. Only half of all children with cleft palates tested so far at St. Luke's Hospital Center have had what we consider completely normal hearing in both ears. Hearing loss in the others was classified as mild to severe.

TYPE AND MECHANISM OF HEARING LOSS

The great majority of hearing losses are of a conductive rather than a neurosensory type. The mechanism of the conductive hearing loss is intimately related to the anatomy and physiology of the pharyngotympanic tube, for the following reasons:

1. In both the normal child and the child with cleft palate this tube is relatively shorter, straighter, and wider than in the adult, so that infection can more readily ascend to the tympanic cavity.

2. A palatal cleft further facilitates the passage of infected material to the tympanic cavity via the tube.

3. For the child with cleft palate, feeding problems put further stress on the pharyngotympanic tube; bottle-feeding in a supine position makes it even easier for food to enter the nasopharynx and pharyngotympanic tube. Incidentally, this mechanism applies to a lesser extent in the normal child. When any infant suffers from recurrent otitis media, one of the physician's first inquiries must be about the feeding method. All children should be held in a semierect position during bottle- or cup-feeding.

4. The tensor and levator veli palatini muscles play an important part in controlling patency of the pharyngotympanic tube; abnormalities of these muscles in the child with cleft palate probably result in increased patency.

IMPORTANCE OF EARLY DIAGNOSIS

The child's ability to recognize and interpret sound, which leads to the evolution of speech, develops principally during the first year of life—called the "readiness to listen" period—and diminishes rapidly thereafter. If a child with an uncorrected hearing problem has not undergone auditory training by the time he reaches the age of 5, it is almost impossible to educate him by means of hearing. The period of "readiness to speak" extends from about 12 to 18 months. It is obvious that speech development is predicated on adequate reception of speech sounds; adequate hearing, especially up to the age of 2, thus becomes most important. Diagnosis of a hearing problem at the earliest possible moment is essential even in an otherwise normal child; it is indeed essential in a child with cleft palate, who has a potential speech problem due to the abnormality. Failure to recognize and promptly treat a hearing problem will greatly handicap the child's entire speech rehabilitation program.

At St. Luke's, we attempt to diagnose any hearing problems before the age of 18 months or even before closure of the cleft. This schedule gives us an opportunity to determine the possible effect of any particular surgical procedure on existing conductive hearing loss, middle ear pathology, or physiology of the pharyngotympanic tube.

HEARING ASSESSMENT

The many difficulties attending the diagnosis of hearing loss before the child reaches 18 months are well known. We arrive at the final diagnosis on the basis of several factors rather than a single test. It should be emphasized that members of a cleft palate team must strongly suspect that a child with cleft palate may have a hearing loss.

The following factors are equally important in evaluating hearing in this group: (1) history; (2) ear, nose, and throat examination; and (3) hearing tests.

History

The history elicited from the mother or information volunteered by her is often extremely valuable. This is especially true if she has older children with normal hearing. Her impression that the child is not hearing well should be accepted until the contrary is proved.

The history should cover a number of points, including:

1. Does the infant's hearing seem normal?

2. Does he appear to respond to sound, especially to the mother's voice, by turning, or smiling, or reaching toward her?

3. Does he make an effort to produce sound himself? Babbling in the early months and disappearance of these sounds at approximately 9 months, with no further speech development, would suggest a hearing impairment.

4. Does the child seem unaware of activities, especially those associated with sound, taking place around him?

Information should also be sought concerning signs, symptoms, and events indicating recurrent attacks of acute otitis media or chronic otitis media. These range from unexplained crying spells as if the infant were in pain or frequent pulling on the ear lobe indicating possible earache, to frank otitis media with purulent otorrhea, several myringotomies, previous diagnosis of acute otitis media by the pediatrician, and so on.

A carefully taken history frequently points strongly to a hearing problem. It should be borne in mind that a hearing child responds to the human voice by 1 year of age and often talks at 2 or earlier.

Ear, Nose, and Throat Examination

At St. Luke's every infant and child with cleft palate has a routine ear, nose, and throat examination with special attention to the ears and tympanic membranes. The child should be in an upright position on the mother's knee rather than lying down; the latter position makes it easy to overlook a fluid level behind an intact tympanic membrane resulting from a serous otitis media.

Any change in appearance of the tympanic membrane should be considered evidence of conductive hearing loss until proved differently. The changes may range from absence of light reflex or retraction of the intact membrane, or serous otitis media with fluid level and mild inflammation, to acute otitis media with inflamed, bulging membrane, or the chronic suppurative form with perforation of the membrane. The patient must be examined more than once as the appearance of the tympanic membrane changes from time to time. With accurate evaluation of the history and an adequate ear, nose, and throat examination, it is frequently possible to draw a conclusion regarding the presence or absence of a hearing loss.

Hearing Tests

The details of particular hearing tests can be found in any standard textbook on the subject and will not be included here. The hearing of infants and young children should be evaluated by experienced audiologists, preferably those who have had special training with this age group and can properly interpret not only the consistent responses but also the random and even lacking responses to test stimuli.

The patients are divided into two groups—below and above the age of 2—largely because different types of tests are required.

TESTS IN CHILDREN UNDER TWO

Although it is very difficult to assess the auditory threshold accurately in a child under 2, every effort must be made toward this end. The methods commonly employed are: (1) testing responses to loud noises (e.g., made by drums or other loud toys, with the noise level reaching at least 75 decibels); (2) testing responses to quiet unfamiliar and familiar sounds (e.g., tapping a cup with a spoon, music boxes, soft high-pitched rattles, rustling papers, bells, and—probably the most important—the voice of the examiner or the mother); and (3) pure-tone audiometry.

Testing is first carried out in a quiet open room in an attempt to learn whether the hearing appears to be normal. The child sits on the mother's knee. Two examiners are necessary: one controls the test sounds, usually from a position behind the infant to avoid giving visual or other clues, and the other watches the responses from a position in front.

If the infant is found to have essentially normal hearing, no further testing is needed. If his responses indicate some hearing impairment, however, the tests are repeated in a soundproof room. The audiologist checks the child's reactions through an observation window while the test sounds are repeated in a free-field situation with the sounds transmitted via a good-quality amplification system permitting control of sound intensity.

This method of testing has been criticized, principally because with noisemakers such as rattles and drums, music boxes, and other apparatus, the frequency span is wide rather than limited or discrete. This criticism is valid, but we have yet to find a more satisfactory testing method, except perhaps pure-tone audiometry.

The following are typical responses in a child with normal hearing:

1. Loud Sounds. The response varies with the child's age. Up to 3 months, a sudden loud sound elicits the so-called startle response, consisting of a general acoustic muscle reflex and a cochleo-palpebral or blink reflex. The infant adapts rapidly to this test so his first response must be carefully observed.

From 3 to 9 months, the startle response becomes progressively milder; sometimes the only evidence is a slight movement of the eyes, not always toward the sound source. Here again, repetition of the test tends to produce no response.

After 9 months, the startle response is replaced by turning the head and eyes toward the sound source. The child may respond more actively to voices and to quiet meaningful sounds than to loud noises.

2. *Quiet Sounds.* The response to quiet sounds also varies according to the child's age. Up to 3 months, there is usually no consistent response.

From 3 to 9 months, the infant looks in the direction of an unfamiliar sound. If it is repeated, he does not usually respond further. On the other hand, he quickly turns his head and eyes toward the source of familiar sounds such as those associated with feeding, familiar toys, and voices; this reaction is repeated on repetition of the sound. He responds to such sounds at about 25 to 30 decibels above his threshold level.

When the child from 9 to 18 months old hears soft familiar sounds, he immediately turns his head and eyes in the direction of the sound, a response that is again most marked to a familiar voice. At this age he also begins to understand simple commands.

From 18 months to 2 years of age, the child responds to even very faint sounds, localizing them accurately and quickly. He is developing speech and may use simple words and sentences.

These tests must be amplified (approximately 25 to 30 decibels above his threshold) in a child with a hearing impairment. Without amplification, the responses expected for the particular age group will be altered or perhaps lacking entirely, for example: (1) persistence of the startle response beyond the usual age of 9 months; (2) a continuing response to loud sounds only, no response to quiet sounds at the expected time; (3) response to familiar sounds as if they were unfamiliar; (4) apparent response with one ear only, as in unilateral hearing loss; and (5) failure to localize sound.

The above testing usually reveals a hearing impairment. When it is suspected, testing is continued in a soundproof room with calibrated amplification of the sound. Under these conditions, we can usually assess the child's hearing threshold, at least roughly, on the assumption that he will respond to the test sound at about 25 to 30 decibels above his threshold.

The main disadvantages of this entire test set-up is the free-field situation, whether in an open or soundproof room. With both ears being tested simultaneously, a unilateral hearing loss may be missed. Another drawback is the difficulty of diagnosing a relatively mild hearing impairment which still requires correction and follow-up. We

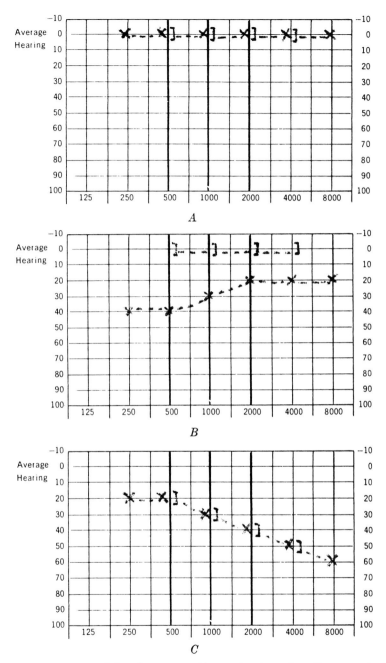

FIG. 18-1 A. *Normal hearing.* ✕ = *Air conduction;*] = *Bone conduction*
B. *Conductive hearing loss in left ear.* ✕ = *Air conduction;*] = *Bone conduction*
C. *Neurosensory hearing loss in left ear.* ✕ = *Air conduction;*] = *Bone conduction*

are therefore relying more and more on pure-tone audiograms for this age group.

3. Pure-Tone Audiometry. For children under 2, pure-tone audiometry was previously considered very difficult and the results inaccurate. If the method could be carried out, it would have the great advantage of permitting individual testing of each ear by exposing it to discrete pure tones rather than to the wide frequency range encompassed by most noisemakers. We are therefore attempting pure-tone audiometry in all infants and children. In common with other centers, we consider it imperative to have the tests given by a skilled audiologist who has had special experience with this age group.

The child must be carefully observed for blinking, eye movement, and other changes in activity while the pure tone is presented to each ear. We concentrate principally on the three middle frequencies—500, 1000, and 2000 cps—and employ the usual headphone set if tolerated by the infant. Otherwise, the mother or an examiner holds an individual ear phone as close as possible to the infant's ear without distracting him.

Basic tests are carried out by air conduction and, in the case of extremely cooperative children, also by bone conduction. It is assumed that any hearing loss revealed by air conduction represents a conductive rather than a neurosensory impairment, and it is treated as such in the child with cleft palate until proved otherwise.

In the hands of a skilled audiologist, reasonably accurate and reproducible pure-tone audiograms appear feasible in this group, although our experience to date is admittedly limited (Fig. 18-1).

TESTS IN CHILDREN OVER TWO

By the time a child has reached the age of 2, surgery for closure of the cleft palate has usually been completed. At St. Luke's this occurs at the age of 1. The child has had audiometric tests and is being followed routinely for one of the following reasons: (1) to confirm a provisional diagnosis of hearing impairment; (2) to confirm the original evaluation of normal hearing; (3) to assess any change in hearing (whether previously considered normal or abnormal) so that necessary treatment can be promptly instituted; and (4) to reveal any improvement in hearing following such measures as cleft palate surgery, local ear treatment, ear surgery, and adenoidectomy.

By the time of follow-up, the child is much more cooperative and can respond more accurately to test situations. Since the testing is easier, the procedures can be more exact and complex. It is relatively easier to assess hearing in each ear separately. In fact, we are convinced that some form of pure-tone test is now feasible.

We employ a form of audiometry based on play or a peep show, details of which are given in most standard textbooks. It has long been argued that since pure tones are not meaningful to young children, the responses cannot be accurate. Our center and others try to impart meaning to the pure-tone test for the older group, e.g., by likening the low pure tones to fog horns and the high pure tones to whistles. The children appear more eager to respond to such a play situation. Accurate, repeatable audiograms are usually obtained in children over 2.

In summary, the cleft palate team must be alert to the ever-present possibility of a hearing impairment in a child with this anomaly. Final diagnosis is based on the history, ear, nose, and throat examinations, and hearing tests. In a child under 2, tests showing normal hearing should be repeated if either the history or physical examination or both strongly suggest a hearing impairment. A skilled audiologist is essential to successful testing and rehabilitation measures. When attempting to test hearing in a child under 2, he will probably require several sessions to decide whether the tests are reliable.

Pure-tone audiometry in infants, recently introduced at St. Luke's Hospital Center, has yielded encouraging results thus far, but its reliability for this age group is yet to be established.

CHAPTER 19

Airway
Obstruction

EDWARD G. STANLEY-BROWN

Since the inception of the St. Luke's Cleft Palate Clinic in 1956, three patients have required a tracheostomy to relieve airway obstruction following cleft palate or lip repair. Two of these children are living and well; one died. Airway obstruction, a terrifying complication, and its management warrant a chapter of their own.

As noted elsewhere in this volume, cleft palate repair is usually performed when the infant is about 1 year old. Endotracheal anesthesia is virtually mandatory to provide a safe airway without interfering with the surgeon's operative field. Our anesthesiologists deserve high praise for their careful and successful management of the very large group of patients who experience no respiratory difficulties following cleft palate or lip repair. The dangerous combination of a receding, underdeveloped mandible, backward displacement of the tongue, and cleft palate (the Pierre Robin syndrome) was present in two of the three patients who required tracheostomy. The third patient had undergone a tracheostomy for severe infectious croup before coming to our hospital for cleft palate repair.

There follow brief clinical summaries of the three patients whose respiratory distress became so severe that tracheostomy was necessary to relieve obstruction of the airway.

J. K. K., No. 45-89-46

At age 12 hours this Negro male underwent primary repair of type III B atresia of the esophagus with tracheoesophageal fistula. The patient's mother had polyhydramnios, and the infant's associated congenital anomalies included cleft palate, micrognathia, and preauricular tabs. Palatoplasty with a primary pharyngeal flap was carried out at age 1 year. Respiratory distress, which was moderate in the recovery room, became increasingly severe over the first 48 postoperative hours. Fever to 103° F., tachypnea, and signs of exhaustion were progressive despite high humidity, oxygen, and judicious oropharyngeal suctioning. Tracheostomy was performed 48 hours after repair of the cleft palate, with immediate relief of symptoms. The tracheostomy tube was removed 4 days later, but respiratory distress recurred and a second tracheostomy was necessary 5 days after removal of the first tube. Steroid therapy was started (hydrocortisone, 40 mg. intramuscularly) and the respiratory difficulties were completely relieved. The tracheostomy tube was removed 6 days later. This patient is now making excellent progress and enjoying robust health.

S. G., No. 47-36-25

This 15-month-old white boy had suffered two severe episodes of infectious croup in the first year of life, and a tracheostomy was performed in another hospital during the second episode. (Details of the procedure were not available.) The patient's cleft of the palate was repaired, with a concomitant posterior pharyngeal flap, at St. Luke's Hospital at age 15 months. In the recovery room laryngeal stridor started as the patient regained consciousness, and despite a croup tent, penicillin, aminophylline, vaponefrin, and intravenous hydrocortisone, respiratory distress became progressively worse. Fever rose to 102° F., and increasing tachypnea and stridor continued until 72 hours after the palatoplasty, when tracheostomy was performed. The patient, exhausted, flaccid, and cyanotic, was immediately relieved and fell asleep for the first time in 48 hours.

Attempts to diminish gradually the lumen size of the No. 0 tracheostomy tube were unsuccessful. After 12 days direct laryngoscopy was performed under general anesthesia. The endoscopist reported laryngomalacia and tracheomalacia with no subglottic changes. Despite intensive medical and nursing care, further respiratory distress occurred 27 days following the tracheostomy. The patient quickly responded to a second course of steroid therapy. The tracheostomy tube was removed after a total of 32 days. The boy is well and healthy at this time.

K. H., 45-51-10

This 3-month-old white girl had microcephaly, micrognathia, brain damage with spasticity and mental retardation, probable blindness, and a median cleft lip and palate. This patient falls into the group with arhinencephalia and median cleft lip. Convulsive seizures had been partially controlled with phenobarbital. A cheiloplasty was performed under local anesthesia at age 3 months.

Cyanosis, apnea, marked retractions, and progressive respiratory distress characterized the 48-hour interval between operation and death. Treatment consisted of oxygen, high humidity, intravenous antihistamine preparations (Benadryl), and, finally, a tracheostomy performed 30 minutes before death. Chest X-ray on the patient's last day of life showed signs of pneumonia. No autopsy was performed.

The first patient was given no drugs prior to the tracheostomy. In seven recent pediatric patients undergoing surgery for conditions other than cleft lip or cleft palate, we have administered a maximum dose (100 mg.) of hydrocortisone intravenously, with sufficient relief of respiratory distress to avoid tracheostomy altogether. A dramatic anti-inflammatory response usually occurred within minutes after administration of the drug. Massive doses of antihistamine preparations have been given to six patients with respiratory distress in the immediate postoperative period with good and bad results equally divided.

Respiratory obstruction is infrequently encountered early after operations performed under general endotracheal anesthesia in children between 2 and 4 years—an age group particularly susceptible to croup or acute spasmodic laryngitis. It occurs rarely in children 5 or 6 years old. Certain children, especially those with a nervous disposition, appear more prone to this condition. For example, patient S. G. was quite tense.

The clinical manifestations of respiratory obstruction usually start with a hoarse, croupy cough, an increased respiratory rate, and low-grade fever. Increasing dyspnea, stridor, and suprasternal and infrasternal retractions are seen, along with restlessness which, in a small child, may be one of the earliest manifestations of air hunger. Untreated, the patient progresses to frank respiratory obstruction with cyanosis, exhaustion, minimal air exchange despite rapid, labored breathing and finally, extreme pallor and/or cyanosis and prostration.

Treatment should start as soon as the child begins to cough. An atmosphere of high humidity is vital to maintain thin, liquid, tracheobronchial secretions. Use of the Isolette or Croupette* permits saturation of the inspired air. Oxygen should be provided if the patient uses any of the accessory muscles for respiration. Oxygen therapy

* Air-Shields Corporation, Hatboro, Pennsylvania.

should not be delayed until cyanosis develops. There are several commercial devices which mechanically vaporize cold water and saturate the inspired air; however, the child will commonly turn his face away from the nozzle of these "cold steam" machines. The Croupette or oxygen tent is a more certain means of assuring high humidity of the inspired air.

Careful and judicious suctioning clears the nose and oropharynx of secretions. Too frequent suctioning is dangerous and most disturbing to the patient. For the child who has had a posterior pharyngeal flap operation with repair of the cleft palate, the greatest care must be exercised in passing suction catheters through the nose and mouth lest the pharyngeal flap be disturbed. The surgeon should mark the suction catheter himself at a safe length beyond which it must not be inserted.

At this stage of treatment the question of drug therapy is raised. Opiates and atropine are never indicated as they tend to dry secretions as well as diminish the cough reflex. While sedation in the form of phenobarbital is commonly prescribed, it is well to bear in mind constantly that restlessness may indicate air hunger as well as postoperative discomfort.

As mentioned previously, we have had limited success with intravenous antihistamine preparations. If these are ineffective and the patient appears to have increasing difficulty in breathing, intravenous steroid therapy is well worth trying. We have used 100 mg. of hydrocortisone as an immediate dose followed by continuous intravenous administration of hydrocortisone mixed with glucose and one-third or one-fourth normal saline.

If these measures do not help and the patient's breathing difficulty continues or increases, the question of when to perform a tracheostomy is raised. Our surgical residents learn early that for the adult with airway obstruction the time for the tracheostomy is when one first thinks of it. This axiom does not apply to the infant or child with respiratory difficulty in the postoperative period. In fact an appropriate rule to follow with the infant is: "Don't just do something—continue to stand there." When a tracheostomy is first contemplated for an infant or child the over-all picture should be carefully evaluated, as it is a serious procedure in this age group.

First, tracheostomy in the infant may be a difficult technical undertaking. The short, fat neck and tiny, soft trachea conspire against the surgeon. Pneumothorax on one or both sides may complicate an emergency procedure done at the cribside. It is generally safer to pass an endotracheal tube, thus overcoming the urgency of the problem, then perform the tracheostomy at leisure in the operating room with proper lighting and assistance.

The tiny tracheostomy tube is easily plugged by a bit of secretion or fleck of mucus, and constant nursing observation is mandatory. Too long a tracheostomy tube may occlude a main stem bronchus, while too short a tube is difficult to keep in place. If the curvature is the same as for an adult-sized tube, the tip may erode the posterior wall of the trachea causing ulceration, bleeding, and, later, possible stenosis.

Finally, "corking" or gradually diminishing the size of the lumen of a No. 0 or a No. 00 tube is difficult at best, and extubation may require weeks or even months.

It appears that our medical staff had these possible complications in mind, for in the three patients reviewed there was a delay of 48 hours in two instances and 72 hours in the third before tracheostomy was finally performed.

Despite the serious consequences and possible dangers attendant on tracheostomy, it is always a great relief to observe the infant or child breathing slowly and easily through the tracheostomy tube, often falling asleep for the first time after hours of a gasping, exhausting struggle to breathe. One is invariably left with the impression that the tracheostomy should have been performed hours earlier.

At St. Luke's the crucial decision to perform tracheostomy is usually arrived at through mutual agreement between pediatrician, anesthesiologist, plastic and pediatric surgeons, and our experienced nurses.

A brief account of the technical details of carrying out a tracheostomy seems appropriate. The conventional tracheostomy is performed under local anesthesia and, as previously suggested, should be done in the operating room. If an endotracheal tube or a bronchoscope has been passed to reestablish the airway, general anesthesia may be necessary. While passage of an endotracheal tube is not vital for older children, it is invaluable for infants. The presence of an intratracheal splint permits easy location of the tiny trachea and simplifies the actual tracheostomy into this flaccid, collapsible structure.

The midline incision is placed in the center of Jackson's triangle. Although a horizontal incision in an adult will be little noticed, the slight advantage of exposure afforded by the vertical incision is needed in the infant or child. The steps of the operation are clearly illustrated in Figure 19-1. With proper light and adequate exposure, bleeding is rarely a problem. A skin hook is perhaps the most helpful instrument for grasping the trachea and holding it steady. The proper size tracheostomy tube must be selected to ensure a proper fit (Table 19-1).

Gauze treated with petroleum jelly may be packed loosely into the skin incision and the tracheostomy tube securely held in place

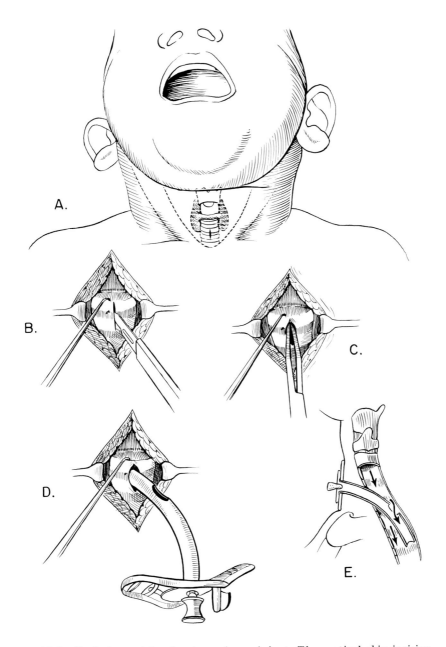

FIG. 19-1 *Technique of tracheostomy in an infant. The vertical skin incision is centered in Jackson's triangle and deepened through subcutaneous tissue, and platysma muscle in the midline. Blunt dissection exposes the trachea, which is seized with a skin hook. A slit incision is made into the trachea and spread open with a mosquito forceps. While the trachea is still held with the skin hook, the tracheostomy tube is inserted after the bronchoscope or endotracheal tube has been withdrawn.*

TABLE 19-1 SIZE OF TRACHEOSTOMY TUBE
SUITABLE FOR CHILDREN
OF VARIOUS AGES

Age	Size of Tube
Newborn	00
6 mo.	00–0
12 mo.	0
18 mo.	0–1
2 yr.	1
3 yr.	1–2
4 yr.	2
5–7 yr.	2–3
8–12 yr.	3–4

with strips of umbilical tape, encircling the patient's neck and tied to the plate of the silver tube.

Postoperative care of the infant or child with a tracheostomy demands constant nursing observation, high humidity of the inspired air, and judicious suctioning. Use of a Y-tube catheter, illustrated in Figure 19-2, is helpful.

It is well to bear in mind that the suction catheter removes air along with mucus and other secretions. Thus, intermittent suctioning is preferable to long continuous periods.

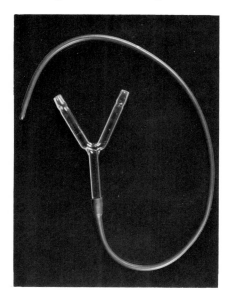

FIG. 19-2 *Y tube for suctioning a tracheostomy. The suction source is attached to one limb of the Y, and the nurse obtains intermittent suction by intermittently occluding the other limb of the Y with her thumb.*

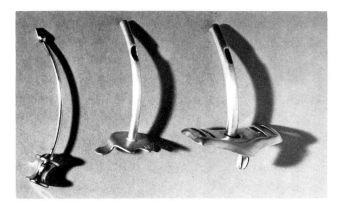

FIG. 19-3 *Tracheostomy tube prepared with fenestration in outer tube and inner cannula. With the tube corked the airway is provided by this fenestration.*

A chest X-ray is advisable to assure proper positioning of the tracheal tube. It must be in the trachea, and not too long, lest it enter either main stem bronchi.

The older child may be terrified to discover that he cannot speak unless the lumen of the tracheostomy tube is temporarily occluded. This maneuver should be demonstrated to him as soon as is feasible after construction of the tracheostomy.

The inner cannula of the tracheostomy tube must be removed and cleansed from time to time since the very small lumen is easily obstructed by a bit of dried mucus or other secretion. After the fourth or fifth day the outer tracheal tube should be changed daily by a physician, to permit cleaning and sterilization.

In infants, gradual removal of the tracheostomy tube is best accomplished by changing to tubes of decreasing diameter. Finally, the smallest tube is corked for short periods. When the patient can tolerate occlusion for many consecutive hours, complete removal may be contemplated. With the smallest tubes and youngest patients, a helpful technique is to pass a specially drilled tube which provides an airway despite the corking (Fig. 19-3). Final removal of the tube should be done during daylight hours with a full complement of medical and nursing staff on hand. In one tragic instance at another institution, the tracheal tube was removed late in the evening. In the small hours of the morning when respiratory obstruction recurred, tracheal reintubation was delayed and the patient died.

In summary, tracheostomy in the infant, though, life-saving, is not without its complications and should not be entered into lightly or inadvisedly.

CHAPTER 20

Language
and
Speech
Development

JANE DORSEY ZIMMERMAN

WILLIAM H. CANFIELD

Since speech problems of patients with cleft palate differ largely in degree, not necessarily in kind, from those of other speakers, a discussion of general language and speech development and disabilities is a prerequisite to the examination of the speech problems of patients with cleft palate. After this discussion, our specific concern will be the rationale of speech therapy at St. Luke's Hospital Center for patients with cleft palate.

NORMAL LANGUAGE AND SPEECH DEVELOPMENT

Language and speech normally develop during the first 2½ years of life. The young child starts with reflexive vocalizations which are gradually turned into oral communications; he progresses through crying, cooing, gurgling, babbling (accidental repetition of speech sound syllables that give him pleasure), lalling (repetition of heard syllables) and echolalling (repetition of another person's repetition of his lalling), to the reduction of these syllables into "real" words such as "mama" and "dada." These words produce desired results when associated with persons, objects, and experiences. Single real words, which may appear at from 8 to 12 months, can have different but related meanings. For example, "mama" may express various desires such as, "Mother, pick me up," "Mother, feed me," "Mother, take me out," or "Mother, I want your attention." During the next 12 months he repeats and learns to use more and more single words to satisfy his needs and desires, gradually adding utterances of two, three, or more words. At 24 months he may be using sentences.

Most children go through similar stages in speech development from the earliest cooing and babbling to words learned for everyday speaking. Although they usually go through these language developing periods at about the same ages, their prespeech and early speech utterances vary considerably. Children make the greatest strides in speech learning during the second year. Early attempts may result in errors in pronunciation (i.e., the common type of baby talk) and in grammar or word usage. Much jargon and jabbering are interspersed with actual speech, but children learn to control their speech mechanism and thinking-speaking processes more precisely through this practice. A 2-year-old does not, however, learn to verbalize his responses unless he has been stimulated to do so from the time his first real words appear. The most important single factor in speech development is probably the child's realization that he *must* talk.

All aspects of language and speech facility are strongly influenced by the child's and family's backgrounds—their health, education, and general mental and emotional states. Although no single factor is in itself decisive, all bear on the rate and extent of learning and the manner of speaking. Specific factors affecting the types, amount, and time of language and speech development include physiological, intellectual and social maturation; normal structure and adequate neurosensory-motor function of the organism (i.e., perception of language and speech through auditory, visual, tactile, kinesthetic, and proprioceptive stimuli, and expression through gross and fine motor coordination and action); intelligence; and environmental stimulation toward speech practice. Normal development presupposes normal structure and functioning. The stimulation offered by family and friends, essential to the child's early over-all development, continues to be an important part of the learning-speaking process throughout his years, in school and out. For those with major disabilities, practice, reevaluation, and continued therapy may be required for many years.

The following material on the production of language and speech elements may be helpful in our later consideration of these factors in speakers with cleft lip and palate.

LANGUAGE

Language is any system used for communication. It may be spoken, written, gestured, or indicated in other ways. Speech is the means of associating spoken symbols of language with ideas or meanings. Perception and association of written and/or spoken symbols with objects, ideas, concepts, or meanings are necessary to use language receptively for reading and listening and expressively for speaking, reading aloud, and writing. Some modalities of expressive language are naming, repeating, counting or other serial language, and calculating, as well as organizing and formulating independent utterances.

The ability to form and use concepts enables one to associate and integrate words as language symbols with ideas. Intelligence and language development are also interrelated, but in a way as yet only partially understood; intelligence is only one item affecting the development and use of language.

SPEECH

Speech, here considered as oral language, may be viewed as a composite of voice, pronunciation, rate, and rhythm, including stress and phrasing—all interdependent. The production of speech is accomplished by the actions of a mechanism that is in a real sense the whole human body. Its over-all contribution to the oral language process provides the requisite balance and coordination which permits the freest and most efficient functioning of all its parts from the beginning to the end of each speaking act through control of the gross muscles for assuming and maintaining good posture, through contraction of the lower abdominal muscles which transforms passive exhalation into active potentials, thus ensuring the slight increase in air pressure needed to help set the vocal cords into vibration and producing voice. This action, with that exerted on the vocal muscles by the laryngeal nerves, is required to initiate and keep flowing smooth, strong tone throughout each sense group of words spoken. In addition, the slowly released contraction of the inhalatory muscles, the diaphragm, and the muscles of the thorax assists in the phonatory process. Such action of the gross muscles is also essential to effect proper tension of the muscles of the larynx, mouth, and oral and nasal pharynx.

VOICE

Voice, the element of speech recognized as tone, produced in the larynx by adjustments of the vocal cords and reinforced in the resonating oral, pharyngeal, and nasal cavities and surfaces, has three physical aspects: *loudness*, *duration*, and *pitch*. Each of these aspects results from the total action of the speech mechanism.

Loudness of voice depends on amplitude of the vocal cord vibrations produced and their reinforcement through resonance. Adequate volume, an important factor in voice projection even for short distances, is necessary for oral communication.

Duration, the time element of voice, results from the sustained production of speech sounds, syllables, words, phases, or sentences. Closely related to duration is the rhythm of speech, which includes both word stress or accent and the rhetorical stress given to important words in a sentence, and varies with the purpose, meaning, and importance of what is said, as well as with the sounds themselves.

Pitch, perceived as the highness or lowness of tone, relates directly to the frequency of vibration of the vocal cords. Vocal pitch includes *key* (the average or base level from which the voice rises or falls), *inflection* (change of pitch within an accented syllable or word), and *intonation* (changes of pitch within a phrase or sentence). Age, sex, education, culture, and the language spoken are among many factors which determine the appropriateness of the speaker's habitual pitch level and "tunes."

Although some sound-producing mechanisms may vibrate at one pitch only, vibrations produced in the larynx are quite complex, with a fundamental frequency of pitch accompanied by a number of different vibrations known as partials or overtones. All these pitches sounding together produce a tone complex known as *quality*. Descriptive terms of voice qualities are usually impressionistic labels, although investigators frequently try to measure qualities objectively through instruments. Results of such attempts are generally inconclusive. Some of the terms used to describe adequate voice qualities are *clear*, *melodious* or *musical*, *full*, *firm*, *rich*, and *resonant*.

These positive voice qualities result from the interaction of the fundamental frequencies produced at the larynx and the selective reinforcement or damping out of partials by the action of resonating cavities and surfaces above, and perhaps below, the vocal cords. The resonating process modifies the tones and imparts to the listener the acoustic impression of quality. The tonal quality depends on the number and relative frequency and strength of the partials. The size, shape, and surface texture of the three principal human resonators (oral, nasal, and pharyngeal cavities) and their openings determine the type and amount of modification and reinforcement of the original laryngeal tone.

Speech Sound Production

Combinations of pitches account not only for voice qualities but also for some of the sound units spoken together to form words. Units formed by some restriction of the outgoing air are *consonants* and are *articulated;* those formed with little or no restriction are *vowels* and are *enunciated*. Two vowels sounded sequentially in a single syllable form a *diphthong*.

Most speakers are aware of these sound units only insofar as they are a part of the pronunciation of a word. *Pronunciation*, however, as considered here, means the sounding together (as words) of consonants, vowels, and diphthongs with level, downward, or upward inflections and with word stress or accent.

Articulation, literally jointing, refers to approximation of speech organs to produce consonants, but here includes descriptions of vowel sounds as well. The articulators are the mandible, lips, teeth, hard palate, velum, and tongue. As these organs meet and move from position to position, stopping or otherwise restricting the breath stream, consonant sounds result. Various adjustments determine the *manner* and *place* of production of speech sounds. If the vocal cords vibrate, the speech sounds are *voiced*; if they do not vibrate, the sounds are said to be *breathed, voiceless,* or *unvoiced.* It should be noted that there is some adjustment in the larynx when any speech sound is produced, whether voiced or voiceless.

Every audible English speech sound, whether voiced or voiceless, has mouth (oral) reinforcement. Vowels, diphthongs, and all the consonants except the final sounds in *hum, spin,* and *sing* resonate primarily in the mouth and throat; but /m/, /n/, and /ŋ/,* which also have some mouth and throat reinforcement, resonate primarily in the nasal passages. Closing the nostrils tightly during the production of any one of these nasal consonants stops the continuation of the sound.

CONSONANT SOUNDS

Consonant sounds result from (1) stoppage of the outgoing voiced or voiceless air, as in plosive sound production; (2) emission of air through the nasal passage to produce nasal consonants; (3) release of the breath stream orally over the sides of the tongue, with its tip held against the upper alveolar ridge for the lateral sound; or (4) restriction of the outgoing voiced or voiceless air in the vocal tract which produces fricative sounds.

Plosives. Plosive sounds made in isolation have three identifying characteristics: (1) a stop, (2) a hold (compression), and (3) a release (slight explosion) of air in the mouth with the velum raised. Plosives formed by the two lips are /p/ and /b/; those formed by the tongue tip against the upper alveolar ridge are /t/ and /d/; and those formed by the back of the tongue against the velum are /k/ and /g/. The first sound in each of these pairs is voiceless and the second sound is voiced.

Nasals. Nasal sounds are made when the velum lowers and voiced air escapes through the nasal passages. In English, the nasal consonants are /m/ formed by the lips, /n/ formed by the tongue tip against the upper alveolar ridge, and /ŋ/ as in *sing* formed by the back of the tongue against the velum, with the tongue tip against the lower

* This symbol and others to follow, which represent phonetic symbols (some are different from the letters of the alphabet), appear in Table 20-1 (page 248) with illustrative words.

gum ridge. The nasal sounds are voiced except when preceded by /s/, as in *smile* and *snow.*

Lateral. The lateral sound /l/, formed when the tongue tip, held against the upper alveolar ridge, permits the air to pass over the sides of the tongue. The velum is raised, and the sound is voiced except when preceded in a word by /p/, /f/, /s/, or /k/ as in *pleat, fleet, sleet,* or *klieg.*

Fricatives. Fricative sounds result when the speech organs restrict the outgoing air with lips rounded to form /ʌ/ as in *where,* and /w/ as in *wear;* with the lower lip against the lower edge of the upper teeth to form the two *th* sounds (as in *thin* /θ/ and *then* /ð/); with the tongue tip (apex) at the upper alveolar ridge to form /r/, /s/, and /z/; with the blade of tongue raised to form /ʃ/ as in *shy* and /ʒ/ as in *azure;* with the tongue tip low and the front of the tongue raised to form /j/ as in *hallelujah;* and with the vocal cords somewhat approximated to form /h/ as in *hand.*

VOWEL SOUNDS

Vowel sounds are produced by relatively unrestricted, vocalized air modified during emission by various adjustments of the pharynx, tongue, and lips. The classification of these sounds as front, middle, and back depends on the activity of the part of the tongue used in their production; as tense or slack, according to the height and tenseness or slackness of the active part of the tongue; and as rounded or unrounded, according to the position of the lips. Back vowels, made with the back of the tongue moving from a high position toward the hard palate to a low position in the oral cavity, are /u/, /ʊ/, /o/, /ɔ/, /ɒ/, and /ɑ/. The lips, pursed for the first two, have open rounding for the third, an oval position for the fourth, slightly rounded for the fifth, and an open unrounded position for the last. Front vowels /i/, /ɪ/, /e/, /ɛ/, /æ/, and /a/ are those made with the front of the tongue moving from a high to a low position in the mouth, and with unrounded lips in isolation, but with lip rounding following a lip-rounded consonant in the same syllable, as in the word *she,* compared with the unrounded vowel, as in the word *see.* Midvowels, made with the central portion of the tongue midway between high and low and front and back positions in the mouth, are /ɜ/, /ʌ/, and /ə/.

DIPHTHONGS

Diphthongs, two combined sounds enunciated within the same syllable, can consist of any two vowels, with one sound serving as on-glide or off-glide of the other. In English, the regularly listed diphthongs are those with /ɪ/ as an off-glide—/eɪ/, /aɪ/, and ɔɪ/; those with /ə/ as an off-glide—/ɪə/, ɛə/, /ɑə/, /ɔə/, and ʊə/; and those with /ʊ/ as an off-glide—/aʊ/ and /oʊ/. Some authors believe that in American English all vowels spoken in stressed or accented syllables have on- and off-glides.*

Rhythm and Synthesis of Speech

The above described consonants, vowels, and diphthongs form syllables and words when blended together in units such as phrases, clauses, and sentences.

All words spoken individually or separately, as in a word list, receive "word" stress. Certain words selected by a speaker to carry the major portion of his meaning are "key" or "content" words and receive sense or sentence stress. These "key" words are usually noun subjects and objects, verbs of action or being, and modifiers such as adverbs and adjectives. In addition, sense groups contain auxiliary, "function," or "form" words: conjunctions, articles, prepositions, pronouns, etc. "Helping" words pronounced individually or used for emphasis may become "key" words, which have strong forms and receive stress. In conversational speech, these words generally have weak or reduced forms.

Sense stress, the prominence given to important monosyllables and accented syllables of polysyllabic words in speaking, results from such techniques of emphasis as an increase in force, or a change in pitch, or an extension of time on these syllables. Such thought-bearing words and syllables of important words also stand out because the "helping" words and nonaccented syllables of the "key" words stand back, as they receive less force and/or time or tone.

The alternation of stressed and unstressed words and syllables recurs regularly and furnishes the essential rhythms of English speech. There is much diversity within the limits of acceptable and appropriate rhythm patterns of the language, as used by the same speaker at different times and as used by different speakers.

Although the time used to utter a phrase or sense group of words may change considerably from one occasion to another or from one speaker to another, the general rate depends primarily on the speaker's habitual tempos and rhythms. Such factors as the speaker's meaning, the speaking situation, the word and sense stress determined by the choice of words, and the phonetic structure of the speech sounds making up the spoken words also determine the rate and rhythm of speech. Moreover, the rate, rhythm, and stress affect the production and use of speech sounds in contextual speech patterns.

The place and manner of producing all sounds used in English

* See Table 20-1.

change to some degree according to their use within a syllable or word or phrase. Speech sounds also influence one another as they occur in connected speech, and this assimilation of sounds influences the phonetic result.

The blending and linking of sounds, syllables, and words in sense groups modifies the sounds themselves as they react upon each other. Consequently, a sound produced in isolation may differ in several respects from the same sound produced in a word or phrase. Speech synthesis therefore results from the dynamic and ever-changing interaction and interrelation of language with the production of voice, pronunciation, and rhythm of speech.

Changes in sound production during the flow of speech may result in the substitution of one sound for another, and/or the omission of a sound or sounds. The following are illustrations of these changes in both "form" and thought-bearing words: (1) The sound /z/, represented by the letter *s* in the form word *is*, is pronounced /z/ in its strong form in such a sequence as "the cat (or dog) is here," but becomes /s/ in the contracted form, "The cat's here," with the vowel /ɪ/ omitted. In the sentence, "The dog's here," the vowel in *is* is omitted but the consonant remains /z/. (2) The sound /t/ is substituted for the letter *d*, with the *e* omitted, in such words as *asked* or *stopped* (/stɒpt/). (3) /æ/ as in *cat* and /ɑ/ as in *calm* may be substituted for /a/ in the so-called *ask*-words—*asked, cast, aunt, dance*, etc. (4) The sounds /ɔ/ and /ɒ/ are both heard in the words *coffee, orange*, etc., also pronounced with /ɑ/ by some speakers. (5) *Root, room*, etc. heard commonly with an /u/ vowel, as in *rude*, may have /u/ substituted by /ʊ/, the vowel in *look*.

Other substitutions may be /v/ for /f/ in *nephew;* /ŋ/ as in *song* for /n/ in *conquest;* and /gʒ/ for /kʃ/ for the *x* in *luxurious*.

Sounds omitted acceptably in some words, as in the omission of /p/ in *empty*, may be acceptable additions in other words such as *comfortable* with the /p/ inserted between /m/ and /f/. The omission of /t/ in *cents*, and its addition to *sense*, and the omission of /d/ in *finds*, and its addition to *fines*, cause a reversal in the pronunciation of each of these two groups of words. It must be noted, however, that many or even most speakers pronounce alike the two words in each of these groups, with /t/ omitted or included in both *cents* and *sense*, and with /d/ omitted or included in both *finds* and *fines*.

LANGUAGE AND SPEECH DISABILITIES ASSOCIATED WITH CLEFT LIP AND PALATE

The language and speech of those born with cleft lip and/or palate, as in the population at large, range from "normal" to severely impaired. This is true of children and adults referred to the St. Luke's Hearing and Speech Department from the Cleft Palate Clinic. Some of them have little or no speech disability; others have severe disorders of one or more of the communication modalities of language and speech.

The specific language and speech problems discussed here include an overview of the language, voice, articulation, and rate and rhythm disorders presented generally by the many patients diagnosed and treated at St. Luke's. Since these types of oral communication disorders vary considerably from one person to another, individual case histories of patients will be given later, representing those who had (1) no surgery; (2) primary pharyngeal flap surgery before speech development (speech adequate); (3) secondary pharyngeal flap surgery after speech development (speech adequate); (4) primary pharyngeal flap surgery after speech development (speech inadequate); and (5) secondary pharyngeal flap surgery after speech development (speech inadequate).

Language Problems

Language problems may be receptive and/or expressive. Of the patients with cleft lip and palate referred for speech and hearing services at St. Luke's language disabilities are not as prevalent as are certain speech problems; however, in patients with multiple handicaps both language and speech may be impaired.

Receptive language problems of some children referred from the Cleft Palate Clinic appear to stem not from an inability to comprehend language but from not having learned to pay attention to oral language. The physical needs and problems of these children often require so much of the parents' attention and energy that their language needs and home stimulation have been neglected.

Receptive language problems in this group may arise, however, because of a hearing impairment. If a child has a hearing loss, he may also have difficulty in language learning, since he is unable to hear the words and patterns needed. Children who acquire language skills and subsequently develop a hearing impairment may have no difficulty in learning to understand written language at a later time. Their problems in comprehending spoken language may be related to loss in auditory reception rather than to any inability to interpret what they hear. Children with severe hearing loss often display reduced oral communication skills in vocabularly development, grammar, sentence structure and length, etc., as well as in voice, articulation, and rate and rhythm of speech.

If children can make their needs known by crying or other nonverbal means, or if mothers satisfy these needs either by anticipating them before they are expressed vocally or by responding to the vocalizations without demanding that the children use conventional language, then the children will not develop speech at a normal rate.

Another factor in delay is the shy, withdrawn personality displayed by some children who seem embarrassed by their appearance. This is especially true of those with a cleft lip, because of the obvious anomaly. Many of them make only limited attempts to verbalize, primarily because of reluctance to call attention to their physical appearance rather than because of inability to do so.

Some language problems encountered in patients from a large metropolitan area, such as New York City, arise from their difficulties in learning English as a second language. Many children growing up in a bilingual environment take in stride a second or even a third language, but others do not. It is often hard to assess the language skills of those who speak little or no English. Their problems tend to be due less to their physical anomalies than to a lack of knowledge of English or of facility in using this language and to an environment offering scant opportunity for practicing oral language. Bilingual parents frequently report that their children who are delayed in learning English are retarded in use of their native tongue as well.

A number of children with cleft lip and palate seen for language and speech evaluations appear to be somewhat slower in developing expressive language than are other children of comparable ages. In a group of 16 children with mean age of 3 years who underwent pharyngeal flap surgery before development of the first meaningful speech, language evaluation revealed some delay in developing and using oral language in almost 50 per cent of the group.

Fortunately, most children delayed in language development, including those with cleft lip and palate, eventually catch up to other children of the same age group and general intelligence if adults require them to use conventional language rather than mere cries, grunts, and gestures. Long-term follow-up evaluations of children undergoing primary pharyngeal flap surgery prior to the development of language indicated that by the time they were 5 years old they compared favorably in language usage with the average of their age group.

Voice Problems

Voice disabilities found among children and adults with cleft lip and palate, as well as in the general speaking population, may include those related to one or more physical aspects of tone, i.e., pitch (including quality), loudness, and duration, each varying in degree from mild to severe. Furthermore, a fault in one voice aspect may give an impression of inadequacy in others.

Faults in pitch are those in which tone is too high or too low in base or key pitch, monotonous, too varied, or stereotyped in the use of inflectional patterns (within words) and intonation patterns (within phrases). The speech of some referred patients was characterized by excessively high-keyed pitch with an even higher rise to stress the important words.

Closely associated with faulty pitch and commonly noted in persons with speech difficulties are disorders of *quality*. Among those heard in patients referred were breathiness, huskiness, harshness, hoarseness, flatness, stridency, and nasality, which ranged from the hyponasal (rhinolalia clausa) to the hypernasal (rhinolalia aperta). Hyponasality or denasalization is sometimes called the "cold-in-the-head" quality. Excessive denasalization heard in the speech of many of these patients caused blurring throughout, along with a muffled thickness of voice quality during at least part of the subject's utterances. Other patients had different types of hypernasality with equally severe quality deficiencies, e.g., nasally overaspirated voice production (sometimes labeled "nasal snorting"), so-called "relaxed soft palate" nasality associated with hypotonus or other inadequacies of the velar muscles, and a nasal twang produced by hyperconstriction of the throat and/or the nasopharyngeal muscles. Flatness and a hypertense "throat-squeeze" called "glottal or vocal fry" were also evident.

Disorders associated with volume included some voices overly loud and others so weak as to be almost inaudible. Certain patients expend all their energy on the first syllables or words, forcing them out with too much intensity, and then fade out at the ends of phrases or sentences to complete inaudibility. Weak volume and lack of projection were more commonly encountered than overloudness.

Faults associated with duration of tone included jerky, choppy, arrhythmic, cluttered utterance with rate too fast for intelligibility, or very slow and hesitant, sometimes drawled and sometimes scanned. These faults may be closely related to certain other aspects of speech disorders, e.g., articulation, rate, and rhythm, as well as to voice production. Some problems of duration result from or influence the rate, rhythm, and phrasing; others are associated with sustaining tone and thus determine how a speaker produces or uses vowel and consonant sounds. Such problems can be noted when consonants are confused, e.g., /v/ becoming unvoiced, or when a type of glottal stop sound is substituted for a postvocalic consonant, e.g., *hat*/hæt/ becoming /hæʔ/. Numerous faults are heard in connection with fading volume of voice at the end of phrases, with the omission of final sounds, and with the lack of a sustained and continuous flow of tone throughout thought groups.

Articulation Problems

Articulation problems often create the most difficulty for those with cleft lip and palate and are also the most obvious oral communication deficiencies. They occur in conjunction with other voice and speech production faults, often in direct proportion to the speaker's over-all speaking disabilities. Some patients with cleft palate have little or no trouble in producing intelligible speech, while others have many and severe types of misarticulation, including omissions, substitutions, additions, and/or distortions of speech sounds, which interfere with their ability to produce acceptable, understandable speech.

Among numerous factors that may influence the type of articulation patterns are the condition of anatomical structures used to articulate speech sounds, the amount of sphincteric action present in the velopharyngeal mechansim, the suppleness and flexibility of lip and velum, the nature and extent of surgery, and the patients' age at the time, as well as the psychological, intellectual, cultural, and educational influences that contribute to language and speech development and usage in all human beings. A most important factor influencing articulation patterns in children with cleft lip and palate is the manner in which they receive early language and speech stimulation from family, friends, and teachers. Many articulation problems grow out of the child's compensatory actions when well-meaning but oftentimes misguided parents and teachers urge him to make his speech clear. The resulting overenergized attempts to produce clear speech sounds become incorporated into his everyday speaking habits. Evaluation of the speech habits and patterns of children and adults with cleft palate who have articulation disorders frequently seems to indicate that their speech habits interfere more with general intelligibility than does the cleft itself, whether repaired or not. Some persons with a sizable unrepaired cleft can easily control the air pressure needed for use in speech sound production, while others with smaller clefts experience much more difficulty in this respect. Tape recordings of sounds made by infants born with cleft lip and/or palate at St. Luke's Hospital reveal little or no distortion of vocal quality during babbling, lalling, echolalling, and other types of vocal play even before surgical repair.

The following case is illustrative:

R. S., No. 48-84-48

Born with a median cleft lip and cleft palate, R had a cheiloplasty 13 days after birth, and upper lip revision 3 months later; palatoplasty and closure of the oral-nasal palate 9 months after that; secondary cheiloplasty at about age 3 years: rhinoplasty at age 5 years.

Sampling of Cries Recorded Follows

Quality of voice was husky and oral, not nasal; volume strong, although vocalizations varied from loud to soft; utterance was staccato.

Vocalizations

Age 5½ months. *Crying:* ?ɑ?ʌ| ?ʌ...?ʌ| ?ɑ?ʌ?ʌ‖; ?ɑ...?ʌ...
?ʌ... *ends with rising inflection, then goes immediately into
smooth, sustained crooning:* ʌ...ʌ...ʌ...‖. *Crooning continues:*
ʌ... *pitch rises... then falls...*‖. *Crying again:* ?ʌ...?ʌ‖ *rasping,
raucous:* ?ʊ...?ʊ‖ *more raucous, ends with falling inflection from
a low pitch;* ?ʌ?ʌ?æ|?ʌ?ʌ‖ *loud, forced, hard quality. Almost
singing: tone high and clear:* ʌ *falling inflection,* ʌ *continues with
rising pitch,* ʌ *falling* ʌʌ *rising* ʌʌ *falling*‖. *Panting,* then *crying*
in a strong, rasping voice on a low pitch, as though in anger,
and then without interruption, changing to quiet crying.
Although the crying sounds were often nasal and/or flat, there
was no evidence of snorting.

Age 1 year. *Crying:* The crying was more sustained throughout, was frequently nasal, and varied in sounds from/?ʌ/ to
/?æ/ to /?ε/.

Age 2 years, 8 months. *Voice production:* Often flat and nasal,
but there was no sound of unphonated breath escaping, and
no snorting.

Age 3 years, 3 months. *Voice production and consonant
articulation:* Nasality and flatness persisted, but at intervals
the voice was clear. Consonants were missing occasionally in
initial position, and had glottal stops (rarely glottal plosives)
substituted for them in final positions of words or sense groups,
and in combination with other consonants. Some consonants
were pronounced adequately, especially in words recently added
to everyday speaking.

Age 5½ years. R had some very smooth productions of voice,
some throaty to husky, some flat and nasal, and with an excessively high pitch when excited, which is often; no snorting. All
the speech sounds are made adequately in some words where
they belong, but also in some words where they do not; there
remain omissions and substitutions in words learned early.

Speech Sample

Age 6 years, 2 months. aε seɪ 'dðɪs‖ 'haɪ 'dɪdu 'dɪdu| ə 'kæ?
ɪn ə 'fɪʊ‖ ə 'kaʊ 'dʒʌmp 'oʊvə dðə ' mun‖ dðə 'lɪtə 'dɔ? 'læəf|
tʊ ' si 'sʌ? 'spo?| dðə 'dɪʃ 'rʌn ə 'weɪ wɪ? ə dɪʃ| a 'min 'spun‖.

Recent Interview

Age 7½ years. R was friendly, but shy, having just returned to
New York to live, and perhaps feeling a little strange. Her voice
production was sometimes breathy, and always a bit husky, but

there was less evidence of nasality than is average in this country. Her articulation was adequate and, for the most part, accurate. There remained some glottalizing of stressed vowels, as for instance she said |ˀʌˀɛəpleɪn| for *an airplane*. She still slighted or omitted some final consonants, such as the /g/ in *dog*, and a few initial sounds such as the *a* in *arithmetic*. When asked what she does in school she said, "We write and do 'rithmetic. We take away and subtrac'."

R has a devoted and resourceful mother who babbled and crooned with her when she was an infant, vocalized with her as she was developing speech, and can be counted on to help her in the speechways that will hold her interest and will be most useful to her.

Some of these same youngsters develop articulation disorders later, however, as they learn to talk.

Patients with repeated surgery on the lip or velum often seem to have a less flexible articulatory mechanism and many articulation deviations because of the considerable scar tissue that is present. Children who have only cleft lip seem generally to have fewer and less severe articulation difficulties than do those with cleft palate as well. Their difficulties are primarily with sounds formed by one or both lips, such as /p/, /b/, /m/, /f/, and /v/, or by some lip-rounding, such as /w/, /ʍ/, /ʃ/, and /ʒ/, and the so-called lip-rounded vowels. Distortion of these sounds, along with others, may be due to asymmetry of the lips, collapse of the alveolus, immobility of the lips either from habit or extensive surgical repair, missing teeth, or malocclusion of the mandible. Immobility and stiffness of the upper lip may result from anatomical and physiological factors, but can also be attributed to the speaker's tendency to hold the upper lip tightly and rigidly against the upper teeth, thus interfering with accurate and clear articulation of labial and other sounds.

When structural anomalies extend to the teeth and alveolus or involve function of the tongue muscles, proper articulation of tongue-tip–alveolar-ridge sounds may be affected. Consonant sounds formed by the tongue tip and teeth (/θ/ and /ð/), the tongue tip and alveolus (/t/, /d/, /l/, /s/, /z/, /r/, and /n/), and the blade of the tongue and alveolus (/ʃ/, /ʒ/, /tʃ/, and /dʒ/) occur the most frequently in every-day speech and are of the utmost importance to intelligibility. Many patients distort such sounds, as they seem to retract or bunch the back of the tongue during speech in an effort to gain better control of tongue and velopharyngeal musculature. Patients with cleft palate may have additional problems of misarticulation. The palate's neuromuscular functioning can be impaired, as well as the anatomical structures making it difficult for the speaker's velopharyngeal and articulatory mechanisms to perform rapidly and with precision during speech. Difficulty in articulating speech sounds may be due not only to the cleft itself but also to the paucity of tissue in the hard palate and velum resulting from a total, subtotal, or submucous cleft. These patients may distort by a blurred or snorted production, or substitute some other sound such as the glottal stop /ʔ/ for many of the consonants, particularly as they occur in final positions of words or phrases.

The manner of producing speech sounds may also be affected by both lip and palate clefts; the speaker sometimes cannot produce needed sounds at all, or does so with such effort as to distort them to the point of unintelligibility. Some of the omissions, additions, substitutions, and distortions of speakers with one or both anomalies seem to bear little or no relation to the anomalies. Rather, they are habitually used by most native speakers. Examples of common deviations are:

1. Omission of such final consonant clusters as *ts* in the word *lists*, *t* in the word *kept*, or *k* in the word *asked*

2. Substitution of voiceless for a voiced sound such as /b̥/ for /bᵊ/ in the word *cab* (not to be confused with the non-native substitution of /p/ for /b/ which makes *cab* sound like *cap*); substitution of a stop sound for *th* as in *thing* and *then*, of /n/ for /ŋ/ in *coming* and *going;* uni- or bisubstitution of a glottal stop sound for a final consonant, such as /lɪʔ/ for the word *live;* substitution of a vowel for a postvocalic /l/, such as /mɪɔk/, or /mɪʊk/ for the word *milk*

3. Distortions which result in variations of place and manner of production of /s/, /z/, /ʃ/, and /ʒ/, generally designated as interdental, uni- or bilateral, labiodental, blade-of-tongue (thick), nasal, or pharyngeal lisps; blade-of-tongue articulation of tongue-tip–alveolar-ridge sounds often designated as dentalization; overaspiration of breathed stop sounds /p/, /t/, and /k/, and many voiceless fricative sounds, especially /h/ when used initially in stressed syllables; and the distortion of vowels and diphthongs generally designated as nasal and/or "flat"

4. An addition such as the glottal plosive to words beginning with stressed vowels such as /ʔæd/ for *add* and /ʔaɪs/ for *ice;* and addition of vowel elements to monophthong vowels to produce diphthongs, such as /mæan/ for *man.*

Patients with cleft palate who have articulation problems have most of the common deviations described above. Although physiological or anatomical disorders compound the difficulty of producing clear and acceptable speech, their articulation errors per se seldom differ from those of numerous native-born American speakers. The differences relate to the degree of severity, complexity, and number of articulation problems rather than to specific types. The "cleft palate speech" syndrome usually refers to difficulties in controlling air pressure for producing plosive and fricative sounds, to nasal or pharyngeal lisps, to nasal snorting on stressed syllables, and to substitution of glottal stops for consonants. Another problem often noted in many of these patients is the blurring of sounds in connected speech. Their attempt to gain control of the velopharyngeal mechanism during speech may cause nasal or oral blurring which is also due to habitual uncontrolled movement of the tongue, retraction of the back of the tongue, or even to a general lack of tongue movement. The telescoping of sounds, syllables, and words produces both blurred vocal quality and indistinct articulation.

Both children and adults seen at St. Luke's have these various difficulties, which may be related to many factors. Children undergoing primary pharyngeal flap surgery before the onset of speech, however, seem less inclined toward nasal snorting and glottal stop substitutions for other consonant sounds than do those who have the secondary palate repaired after speech develops or after unsuccessful palatal surgery. The ratings of articulation of this group at St. Luke's were generally "average." Their misarticulations consisted mainly of the usual omissions and sound substitutions heard in many children of comparable age. In addition, they appeared to have less blurring, unintelligibility, and inaccurate sound production than did others not yet operated on or operated on after speech developed.

Another factor hindering the development of adequate articulation and sometimes creating other errors is the tendency of the individual with cleft palate to overenergize speech production, causing extreme constriction of the voice and speech mechanism. This manner of speech production often results in overaspiration of speech sounds and nasal snorting. A forcing, pushing, or collapsing (letting go) may compensate for the speaker's lack of flexibility, firmness, and precision in use of his articulatory organs during speech. Forcing and "pounding out" sounds and words also create faults of voice production, rhythm, and speech stress.

The speech patterns of these subjects, regardless of their obvious misarticulations, show a wide range of use and production of speech sounds. Even those having specific difficulty with a sound or with one or more types of sounds, such as plosives or sibilants, are usually able to form them fairly clearly in certain sequences of speech, depending upon the context, the adjacent sounds, the position of the sounds in the syllable, word, or phrase, and the length and rhythm of the word or phrase in which the sound appears. Most of St. Luke's patients who had trouble forming consonants at the beginning of stressed syllables pronounced these sounds clearly and without undue effort in other positions and contexts within thought groups. For instance, a child considered to have difficulty with plosives could not produce the /p/ adequately in the word *pie* but managed the word *spy* quite clearly.

A comprehensive and accurate estimate of each patient's overall articulation disorders and potential for habilitation or rehabilitation must always include a detailed analysis of all sounds defective in certain word positions and of his recurring patterns of voice, articulation, and rate and rhythm.

Problems of Rate and Rhythm

Irregularities in rate and rhythm of speaking do not usually affect understandability of those with cleft palate nearly as much as do other aspects of their voice and speech production. Any such problems are likely to be directly proportional to other speech disabilities, e.g., in voice and articulation, and may, in fact, be directly related to them. Unless the problem is extremely grave, it may not interfere with intelligibility. On speech evaluation at St. Luke's, most children who had had primary pharyngeal flap surgery received ratings of average or above in such categories as phrasing, rate, rhythm, and stress (word and sentence). Rate and rhythm deviations in the speech patterns of both the children and adults were similar to those found among many speakers in the general population, varying widely in type and severity. The faults include tempo that is too fast, too slow, or even labored; a "choppy" or arrhythmic flow of speech; too short, too long, or stereotyped phrasing of words into thought groups; and inaccurate stress of words and/or sentences. Persons who speak very rapidly usually display slack articulation, omit many sounds, and do not use a strong voice or sustain the tone properly through the ends of thought groups; their rapid speaking rate does not allow enough time to produce speech sounds adequately and to sustain phonation. Conversely, persons who speak very slowly often have as much difficulty in forming speech sounds clearly and precisely; at the same time, they produce distorted qualitites of voice, e.g., nasality, huskiness, breathiness, by forcing and thereby constricting the speech organs. They often develop an exaggerated "scanning" type of speech, giving equal time, tone, and stress to every syllable in the phrase or sentence, to the stressed and unstressed syllables of important thought-bearing words, and to the auxiliary words used to aid understanding. In such utterances the sense or meaning may be distorted, and the choppy or even staccato rhythm of speech may be characterized by inappropriate grouping of words to express ideas or thoughts.

CASE HISTORIES

UNOPERATED CLEFT PALATE

Mrs. F, No. 43-15-53, born in Puerto Rico, was 52 years old when first referred to our Hearing and Speech Department. She had a unilateral subtotal cleft of the primary palate and a total cleft of the secondary palate. Cheiloplasty was performed in Puerto Rico when she was 8 years old, but the secondary palate had never been repaired. Because of her age and associated cardiac history, she did not have palatoplasty. Urged by her family, however, she agreed to have secondary cheiloplasty and rhinoplasty and was eventually fitted with an obturator. She had a moderate, bilateral, mixed type of hearing loss. This pleasant and some-what placid woman had had little formal education. She appeared to be unconcerned about her anomaly and its effect on her appearance and communicative skills.

Language and Speech Skills

Mrs F spoke Spanish exclusively; her family and friends reported great difficulty in understanding her. When using her few English words or phrases, Mrs. F's speech seemed more intelligible and her voice clearer than when she spoke Spanish. She was not very talkative, even in her native tongue. The following are excerpts from an evaluation of her voice and speech patterns.

Volume. Adequate to weak, fading at end of phrases.

Pitch. Appropriate in key, somewhat restricted in range and variety of intonation patterns.

Quality. Breathy, husky, denasal, nasal with much snorting, extreme nasal and denasal blurring; tone clearer when laughing and singing.

Articulation. Words often unintelligible, very slack tongue and lip movements for the most part, blurring of the majority of sounds. Substitution of /ʒ/ for /dʒ/ and /ʃ/ for /tʃ/, or glottal stop for many consonants, especially for intervocalic plosive sounds; implosive or fricative production of breathed and voiced plosive sounds as well as nasal snorting on these sounds in prevocalic positions of syllables; distortion of the vowel sound /ɜ/; nasal overaspiration on initial plosives and fricatives, especially /s/ and /z/; used blade of tongue for articulation of most tongue-tip–alveolar-ridge sounds; tongue often protruded interdentally for many consonants. Omission of most final consonants and postvocalic nasal sounds /m, n, and ŋ/ and often of /s/ and /z/. Addition of glottal plosive on initial stressed vowels.

Rate and Rhythm. Choppy, word-by-word utterance with inaccurate word and sense stress, rapid tempo.

Mrs. F's voice and speech were somewhat clearer after she was fitted with an obturator, but she still maintained many previous speech habits. She received some speech instruction at each of her periodic appointments for reevaluation and showed some improvement in practice. She did not wish to receive speech therapy, being satisfied with the improvement brought about by the obturator.

PRIMARY PHARYNGEAL FLAP SURGERY BEFORE SPEECH
DEVELOPMENT (SPEECH ADEQUATE)

V. C., No. 278-272, born with a total cleft of the secondary palate, was referred to us at 19 months of age, 5 months after she had had a primary pharyngeal flap and von Langenbeck palatal repair at St. Luke's. Her hearing was essentially normal. During her first evaluation, V. C. responded well, engaged in considerable vocal play stimulated by her mother, with adequate articulation of the speech sounds employed and clear vocal production except for slight denasalization. After the first year year, she returned periodically for reevaluations and received speech therapy.

Language and Speech Skills

V. C., always lively and responsive, showed good development of receptive and expressive language. The following observations were made during periodic evaluations of her voice and speech patterns following surgery.

Volume. At first audible but weak, stronger in later tests, and adequate in last evaluation.

Pitch. Generally appropriate.

Quality. Breathy and denasal in early evaluations; later, still breathy to husky, singing quality clear; last rating, slightly breathy and mildly nasal and denasal.

Articulation. Consonants in initial positions reasonably clear except for some overaspiration which diminished later; omission of /l/ noted in an early evaluation and of many consonants in final positions, with a glottal stop substituted for some of them; a glottal plosive persisted as an added sound in the initiation of vowels.

Rate and Rhythm. Slow rate and staccato rhythm in the early evaluations, changing to normal rate with maintenance of the staccato rhythm.

This child's language and speech development continued to improve; voice and speech characteristics usually associated with cleft palate have been eliminated.

SECONDARY PHARYNGEAL FLAP SURGERY AFTER SPEECH DEVELOPMENT (SPEECH ADEQUATE)

Mrs. T. H., No. 48-07-90, a 36-year old graduate student from the Far East, was referred by an instructor in voice and speech at her university. Three repairs performed abroad for a total cleft of the secondary palate, during her fifteenth, twenty-seventh, and thirtieth years, were unsuccessful. She had no hearing difficulty. At St. Luke's she underwent secondary pharyngeal flap surgery and closure of an oronasal fistula.

This woman was very intelligent, pleasant, and cooperative; she received speech therapy for 2 years.

Language and Speech Skills

Mrs. H was trilingual and unusually competent in English, which she hoped to teach after returning to her native country. When first seen, reception and expression of English were good, then became better, and, at the last evaluation, were excellent. The following notations are representative of her voice and speech patterns.

Volume. At first audible to fading; stronger following surgery.

Pitch. Keyed high preoperatively, her pitch rose even higher for stress and while striving for audible speech; postoperative pitch generally appropriate, with occasional rise for stress.

Quality. Preoperatively, patient showed both nasal and denasal blurring, slight nasal snorting, some pinching of the nostrils, breathy ("pushed" nasal breath), and glottal (squeezed) quality; postoperatively, much less nasal blurring, some "relaxed soft-palate" nasality, less breathiness.

Articulation. Initial vowel sounds glottalized and nasalized preoperatively, postvocalic nasal consonants slighted or omitted, plosives omitted in vowel plus nasal plus consonant sequences at the end of words, final voiced consonants unvoiced; post-operatively, most of these substitutions, omissions, and additions were still present but much less pronounced. Non-English substitutions were more noticeable than before.

Rate and Rhythm. The same choppy rhythm and non-English

word and sense stress patterns and intonations persisted after surgery.

Mrs. H, with continued practice, showed marked improvement in all respects. When last evaluated, 3 years after secondary surgery, her voice had very little "cleft palate" quality and there was no trace of it in her articulation.

PRIMARY PHARYNGEAL FLAP SURGERY AFTER SPEECH DEVELOPMENT (SPEECH INADEQUATE)

E. W., No. 401-362, age 4 when first referred to our Hearing and Speech Department, had recently undergone pharyngeal flap surgery for repair of a subtotal cleft of the secondary palate at St. Luke's. She also had a moderate unilateral hearing loss. She was attending nursery school when her speech was first evaluated and during the sessions was alert and cooperative.

Language and Speed Skills

This child had no difficulty with the reception and expression of language. The following are typical observations on her voice and speech patterns:

Volume. Adequate.

Pitch. Appropriate general level and good use of inflectional patterns for meaning.

Quality. Breathy, thin, denasal, and nasal with some snorting and blurring, but also some intermittent clear tone production.

Articulation. Unintelligible at times, generally slack use of tongue and lips for speech sound formations; some difficulty with plosive sounds (she held her nose to produce /d/ and /b/). Some problems perhaps related to general speech development with the sounds /r/, /t/, /dʒ/, and /θ/ and /ð/.

Substitution of nasal snort or /n/ for many plosive sounds as well as for /s/ and /z/ in initial positions of stressed syllables, and of a glottal stop /ʔ/ when these sounds occurred intervocalically or in final positions of stressed syllables. Other substitutions included /n/ for /θ/ and /m/ for /p/ and /b/, as well as distortion, overaspiration, and blurring of plosive and fricative sounds. Many variations and inconsistencies in the articulation of consonants.

Omission of final consonants and nasal sounds /m/, /n/ in initial positions, and of many /s/ and /z/ sounds.

Addition of snorted /h/ before many initial stressed syllables.

Rate and Rhythm. Somewhat arrhythmic word-by-word utterances; tempo ranged from appropriate to fast.

E. W.'s voice and speech patterns improved slightly just

after surgery. Her mother received suggestions for language and speech stimulation and practice at home. During periodic evaluation sessions, the child also received instructions for speech practice. She has continued to improve in oral communication skills, voice clarity, and speech intelligibility since that time. It is reported that with continued speech practice, she has made exceptional improvement.

SECONDARY PHARYNGEAL FLAP SURGERY AFTER SPEECH DEVELOPMENT (SPEECH INADEQUATE)

Mrs. B. S., No. A199-678, born in Puerto Rico, was 33 years old when referred to our department. Secondary palatal surgery with a pharyngeal flap and push-back had been performed earlier. She first had oral surgery at age 18 for total cleft of the secondary palate. Her hearing was adequate for everyday purposes. Mrs. S, always seemed alert, pleasant, and cooperative during her few speech therapy sessions.

Language and Speech Skills

Although her first language was Spanish, Mrs. S had good comprehension and command of English. She was somewhat shy, however, and not very talkative in either language. Her voice and speech production was clearer and more intelligible in English than in Spanish. Her voice and speech patterns showed little or no change after surgery, as shown by these notations from evaluation sessions.

Volume. Quiet to fading at ends of phrases and sentences.

Pitch. General level appropriate, with Spanish intonation patterns.

Quality. Denasal and nasal, including blurring and snorting.

Articulation. Too little tongue and lip activity resulted in general over-all distortion and blurring of vowel and consonant sounds.

Substitutions included a glottal stop /?/ and nasal snort with pinching of the nostrils for most plosive and fricative sounds, especially /h/, /p/, /t/, /k/, and /f/; also substitution of unvoiced for final voiced consonants.

Omission of final consonant sounds and consonant clusters, and intermittent omission of intervocalic and postvocalic nasal sounds.

Addition of glottal plosive sounds before initial vowels.

Rate and Rhythm. Staccato, choppy rhythm and slow tempo of speaking; word-by-word utterance with tendency to give all syllables equal stress and duration.

In practice sessions, Mrs. S's voice and articulation were clearer when she used her tongue and lips to form sounds and blend them together in short thought units than in her general speech. She made little progress, however, in carrying over practice techniques into her daily speech.

TABLE 20-1. PRONUNCIATION SYMBOLS*

Symbols	Words	Symbols	Words
ɑ	calm	ŋ	long
ɑə|r	bar	o	hotel
a	ask (also /æ/, /ɑ/)	oʊ	beau, go
aʊ	bough	oə|r	bore
aɪ	buy	ɔə|	
æ	sat	ɔ	bought
b	bat, cab	ɔɪ	boy
d	dad	ɒ	sorry
e	aorta	p	pep
eɪ	bay	r	roar
ɛ	bet	s	sauce
ɛə|r	bear	ʃ	shoe, fish
ɜ|r†	erred	t	tat
ə	above	θ	thin, breath
ə|r†	doctor	ð	then, breathe
f	fife	u	rule
g	gag	ʊ	good
h	hat	ʊə|r	poor
i	pique, peak	ʌ	cut
ɪ	pick	v	vow, five
ɪə|r	beer	ʍ	white
j	hallelujah mute	w	way
k	kick	z	zone, ooze
l	live, ill	ʒ	azure, rouge
m	mum		
n	none		

*The symbols listed here are included in the alphabet of the International Phonetic Association. Additional symbols used in transcriptions are:

1. /ʔ/, called a glottal plosive when it initiates a vowel sound, which it does in the enunciation of most stressed vowels in English which are initial in the syllable; called a glottal stop when it is substituted for plosive or other consonants in final or consonant combination final positions.

2. /~/, indicates nasalization of a sound, |æ̃|, etc.

† The retracted vowel sounds heard in the stressed and unstressed syllables of these key words are represented by the symbols |ɜ˞| and |ə˞| respectively.

CHAPTER **21**

Language, Speech, and Hearing Therapy

JANE DORSEY ZIMMERMAN

WILLIAM H. CANFIELD

The Hearing and Speech Department of St. Luke's Hospital offers hearing, language, and speech testing, diagnosis, and remedial services for children and adults with cleft lip and/or palate referred by the Plastic Surgery Clinic; the Ear, Nose, and Throat Clinic; private physicians; other services within the hospital; city schools and colleges (private and public); the Bureau of Handicapped Children of the Department of Health; other centers, agencies, and institutions; and parents of children so handicapped. Self-referrals are also accepted. Patients receive these services on either an in- or outpatient basis. The inpatients may be newborns, persons awaiting surgery, or those convalescing from surgery. Among the outpatients are those who have had no surgery, who have had primary or secondary repair of either palate, or who are returning for postoperative check-ups.

On the patient's admission to the department, he or a parent supplies a staff member with information concerning the anomaly or the patient's social, physical, and environmental development which may be directly related to language-speech-hearing development. The speech pathologist makes a detailed analysis and evaluation, including a tape recording of language and speech characteristics of the patients referred for speech services, and the audiologist conducts appropriate hearing tests when indicated. Many patients require both types of testing.

A summary report consisting of the test results, diagnosis, and recommendations for further testing and habilitation or rehabilitation services becomes part of the patient's permanent medical record. Copies of the report are sent to the referral source upon request. Samples of test and report sheets appear at the end of this chapter.

HEARING TESTS

The basic evaluation used by the audiologist is a pure-tone audiometer test. It determines the hearing threshold for each ear through both air and bone conduction, from 125 to 8,000 cycles per second (cps) frequency, with special attention to the frequencies most important for understanding and receiving speech (500, 1,000, and 2,000 cps). Bone conduction thresholds from 500 to 4,000 cps are taken for each ear when the air conduction thresholds suggest some hearing difficulty. A threshold difference between ears at any frequency over 25 decibels (intensity) in air conduction or 5 decibels in bone conduction necessitates the use of masking noise. While one ear receives the pure-tone stimulus, the other ear simultaneously receives the masking noise at a higher level of intensity, enabling the audiologist to obtain more accurate hearing thresholds for each ear than would otherwise be possible.

Speech audiometric tests, which are used to confirm or corroborate pure-tone test results, also help the audiologist to choose a proper hearing aid when indicated. Speech audiometry includes determination of speech reception thresholds and speech discrimination abilities. Spondee words (two-syllable words with stress on each syllable, such as *cowboy* and *railroad*) in standardized lists are helpful in determining the threshold of sound intensity needed by the person to understand speech. The phonetically balanced (PB) word lists (monosyllabic words which contain the approximate normal occurrence of speech sounds in conversational speech) are useful in evaluating the subject's ability to recognize and discriminate speech sounds heard. The decibel intensity at which he responds correctly to 50 per cent of the spondee words becomes the speech reception threshold (SRT). The PB word lists help to reveal the percentage of speech intelligible to the subject at a comfortable listening level. A number of other audiological tests and devices may be employed to discover whether a child responds to sound at all. An audiogram containing all hearing test results becomes part of the permanent hospital record.

A child who does not respond accurately or consistently to formal audiometric tests must be conditioned to react visibly in some way to sounds. He may be taught to select a block and place it in a box, string a bead, or perform another action in response to a sound stimulus. By controlling the intensity of the sound presented—either music or speech—the audiologist can determine whether the child hears at all and obtain a general estimate of his sound threshold. All these audiological test procedures take place in a sound-treated room with various stimuli presented through headphones and/or in a free field. If an infant or child does not respond to formal audiometric tests, the audiologist may use such noisemakers as a bell, shaker, or cricket clicker, without the child's seeing the source of the sound, to gain a very general estimate of his ability to hear sounds. The department director, an otologist, receives a report of all audiometric test results and then sends his diagnosis and recommendations to the original referral source and to the parents.

LANGUAGE AND SPEECH EVALUATION

The speech pathologist evaluates language and speech development as well as usage. Periodic tape recordings become part of the patient's permanent record and furnish valuable material for immediate analysis as well as for long-range follow-up study. Test materials used for eliciting language and speech responses vary with the individual patient, according to his age, education, interests, and intelligence. The speech and language test must provide opportunity for each person to display such communication skills or abilities as conversation, reading aloud prose and poetry selections, repeating syllable or speech sounds, or repeating words and phrases. Test procedures range from very informal and indirect methods of obtaining adequate speech samples to the more structured and specific types of responses. The amount and type of speech stimulation provided in each instance depend largely on the patient's speech and language disabilities and capacities.

Language Testing

Among the various language modalities tested are (1) gestures; (2) language formulation including vocabulary, grammar, syntax, and sentence length; (3) speaking-naming, repeating, reading aloud, counting, and conversing; (4) responding to questions (written as well as oral for patients who can read), spoken requests, and directions; and (5) singing. Receptive and expressive language are interdependent: the use of each depends partially on the other as well as on the patient's sensory and motor capacities.

The speech pathologist takes note of the sounds produced by infants with no speech during crying, laughing, gurgling, and babbling. He utilizes toys, games, and picture books as stimuli to encourage young and even older children to "talk" spontaneously and informally. This procedure gives him an impression of the patient's ability to formulate, understand, and use language and speech appropriately. Specific language skills may be tested by asking the patient to repeat short sentences or phrases, words, syllables, or sounds; to name familiar objects; to say a rhyme or sing a song such as "Happy Birthday." The material used for each test must be within the interest and age level of the patient, whether infant or child or adult. Much of the testing may be unstructured, but the speech pathologist must be cognizant of the patient's use of each language skill as well as his ability to integrate it with all others.

In a metropolitan city such as New York a speech and hearing center must have tests available in a number of languages. At St. Luke's, for example, many patients speak little or no English. But this hospital is fortunate to have available employees and volunteers who speak most of the languages needed, and can be called on to assist the speech pathologist in giving the test if a patient comes without a family member or friend who is bilingual. Because we serve a large Spanish-speaking population, most of our language and speech testing materials are available in Spanish as well as in English. Examples of some of the tests given to bilingual children and adults appear at the end of this chapter in both the English and Spanish versions.

Voice and Speech Evaluation

Oral language responses allow the speech pathologist to determine the nature of such abilities and problems as (1) voice production (initiation and flow of tone, and quality, pitch patterns, and volume); (2) pronunciation (articulation of consonants and enunciation of vowels and diphthongs); and (3) rate and rhythm of speaking, including word and sentence stress and phrasing. On the charts for language, voice, and speech evaluation, which list terms describing adequate (or appropriate) and inadequate (or faulty) characteristics, the patient's current assets and liabilities as well as his progress or regression can be recorded.

Language and speech and auditory training and retraining begin when recommended, after test procedures and evaluations have been completed. Regardless of individual speaking difficulties or recommended remedial measures, the basic purpose of training must be made clear to the patient, so that he understands how each step in the therapeutic procedure will help him to communicate more easily and efficiently, and that the particular practice he is concentrating on is part of all other aspects of his voice and speech. When working to improve his vocal quality, for example, he must realize that he will need to improve articulation of the speech sounds which, when blended together to permit him to express his thoughts, make up the flow of voice.

LANGUAGE TRAINING

Language practice is the basic aspect of speech and hearing therapy, since language is the means of using the various speech elements. Many of our referrals from the St. Luke's Cleft Palate Clinic are children who develop language somewhat later than most of their peers; therefore, speech therapy begins with language stimulation and development.

Bilingual youngsters who attend schools where only English is spoken will no doubt benefit most by beginning their language training in English and then learning to relate it to their parents' (and their) native language. A speech pathologist who is multilingual will find many opportunities to stimulate the interest and practice of school-age children through songs, rhymes, and games in their "home" language. With such material, he can also enlist the aid of parents and teachers for home and school practice.

The following notes and transcriptions illustrate language and speech practice carried on with a little boy and, at first, his father, and then the speech pathologist (SP).

W. M., No. 40-66-48

This child, born in Puerto Rico, had a complete cleft of the primary and secondary palates. The lip was repaired in Puerto Rico in infancy; the soft palate was repaired at 3 years of age at Lincoln Hospital, New York City; secondary palatoplasty with pharyngeal flap was done 2 years later; secondary cheiloplasty was done the year following; and columellar advancement and lip repair were done at 8 years of age at St. Luke's Hospital.

Hearing was normal in both ears at 5 years of age; mild conduction loss 2 years later was noted in both ears; 11 months later, the right ear was normal, the left ear still showed mild conduction loss.

W came with his father for the first interview at 5 years of age Spanish is the family language, but both W and his father (F) can speak English. W was very shy and refused to talk to the speech pathologist, who asked the father to conduct the interview, which was tape recorded:

F: (Showing objects to W or
   pointing to pictures of
   objects)*
   ¿Qué es esto?   W: (No response).
F: (Naming object)
   pantalón.   W: ?a?lõ.*
F: Camisa.   W: ?ami?a.
F: Pelo.   W: peɔ.

* Each of F's stimulus words is repeated by W before F gives the next.
† W's responses are transcribed into phonetic symbols to illustrate his pronunciation patterns. F's questions and directions, which vary from English to Spanish are given in their spelling forms.

F: Uno.† Dos. Tres.	W: uno. do. hrɛ.
F: Cuatro. Cinco.	W: kwɑʔo. ʔĩʔo.
F: Bueno. Ahora inglés. One.	W: wʌʔ.
F: Two. Three. Four.	W: tu. ʒtri. fɔi.
F: Five. Six. Seven.	W: faiʔ. hıks. 'sɛvi.
F: Eight. Nine. Ten.	W: eıʔ. jaiʔ. (skipped ten).
F: That's good. Adios mama.	W: ɑʔio mɑ.
F: Adios papa.	W: ɑiʔo pɑpɑ.
F: guʔ bai (good bye).	W: gʊm ai.
F: So long. I see you	
tomorrow.	W: nɔŋ. si jə.

The speech pathologist observed the session, complimented the father and W, and urged them to continue to play their speech game at home. W must practice both Spanish and English, Spanish to speak with his mother at home, for she speaks only Spanish, and English for school. It should be said. however, that W's use of both languages is limited to one- or two-word responses at this time, and even those only with his father or brother.

As can be noted in the transcription above, he omits most final consonants, substituting a glottal stop /ʔ/ for most of them; nasalizes vowels, such as /ʌ/ in *one;* and snorts *s.* His voice quality is breathy, nasal and squeezed.

The following excerpt is from a practice session tape recorded 6 months later with the speech pathologist. They used a toy telephone:

SP: Shall we call some one	
on the telephone?	W: ʔɛʔ (yes).
SP: Very well, let's call your	
Dad. Say to him in	
Spanish "ɑlo pɑpɑ."	W: ɑlo pɑpɑ (in a husky voice).
SP: Say to him in English	
"how are you?"	W: ha ɑ jə?
SP: Tell him "I'm fine."	W: ai fai.
SP: When you hang up say	
"good bye."	W: bai (voice is still husky).

Four years later, when W is 9 years old, he is much more active and responsive in practice. He goes to school where he speaks English, but he continues to speak Spanish at home and with some of his friends. At this session he comes into the practice room, goes to the cupboard, and takes out the materials the speech pathologist tells him they will use for this lesson.

He is singing and humming "Camptown Races," the tune is correct, and his singing voice is clear, smooth and varied in quality. There is no snorting, no huskiness as he sings/ɑ-li-ɑ-lɑ-vɑ-li-i/.

SP: What's that you're
singing?　　　　　　　　W: (Sings again) ɑ-lɛ-lɛ-lɛ-lɛ-lɛ-ɑ.
SP: Sing the chorus.　　　 W: (Sings it).
SP: Where did you hear
that song?　　　　　　　 W: æt maɪ haʊʔ ɔn ðə ti vi.

W starts to sing and hum again. The speech pathologist helps him with some of the words he hasn't yet learned, and he seems pleased with his accomplishment. He can now produce all the sounds in both Spanish and English correctly, but he omits many of the final consonants, or continues to substitute a glottal stop or plosive for them.

The following excerpt is from W's last tape-recorded session at age 11 (a mirror is useful in practice).

SP: Will you say "my
name is" and say your
full name, please?　　　 W: maɪ neɪ iz . . .
SP: You left out the *m* in
name. Will you try
name again?　　　　　 W: (Repeats the word clearly this time, sustains a fully resonant *m*, then announces himself again, still nasalizing the *a* but with a good *m*.
SP: What's today's date?　 W: dʒu faɪ tu.
SP: Try June second.　　　 W: dʒu hekən. (markedly over-aspirates on /h/, but no snorting).

SP: Can you make it *second*　W: (Can, but still leaves off the final *d*. Says it again, correcting himself, this time with a sharp *s*, a fully sustained *n* in both *June* and *second* and a good approximation of *d*, although voiceless).

During this practice he works with two other boys his age, and relates well with them. Each boy brought in some words and phrases he is practicing. They help each other over the

"hard" sounds each has trouble with, and they look at themselves and each other to get visual as well as auditory cues.
Some of the words W is practicing are *fork*, which comes out
/hɔk/ until the speech pathologist suggests that he try biting
his lower lip to get an *f* to start the word. He looks at his mouth,
tries a bite, and it comes out right. The other boys give him
some *f*-words to practice. He tries them out, then writes them
in his workbook to practice at home. His fricative sounds, *f*, *s*,
th, *h* are often blurred, but not snorted. His voice quality remains
husky, as it is often in the voices of those born with clefts. There
is apt to be nasality, too, especially in the words learned early.
But W is making steady improvement, and if he keeps up his
practice, he should eventually speak quite clearly. Fortunately,
he remains bilingual, transferring easily from English to Spanish
and back again, especially with his brother. When his mother
comes with him for his lesson, he is careful to translate into
Spanish whatever is said to him in English. They are a devoted
family, and W is a lucky boy to be one of them.

The language stimulation and practice given at home by parents
and others and the language and speech "models" they present are
extremely important factors in the earliest stages of learning and
throughout the child's school life. Babbling, cooing, and otherwise
vocalizing with the infant as he makes at first random and then selected
sounds helps to reinforce these prelanguage activities by providing
him with echoes of his own responses, which he in turn can re-echo.
It must be emphasized that this echoing cycle and other forms of vocal
play do not pass directly into "real" or verbal language, but provide
the substance for later development of words, phrases, and sentences.
They must therefore be practiced, in the same way as real words, as
they are introduced. Conversely, imitation of the child's errors of
substitution and omission during his first attempts to use real words
(baby talk) may create language and speech inadequacies which the
child retains long after the adults stop finding them appealing.

Handicapped children such as those with cleft lip and/or palate
usually need extra attention and stimulation, as well as long-term
continuous practice, for adequate language and speech development.
To pique and hold their interest parents should provide them early in
their infancy with toys that make sounds, and in the later preschool
period supplement these with simple games and phonograph records
for auditory and rhythm training through the singing and saying of
words.

The following notes and transcriptions illustrate some of the
practice procedures used for continuing the language and speech

development and auditory training of a 5½ year old girl, who was first seen when she was 2 years old, just before pharyngeal flap surgery.

M. Q., No. 42-42-47

> This child, born in Puerto Rico, had a secondary cleft palate, bilateral aural atresia, and no external ears. At 2 years of age she had no speech, but she cried lustily, and the quality of her crying voice was clear, with no noticeable huskiness or nasality. There was no discernible response to any of the attempts to test her hearing.
>
> Three months or so later she still had no intelligible language, but tried to express herself with grunting and gurgling sounds, some glottalized vowelizations, and a few gestures. She seemed to comprehend visual cues and responded to them vocally.
>
> Two years later, after a series of otological operations, she started to wear a bone conduction hearing aid with increasingly good results. Within the next year and a half her hearing with the aid improved from a bilateral pure-tone loss of 20 decibels to a loss of 10 decibels in the right ear and 5 decibels in the left ear. Her speech reception threshold loss at this time was 25 to 30 decibels with the bone conduction aid.
>
> Part of a testing and practice session follows. The speech pathologist (SP) shows M various objects or pictures, and asks her to name them and/or talk about them:

SP: What are these?	M: Gabbo.
SP: They're cherries. You can say that. Try it.	M: Cherries.
SP: That's right. I knew you could say that word, we've practiced it lots of times. Here's something else you can say, and it's something you like to eat. What's this?	M: Wa-Wa.
SP: You didn't try very hard on that one, is it a wa-wa or a cookie?	M: A cookie.
SP: Of course, a cookie, and it's for you to eat after the lesson.	M: Well, Well.
SP: What's this a picture of?	M: That's a baby.

SP: That's right, it's a baby.   M: (Repeats) That's a baby.

SP: What's the baby wear-   M: That's the baby shoogah.
ing on her feet?

SP: Pretty good. Look at   M: Oh, yeah.
me when I say it, that's
the baby's shoes. Look:
shoes.

SP: Try it again, that's the   M: Yeah, shoogah.
baby's shoes. Did you
see me say shoes, and
then stop?

SP: Listen, M, are they   M: Shoes.
shoogah or shoes?

SP: Of course, I knew you   M: A coa? (substituting a
could say shoes. What   glottal stop for the *t* which the
else is the baby wearing   SP accepts for the present).
in this picture?

SP: What's the baby wear-   M: Vocalizes a series of sounds
ing on her head?   that are not intelligible.

SP: I don't understand that.   M: Oooooh (as though she just
She's wearing a cap.   realized that she knew how
Try to say cap. Look,   to say it) ca? (substituting
it starts just like cookie   a glottal stop for *p*).
does.

SP: Good. I knew you could   M: Bye-bye (indicating that
say that easy word, *cap.*   she'd worked long enough).

SP: Let's sing a song before   M: Well, come on.
you go.

SP: (Starts to sing) Happy   M: (Singing her own tune)
Birthday to you.   Happy birthday to you
(repeats), happy birthday to
baby (then says) Where's
the baby?

SP: Happy birthday to you   M: (Singing, still with her own
(continues singing).   tune) Happy birthday baby
(repeats four times) then
ends with Happy and a
series of unintelligible words
following her same tune
pattern.

SP: Good, very good.   M: Happy birthday to you.
Good bye, M.

SPEECH TRAINING

Whether dealing with developmental or rehabilitation problems, one should realize that each of the various speech elements has one or more characteristics of the others. For instance, in the sentence, "That word is a noun" the initial and final sound /n/ in the word *noun* offers practice in tone and articulation, while the whole sentence offers training in the rate and rhythm of speaking. Training practices and techniques should be so designed that the oral responses are acceptable and "correct," and thus should deal with each problem according to its importance and effect on the total oral utterance. Training to eliminate a nasally blurred plosive sound, such as *p* in *print*, should provide means not only of correcting the faulty articulation, but also of incorporating the improved sound as improved voice production, inasmuch as the voice quality of the other sounds in the word are likely to be affected. Practice must continue until the new sound becomes habitual in everyday speaking.

At St. Luke's, the speech pathologist's session with one patient or with a small group of children or adults usually begins with greetings; passing the time of day remarks; questions about school, play, home, family, work, or any other topic that leads to an informal discussion. During the "free" conversation in this warming-up period lasting 5 or more minutes, the speech pathologist takes account of (but doesn't mention) details of the language and speech responses—adequate as well as inadequate.

When the session moves into practice conversation on the same topic or another growing out of it, the speech pathologist begins to identify for the patients certain language and speech assets (potential and actual) and liabilities that they might profitably concentrate on at this time. Practice may proceed from a question or answer in the introductory conversation, with attention focused on one or more problems such as (1) inappropriate or incorrect words affecting the meaning; (2) words uttered too quickly or too slowly or scanned; (3) unrhythmical word sequence; (4) too loud or too weak a tone; (5) pitch started at too high a level, with succeeding stressed syllables raised still higher; (6) faulty voice production; and (7) articulation with errors of omission, substitution, and/or addition.

A therapy session has at least one specific goal based on the immediate language and speech needs of each individual but also directed to his over-all oral communication skills. The free conversation suggests areas for concentrated practice, and the speech pathologist then introduces the required practice techniques and procedures.

If, for instance, the goal is to improve an *s* sound which may be snorted or otherwise incorrectly produced, practice may include instruction in the place and manner of articulation, with illustrations of how the sound (1) relates to similarly produced sounds such as its cognate /z/, to others made with the tongue tip on the alveolar ridge, and so on; (2) influences contiguous sounds in syllables and words; (3) affects vocal qualities; and (4) varies according to its context with other sounds and its position in unstressed words or syllables. How many factors can be included in the practice during one session often depends on the severity of the particular fault in the speech of the patient or group, the habitual manner of producing it, and the speech pathologist's judgment of the techniques needed for improvement. Practice techniques provide opportunities for the patient to recognize aurally, visually, and/or tactually the differences between his own incorrect and the correct manner of forming the *s* sound and, most importantly, help him learn to use it when he talks.

Actual practice begins with suggestions for strengthening the potentially good aspects and eliminating harmful or undesirable ones. When a patient's voice fades at the end of a sentence, e.g., "I'm thirsty, please give me a drink of milk," the speech pathologist may need only to say, "That last word is the most important one in the sentence. Make it strong." If this suggestion does not work, "Listen to me, please, as I say the sentence; tell me if you hear every important word clearly including the last one." The patient listens and is then asked to repeat the sentence as said. Both linguistic procedures, of which the second is also auditory and imitative, should be tried many times. For a patient with normal intelligence and hearing who understands how to tell something using his own (or supplied) sentences, these suggestions may be sufficient to help him develop adequate and acceptable speech. Repeating verses or rhythmic prose may reinforce his potentially effective patterns and contribute toward an interest in, and feeling for, words and their production and indirectly help him avoid or eliminate minor faults. Other faults such as starting out on too high a pitch and further raising the level on important words, and speaking in word rather than thought units may be similarly approached.

If the patient is unable to reduce even mild faults in this way, it may be necessary to break up the sentences into phrase, word, syllable, or even sound units in order to provide the specific and detailed sensory-motor stimulation and practice to ensure effective learning and relearning. For practice purposes, the sentence, "I'm thirsty, please give me a glass of milk," may become, "I'm thirsty . . . please . . . give me . . . a glass . . . or give me a glass . . . or a glass of milk . . . or give me a glass of milk." Smaller units usually facilitate the production of a stronger voice, smoother initiation and flow of tone, a more audible follow-through to the end of word groups, and intelligibility. If necessary, the sense group could be divided into word or syllable units—*thirsty, please, glass, milk*—or even into sound units to correct omissions such as /s/ in *thirsty*, /l/ in *please, glass,* and *milk;* or substitutions such as /t/ or /f/ for /θ/ *th* in *thirsty*.

When a child requests something by saying *pease* for *please,* it is sometimes enough to say, "Will you try to say 'please' give me a glass of milk, not 'pease'?" He can later be given a chance to practice saying this in other similar requests. Often he can correct the fault without breaking up the context, but he may have another difficulty with *please,* substituting an interdental unvoiced sound similar to *th* for the final sound pronounced /z/, although spelled with an *s*. If the word has been reduced to sound units and no sensory procedures (hear it, see it, feel it) seem helpful, the speech pathologist may find another word in which the patient pronounces the final /z/ correctly, such as *sneeze* or *squeeze,* where the sound is actually represented by the letter /z/. If this fails, the patient's ability to pronounce the sound adequately in the initial position may be tested in such words as *zoo* or *zebra,* where it is always followed by a vowel and is thus easier to correct. Since the sound is more readily identified in this position, it is also more clearly produced by the one who sets the "pattern," inasmuch as most speakers have a tendency to slough off and unvoice final voiced consonant sounds.

Practice on conversational phrases may continue by means of selections containing similar examples and other related exercises. These may include prose, poetry, stories, and songs on subjects suitable for the patient's age and interests. Practicing a sound, syllable, or word by itself is not sufficient; it must also be tried out in sequences so that the individual will eventually be able to use it in other language patterns and contexts.

Once he attains the required level of proficiency at any particular step, the speech units can be made progressively larger until he can handle the entire phrase or sentence; that is, he puts the sound into the syllable, the syllable into the word, the word into the phrase, and the phrase into the sentence.

The following transcription illustrates some of the practice techniques described above.

B. K., No. 38-79-77

Born in the United States with a complete cleft of the primary and secondary palates, B had a cheiloplasty 5 days after birth, and a palatoplasty with primary pharyngeal flap at 1 year. His hearing is normal.

One of the purposes of B's practice was to enable him to

produce a correct /ʃ/ sound in words he knew and used, but in which he substituted *s* for *sh*. He was cooperative, alert, and eager to learn. The following is an excerpt from a tape recording of a lesson when B was 4½ years old.

SP: (Showing B a picture) What's the boy doing here?

B: Putting on his/suz/.

SP: Yes, he's putting on his *shoes*. Can you say *shoes*?

B: Sure, I can say /suz/ (starts *sure* with *s* also).

SP: Listen carefully, and look at me when I say *shoes*.

B: /suz/.

SP: Look again, and listen to the beginning of *shoes*: /ʃ/. You have to purse your lips: /ʃ/. I raise my tongue, too, but you can't see my tongue, because my lips are close together. You try /ʃ/.

B: /ʃ/.

SP: Do you think you can say it that way in *shoes* now?

B: /ʃuz/.

SP: That's right. Now what's the boy doing?

B: He's putting on his—/ʃuz/.

SP: Very good. Let's see what it sounds like at the end of a word. What's the boy holding in this picture?

B: A /fɪs/.

SP: Is it a /fɪs/ or a /fɪʃ/?

B: It's a /fɪʃ/.

SP: Yes, it's a *fish*.

SP: Do you remember that in "Hey Diddle,

B: A dish (said correctly)* ran away with the spoon.

* B's correct articulation of /ʃ/ in the rhyme provides an exception to the observation made here that faulty sounds are likely to be more easily corrected and firmly fixed in words that are new to the patient, than in words he learned early. The facts that it is a rhyme, and that he liked it when it was first presented, and sang it and said it, not only in the speech class, but at home, no doubt have much to do with his correct pronunciation of the *sh* in *dish*. His production of the rhyme was correct in all respects—sounds, rhythm, and tune—when he sang it.

Diddle," which you
learned a long time ago
something ran away
with the *spoon*? What
was it?

SP: Would you like to say   B: Says the rhyme (comes
    the whole rhyme? Be   out strong, clear and
    careful when you get to   triumphant on *dish*).
    the last line.

SPEECH THERAPY TECHNIQUES

Effective communication requires that persons, when speaking, must continuously adapt themselves to the needs of each speaking situation in their coordination and control of all the parts of the speech mechanism; they must maintain a dynamic posture, healthy emotional and social attitudes, a lively interest, and coordinate all of these factors with linguistic, mental, and neuromuscular processes.

Numerous speech and hearing habilitation and rehabilitation techniques can help patients develop and sustain adequate abilities to communicate orally. Regardless of procedures employed, the patient must practice continually, not only to maintain and improve skills already established, but to develop others. Without a positive conviction that speech can improve with practice, patients will achieve only minimal results despite any and all efforts of the speech pathologist.

Practice may always begin profitably with techniques for developing clear, strong, sustained vocal tone through the use of effective body mechanics. The over-all body tonus needed for efficient voice production influences other motor aspects of speech, thus affecting articulation and timing and rhythm.

Such speech controls are extremely significant, since many persons with cleft palate attempt to compensate for deficiencies in structure and function by overenergizing and forcing out unphonated air during attempts to speak, thus developing throat strain, resulting in husky quality of voice, nasal snorting, or hyper- and hyponasality and overaspiration. These patients, like all other speakers, need a minimal amount of air siphoned through the vocal cords to help produce clear phonation and to sustain a strong tone. By teaching them how to develop proper control of the gross muscles involved in tone production, the speech pathologist has no need to employ the "breathing" and relaxation exercises usually recommended for this control. Those drills are likely to create new voice and speech faults or aggravate existing ones. Patients who are unable to apply the requisite controls while speaking should be referred to a physical therapy department or to other specialists trained to deal with general problems of breathing or relaxation.

Similarly patients who cannot adjust to the social and emotional demands of speaking situations may need the help of a psychological counsellor or even of a psychiatrist. The speech pathologist should know when to make these referrals.

Just how much practice a patient will require to coordinate body mechanics, thinking, and feeling with voice and speech production often depends on his previously established speech habits and the extent of his disability. As he develops the necessary coordination and control, he begins to be able to produce the most efficient motor speech activity possible without excessive effort.

When teaching speech sound production, the speech pathologist continually makes use of as many sensory and motor cues as are needed for clarification. For example, the patient may watch the therapist and/or himself in a mirror while forming a sound. He may need to be made aware of tactile and kinesthetic sensations from placement and movement of the speech organs while he is looking in the mirror and listening to a particular sound. His tape recordings and, for comparison, those of the speech pathologist offer a valuable means of increasing his auditory awareness of correct and incorrect articulations. It is, of course, essential that the speech pathologist articulate clearly, producing good speech models at all times.

It may be necessary to concentrate at first on words that are new to the patient, and return later to correct the mispronunciations learned at an earlier age. For example, a child may omit s in the word *spoon* learned early, but pronounce it correctly in *spic and span* learned later from a TV ad; he may incorrectly pronounce s in *sled*, but learn to say it without difficulty in *slip*. It should be reemphasized that a sound produced in isolation is vastly different from the same sound produced with others preceding and following it in context. Speech sounds appearing in context influence each other in acoustic and phonetic characteristics, depending on the place and manner of articulation, the stress of the syllable in which each sound appears, and its position in the syllable, word, or phrase. Therapy techniques for articulation practice should incorporate sound sequences and patterns of everyday phrases and responses, thus helping the speaker to learn and recognize correct ways of forming and using sounds in oral language responses, rather than as isolated phones.

A cleft of the primary palate may make it particularly difficult to produce labial sounds; therefore, these patients need considerable practice to develop adequate mobility and flexibility of the lips. In addition to practice on phonetic placement of /p/, /b/, and /m/ sounds, the technique of pursing the lips in a whistle position may help to produce the lip rounding also needed for /ʍ/, /w/, /ʃ/, /ʒ/, /r/, and the lip-rounded vowels. This lip-rounding practice facilitates clearer formation of the sounds and increased fullness of tone. This procedure also tends to increase awareness of lip movements and positions during satisfactory sound production, and to help overcome any immobility, flaccidity, or stiffness of the lips caused by scar tissue and the various anomalies of the primary palate. Speech patterns calling for movement from rounded to unrounded lip position, as in the phrases *two by two* or *two by four*, offer excellent practice.

A number of patients with unintelligible speech overenergize greatly in an effort to make their speech understandable, creating muscular hypertension which interferes with clear production of voice and articulation. The word and sense stress as well as the rate and rhythm may become distorted as a consequence. When the muscular hypertension involves the head, neck, and shoulders, the patient tends to produce voice quality that is breathy, husky, nasal, denasal, glottal, etc., and to omit, substitute, or distort the speech sounds he is attempting to articulate. Much practice is needed to promote adequate movement of the tip, middle, and back of the tongue for clear articulation, since lack of tongue activity or retraction of the back (dorsum) of the tongue leads to nasal snorting and/or overaspiration, especially on initial /p/, /t/, /k/, and /h/ sounds in initial consonant plus vowel in a stressed syllable. Practice directed toward firm, precise, and accurate tongue and lip movements to form sounds habitually forced, snorted, blurred, or otherwise emitted nasally in word and phrase sequences is usually much more helpful to the patients than are blowing exercises or tongue and lip exercises as such.

Another common problem of the patients referred from the Cleft Palate Clinic at St. Luke's is the very slack production, slighting, or even omission of the nasal consonants /m/, /n/, /ŋ/ in inter- and postvocalic positions in words or sense groups. This habit produces denasal or nasal voice and slurred articulation. Practice in sustaining these sounds longer than is usual in connected speech can help minimize the faults just mentioned and provide the needed nasal resonance. While giving extra time to all the voiced consonant continuant sounds, the patient develops increased tonicity of the muscles used for their articulation and, by blending them together in phrases or sentences, produces a stronger, clearer voice. Such practice, especially important for voiced consonant continuants that are postvocalic and final, or postvocalic and preconsonantal in the sense group, makes the prolongation of vowels and diphthongs both unnecessary and undesirable, although they are the most sonorous of the speech sounds. Most United States speakers of English seem unable to enunciate vowels and sustain them without diphthongizing single vowels, and triphthongizing the legitimate diphthongs. The attempt to sustain vowels results in a squeezed, "throaty" quality, and the vowels lose their sonority. To maintain their carrying power and their varieties of color when clear, it is safer to say the vowels quickly and to sustain the tone-carrying consonants.

The following transcription illustrates therapy techniques discussed in this section.

K W, No. 42-57-88

Born in the United States with a subtotal cleft of the primary and secondary palates, the child had cheiloplasty 6 days after birth and palatoplasty with superior pharyngeal flap at 10 months of age. When seen by the speech pathologist the first time at 3 years 8 months of age, she did not speak spontaneously. When cajoled into responding, she could produce approximations of a few vowels and the consonants *b* and *m*. Her voice was breathy, with some snorting, nasal and denasal.

The following excerpt is from a practice lesson with tape recording made when K was 4+ years old. The purpose was to help K, who uses language well, develop clear voice production through special practice on the nasal consonants *m*, *n* and *ng* /ŋ/. K pushes out a great deal of unphonated air when she speaks, and her quality is both nasal and denasal. At this session there was no evidence of snorting, although earlier in her practice the breathed plosives, *p, t, k* plus vowels in stressed syllables were approximated with that characteristic.

SP: (Showing K a picture) What's the girl doing here?

K: She's *jump'm* /dʒʌpm̩/ (vowel is nasalized, *m* following vowel is slighted or omitted, and following *p*, m̩ is substituted for *ing*.

SP: Yes, she *jumping*. Try to say it this way, *jumping*, and put a *ping* in it, *jumping*.

K: *Jumpen* /dʒʌpən/. (This time /ən/ is substituted for *ing* /ɪŋ/. I can't say it your way.

SP: Try once more. Let's divide the word. Say *jum*, and hold on to a good strong /m/.

K: /dʒʌmmm/.

SP: Now the second part *ping*, and this time hold on to the end of *ping* /pɪŋ/.

K: /pɪŋŋŋŋ/.

SP: Now let's put the
    word together again
    jumping.

K: (Says it with a fair approximation of *jumping* by
saying /dʒʌmmmpɪŋŋŋ/
with both *m* and *ng* sustained
overlong, and with equal
stress on both syllables,
with a clear production of
voice).

SP: That's fine.

The lesson continues with additional *-umping* words practiced: *dumping, bumping, thumping.* When K pronounced the words or used them in short phrases with exaggerated sustaining of *m* and *ng* her voice was strong and clear. But when she "talked" about the words and said them, *ing* came out /ən/, except in *thumping,* a new word for her, which she said over and over, thumping on the table as she did so. Note that /ɪŋ/ is recommended over /ɪn)/ or ən/ for all such words, /ɪŋ/ more likely to supply more resonance than endings with *n,* as pronounced by most United Statesans.

The foregoing are only a few of many suggestions that may prove advantageous for speech therapy. Speech rehabilitation is usually a long-term process calling for understanding and interest on the part of all members of the rehabilitation team, including families.

The cooperation and patience of the family can help motivate the patient to practice purposefully and to carry over improvements from therapy sessions to his everyday speech. Songs, games, and rhymes are fun and useful, but the real test of speech habilitation and rehabilitation comes when the person starts to talk of things in his own personal world.

THE CHARTS USED BY THE SPEECH PATHOLOGIST IN THE
HEARING AND SPEECH DEPARTMENT FOLLOW AND INCLUDE:

1. Basic Information Sheet
2. Language and Speech Evaluation Test in English for Adults
3. Language and Speech Evaluation Test in Spanish for Adults
4. Language and Speech Evaluation Test in English and
   Spanish for children
5. Language and Speech Evaluation Details
6. Summary: Language, Speech, and Hearing Evaluation and
   Progress.

THE CHARTS USED BY THE AUDIOLOGIST ARE AS FOLLOWS:

7. Auditory History
8. Audiological Evaluation for Pure Tone Testing
9. Speech Audiometry for Speech Thresholds and Discrim-
   inations
10. Hearing Aid Evaluation Form

CHART 1. BASIC INFORMATION SHEET

Hospital No. _____
Service _____

Name _____
Date _____

Last   First

Age _____ Date of birth _____ Sex _____

Address _____ Telephone _____

_____

Parents' names _____ Occupation _____

Referred by: (Dept. & Dr.) _____

Number and ages of siblings _____

Name & address of school _____

Grade _____ Teacher _____ Performance _____

Developmental history:

Uses _____ hand; walked at _____; babbled at _____

Said first words at _____; sentences at _____

Birth history _____

Medical history:

Medical diagnosis _____

Operations _____

Other _____

_____

_____

_____

Speech history:

Speech problems: Voice _____ Articulation _____ Rhythm _____

Language: Receptive _____ Expressive _____

Onset of speech problems _____

Native language _____ Language spoken at home _____

Family speech problems _____

Previous speech lessons _____

General impressions:

_____

Speech Pathologist

CHART 2. LANGUAGE AND SPEECH EVALUATION TEST IN ENGLISH FOR ADULTS

1. Good morning. How are you? I am (speech pathologist gives name and title).
2. What is your name?
3. I'd like to make a tape recording of your speech, please.
4. Will you please say "My name is . . . " and give your full name?
5. Where do you live? Where were you born?
6. Please count from one to ten in a strong voice.
7. Please repeat these numbers: 641; 3142; 572891.
8. Please say this sentence after me: "The sun is hot in summer."
9. Please say these two sentences after me, but wait until I have said both of them: "Walter had a fine time in the country. He went fishing every day."
10. Please say the names of the days of the week, beginning with Sunday.
11. Please say the names of the months of the year.
12. Where did you go to school, and how far did you go?
13. Do you work? What kind of work do you do?
14. How is your speech? Do you have trouble with your speech?
15. Do you see well? Do you hear well?
16. Will you please read the attached short paragraph and answer the questions given below it.
17. Please write your name and address on this piece of paper.
18. Thank you very much.

CHART 3. VALUACIÓN DE LENGUA Y HABLA EN ESPANOL POR ADULTOS (LANGUAGE AND SPEECH EVALUATION TEST IN SPANISH FOR ADULTS)

Preguntas y Ruegos (y Saludos)

1. Buenos días.   ¿Como está usted?
2. Yo quiero grabar su conversación, por favor.
3. Cuente del uno al diez, por favor.
4. Dígame los días de la semana, por favor.
5. Dígame su nombre, por favor. Mi nomi es.
6. ¿Donde vive?
7. Dígame los meses del año, por favor.
8. ¿Cuando llegó a New York?
9. Por favor, repita:
   641 (seis ciento cuarenta y uno).
   3142 (tres uno cuarenta y dos).
   372891 (tres siete dos ocho nueve uno).
10. Por favor repita:
    El sol es caliente en el verano.
    Juan tuvo un tiempo feliz en el campo.
    Fué a pescar todos los días.
11. Escriba su nombre y su domicilio en este papel, por favor.
12. Lea este párrafo, por favor:
    Un fuego anoche quemó varias casas la zona centríca de la ciudad. Demoró un tiempo para que el fuego se apagase. La perdida fuer de más de cien mil dolares, y diez y siete familias perdieron sus hogares. Por salvar la vida a una muchacha que dormía en la cama, un bombero se quemó en las manos.
    Responda estas preguntas, por favor:
    1. ¿ Que clase de accidente ocurrio anoche?
    2. ¿ En que parte de la ciudad se originó el fuego?
    3. ¿ Cuanto dinero se perdió?
    4. ¿ Cuantas familias per dieron sus hogares?
    5. ¿ En que parte del cuerpo se quemo el bombero?
13. Es suficiente, gracias.

Preguntas y Ruegos (y Saludos) Respuestas incluidas.	*Questions and Requests (and greetings) Responses included.*
1. Buenos días. ¿Como esta usted?	Good morning. How are you?
2. Estoy bien, gracias, ¿y usted?	I'm fine, thank you, and you? Good.
3. Me llamo_____ nombre	My name is_____ *or* I am_____
4. Dígame por favor su nombre. (or ¿cual es su nombre? or ¿Como se llama?)	What is your name, please?
5. Aqui está pintures a examin.	Here are some pictures to look at.
6. ¿Que está haciendo el muchacho en este cuadro? ¿En este cuadro? (y así sucesi vamente.)	What's the boy doing in this picture? (and in this picture? etc.)
7. El muchacho está comiendo melón.	He's eating melon.
8. El está saltando.	He's jumping.
9. El está lava la cara o las orejas.	He is washing his face or his ears.
10. ¿Que está haciendo el niño (el bebé) un este cuadro?	What is the baby doing in this picture?
11. El niño está bebiendo leche o agua.	The baby is drinking milk or water.
12. ¿Que es esto? Un aeroplano.	What is this? An airplane.
13. ¿De que color es este balon?	What color is this balloon?
14. Rojo. Verde. Azul. Amarillo.	Red. Green. Blue. Yellow.
15. ¿Que animal es este?	What animal is this?
16. Caballo. Vaca. Perro. Gata. Leon. Tigre. Pescado. Mono. Pollo. Cabra. Puerco. Ave.	Horse. Cow. Dog. Cat. Lion. Tiger. Fish. Monkey. Chicken. Goat. Pig. Bird.
17. ¿Si usted tiene, tres deseos y es possible tener cualqier en el mundo, que desearía usted?	If you had three wishes and you could wish for anything in the world, what would you wish for?
19. ¿Puede cantar?	Can you sing?
19. ¿Sabe la cancion Feliz Cumpleaños?"	Do you know the song "Happy Birthday?"
20. Cantela, por favor.	Sing it, please.
21. Es suficiente, gracias. o, Es bastante, gracias.	That is all, thank you.

CHART 5. LANGUAGE AND SPEECH EVALUATION DETAILS

NO. _____ Date: _____

Name _____ Hosp. No. _____

I. ATTITUDES:	RATING
Pleasant	
Responsive	
Communicative	
Cooperative	
Alert	
Apprehensive	

II. LANGUAGE SKILLS:

Receptive	
Expressive	
Developmental	

III. SPEECH ABILITIES:

A. Rate

Appropriate	
Fast	
Slow	

B. Stress

Accurate word	
Accurate sense	
"Form" word errors	

C. Rhythm

Smooth	
Fluent	
Choppy	
Staccato	
Scanning	

D. Volume

Adequate	
Sustained	
Strong	
Overloud	
Fading	
Weak	

E. Pitch

Appropriate	
High	
Rises with stress	
Inconsistent	
Stereotyped intonation	

III. SPEECH ABILITIES (cont)	RATING
F. Quality	
Clear	
Pleasant	
Resonant	
Breathy	
Husky	
Glottal fry (squeezed)	
Hoarse	
Strident	
Colorless	
Flat	
Nasal (hyper)	
Snorting	
Blurring	
Emission	
Twang	
Denasal (hyponasality)	
Blurring	
Muffled	
Dysphonic	

G. Articulation

Intelligible	
Firm	
Accurate	
Slack	
Blurred	
Slurred	

IV. DETAILS: (list speech sounds affected)

A. Overaspiration _____

B. Nasalization _____

C. Unvoicing _____

D. Addition _____

E. Omission _____

F. Substitution _____

G. Distortion _____

H. Lisp: Nasal ____ Lat. ____ Interdent. __

I. Inadequate use of tongue _____

　　Lips _____ Velopharyng. _____

J. Facial grimaces ____ Nares constr. ____

K. Other _____

L. Blocks _____; hesitations _____;

　　repetitions _____

PATIENT'S EVALUATION OF HIS SPEECH:　　SUMMARY:

CHART 6. SUMMARY: LANGUAGE, SPEECH, AND HEARING EVALUATION AND PROGRESS:

Name _____ Hospital No. _____

Language and speech problems: Lang: Recept. _____ Expr. _____ Devel. _____

SP: Voice _____ Artic. _____ Rate-rhythm _____

Hearing status: _____ Dates of audio test _____

Evaluations and recordings: (give date and file No. of recordings)

1. Initial/preoperative _____

2. Postoperative _____

3. Reevaluation _____

EVALUATION RATINGS:

Key: 1. Considerably above average
2. Slightly above average
3. Average
4. Slightly below average
5. Considerably below average

PROGRESS RATINGS:

Key: A. Improved considerably
B. Improved slightly
C. Maintained status quo
D. Regressed slightly
E. Regressed considerably

	Evaluation No.				Progress		
	1	2	3	4	1 to 2	2 to 3	3 to 4
I. Attitudes							
II. Language skills							
Receptive							
Expressive							
Developmental							
III. Speech Abilities							
Volume							
Pitch							
Quality							
Rate-rhythm							
Articulation							
IV. Hearing							

SUMMARY: (see following page for details)

RECOMMENDATIONS: Postop. reevaluation _____; follow-up reevaluation _____

Speech _____ Hearing _____ Therapy _____ times per wk. at _____

to begin _____.

Date: _____

_____
Speech Pathologist

CHART 7. AUDITORY HISTORY

Name: Date:

Address: Phone: Hospital No.:

Sex: Age: BD: Occupation:

Short history of present hearing difficulty:

Check presence of any of the following in history (past and present) of patient:

Scarlet fever _____   T and A operation _____
Rheumatic fever _____   Acoustic trauma _____
Otosclerosis _____   Medication, such as salicylates, quinine,
Meningitis _____   neomycin, other toxic drugs _____
Meniere's syndrome _____   Wears hearing aid _____
Mumps _____   Previous audiogram _____
Measles _____   Tinnitus _____
Chicken pox _____   Vertigo _____
Diphtheria _____   Other pertinent operations _____
Otitis media _____   Streptomycin: (type) _____
Discharging ears _____   Dosage: _____
Lues _____   Begun: _____ Stopped: _____
Head injury _____   Difficulty c̄ telephone: _____
Neurological disorders _____   Loss of balance: _____
Malaria fever _____
Typhoid fever _____

Family hearing history: Mother _____   Sister _____
                             Father _____   Grandparents _____
                             Brother _____   Other _____

Was mother's pregnancy normal? Yes _____ No _____
During mother's pregnancy, did she have: Measles? _____
German measles? _____ Lues? _____
Medication that might have injured child's auditory apparatus? _____
Rh factor in mother's pregnancy? _____
Was patient birth normal? _____

SPEECH
When did child babble? _____ Start speaking words? _____ Sentences? _____
Any speech defects (patient and family)? _____
Mental condition _____

CHART 8. AUDIOLOGICAL EVALUATION

AUDIOLOGICAL EVALUATION

Name _____

Hosp. No. _____ Nursing Unit _____

Service _____ Classn. _____

Adm. Date _____ Sex _____ Age _____

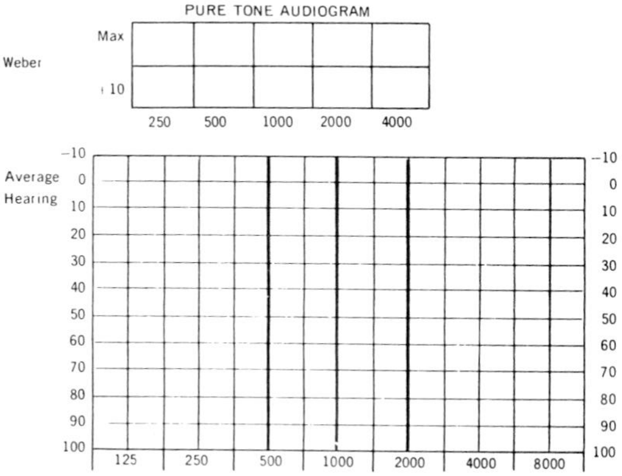

Date _____ Referred by _____

PURE TONE AUDIOGRAM

Weber

Max

ι 10

250 500 1000 2000 4000

Average Hearing

-10
0
10
20
30
40
50
60
70
80
90
100

125 250 500 1000 2000 4000 8000

-10
0
10
20
30
40
50
60
70
80
90
100

Pure Tone Averages:
(500, 1000, 2000)

Right Ear _____

Left Ear _____

Binaural _____

Tinnitus Description:

_____

Location _____

Masking $\bar{c}$ _____

for A C _____

for B C _____

Patient Response

LEGEND FOR AUDIOGRAM

Right Ear (red)

A. C.   o———o

A. C. $\bar{c}$ masking △————△

A. C. not heard

A. C. $\bar{c}$ masking, not heard △

B. C.   [

B. C. $\bar{c}$ masking Ր

B. C. not heard

B. C. $\bar{c}$ masking, not heard ↑

Tolerance Threshold T

Left Ear (blue or black)

A. C.   X----------X

A. C. $\bar{c}$ masking ▽----------▽

A. C. not heard X

A. C. $\bar{c}$ masking, not heard ▽

B. C.   ]

B. C. $\bar{c}$ masking 1

B. C. not heard

B. C. $\bar{c}$ masking, not heard 1

Tolerance Threshold T

Weber Lateralization:

Right ←——Left ——→ R & L ←——→

Not Heard ↓

Abbreviations:

R. Referred to right   B. Referred to both
L. Referred to left   P. $\bar{c}$ pressure on BC oscillator

Loudness Balance:

Better Ear

Poorer Ear

Tolerance Problem:

_____

_____

Remarks: _____

_____

_____

_____

Instrument: _____

Audiologist _____

CHART 9. SPEECH AUDIOMETRY

SPEECH AUDIOMETRY

	RIGHT	LEFT	FREEFIELD (BINAURAL)
SPONDEE THRESHOLDS re: normal hearing	db	db	db
DISCRIMINATION SCORES at + 40 db re: threshold	%	%	%
DISCRIMINATION SCORES c̄ NOISE in contralateral ear at + 40 db re: threshold	%	%	%
DISCRIMINATION at 45 db re: normal hearing	%	%	%
TOLERANCE THRESHOLDS re: normal hearing	db	db	db

SPECIAL TESTS

D – S _____

LOMBARD_____

STENGER_____

BEKESY_____

SISI_____

OTHER_____

HEARING AID PROGNOSIS

GOOD _____

FAIR _____

POOR _____

QUESTIONABLE _____

LIPREADING ABILITY

GOOD_____ POOR _____

VISION IMPAIRED_____

RELIABILITY

GOOD _____

FAIR _____

POOR _____

QUESTIONABLE _____

NOTES· _____

_____

_____

_____

_____

_____

_____

_____

_____

_____

_____

INSTRUMENT _____

AUDIOLOGIST _____

271

CHART 10. HEARING AND EVALUATION

HEARING AID EVALUATION

NAME _____

HOSP. NO. _____ NURSING UNIT _____

SERVICE _____ CLASSIFICATION _____

ADMISSION DATE _____ SEX _____ AGE _____

DATE: _____ REFERRED BY: _____

	UNAIDED	# 1	# 2	# 3	# 4	# 5	# 6
HEARING AID NAME							
MODEL NUMBER OR TYPE AID							
RESPONSE SETTING							
RECEIVER							
BATTERY							
EAR							
VOLUME CONTROL SETTING							
SRT SCORE							
DISCRIM AT + 45 DB							
SUBJECTIVE SELECTION							
OBJECTIVE SELECTION							

RELIABILITY   Good: Fair: Poor:

_____

_____

_____

_____

AUDIOLOGIST _____

MR 132

272

CHAPTER 22

Postoperative Evaluation of Cleft Palate Surgery: Experimental Techniques

R. C. A. WEATHERLEY-WHITE

In a Hunterian Lecture to the Royal College of Surgeons of England in 1928, W. E. M. Wardill precisely defined the priorities in cleft palate surgery: "The greatest item . . . must undoubtedly be the speech results, and considerations . . . largely aesthetic should be given a very low value."

Surgical procedures to correct congenital clefts are truly functional. Success must be gauged by the patient's ability to communicate effectively rather than by elegance of the repair or even by certain physiological criteria that can be measured with numerous sophisticated devices available to the clinician. This assessment is necessarily related to perceptual evaluation, since recognition of human speech or verbal communication needs a listening ear.

With this principle in mind, it is difficult indeed to compare the success of different modalities of treating cleft palate. Several modifications of the classic von Langenbeck procedure have appeared in recent years, e.g., the Veau-Kilner-Wardill retroposition operation, Millard's island flap, and Stark's primary pharyngeal flap. Investigators differ on the value of early surgery, as opposed to prosthetic treatment followed by later palate repair. Can the various treatment modes be evaluated in terms of speech proficiency, leading to a final decision on the optimal approach to cleft palate? Obviously, the simplest and most direct method of comparing postoperative results is critical evaluation of the patient's speech by a trained observer. In the vast majority of reports in the literature, the degree of success achieved by cleft palate surgery is measured by clinical speech evaluation in one form or another. But speech recognition is perforce affected by personal bias; all evaluations of "normal," "acceptable," or "defective" speech are certainly not based on the same criteria. When articles report "85 per cent of the patients achieved normal speech following this type of repair," it is natural to wonder how "normal speech" is defined. Some reports have indicated quite dissimilar ratings of tape recordings in a panel situation by staff members of the same institution. It would thus seem difficult or even impossible to compare the data of different observers on speech proficiency following surgery at different centers.

Attempts have been made in recent years to counter this basic dilemma by introducing objective criteria for comparing postoperative results. Of the two principal approaches, one has borrowed from experimental psychology, making use of scaling techniques, intricate statistics, and computer technology to obtain valid and reliable data from perceptual phenomena. In the other approach, results are calibrated by means of numerical standards obtained from measuring physiological events related to speech production and from acoustic studies of normal and defective speech.

PERCEPTUAL EVALUATION

A detailed description of the complex abnormalities involved in cleft palate speech appears in Chapter 21. However, a brief explanation of the processes developed to ensure reliability of subjective evaluations is necessary to understanding of the present discussion.

In general, cleft palate speech results from the repaired palate's inability to form an effective valve with the posterior pharyngeal wall. When the palate is foreshortened in relation to the depth of the pharynx, a competent velopharyngeal "seal" cannot be achieved; air is constantly emitted through the nose, and the nasal resonating chamber affects all voiced sounds. A scarred and immobile palate is incapable of the rapid muscular action needed for instantaneous coupling and uncoupling of the nasal and oral resonating chambers at the appropriate time and rate. Instead of the wide range of normal nasal resonance and full oral tones which lend contrast and brilliance of normal speech, we have the flat, monotonous voice quality typical of cleft palate victims with poor speech. Compounding these factors are the patient's attempts to compensate for his inadequate anatomical equipment, e.g., by the "glottal stop"—obstruction of the air stream at the glottal level to obtain the breath pressure necessary for pronouncing /k/ and /g/.

These physiological defects result in abnormal articulation as well as voice quality. Correct pronunciation—particularly of the plosives, fricatives, and affricates—depends on impounding adequate breath pressure within the mouth. When breath pressure escapes nasally through an incompetent velopharyngeal valve, such sounds are weakened or lost. The voice quality defect, generally classified as hypernasality, is more subtle. It was long assumed that the abnormal nasality resulted from a constant overlay of nasal resonance because the palate could not exclude the nasopharynx from the resonating system. Recent observations, however, indicate that a person with nasal speech can simultaneously have hyponasality—adenoidal speech in which /m/ becomes /b/, /n/ becomes /d/, and /ng/ becomes /g/. The two defects, hitherto regarded as mutually exclusive, are therefore not necessarily at opposite ends of a voice quality spectrum. Furthermore, such variables as huskiness, breathiness, and throatiness may adversely affect the voice quality to some degree.

Defective articulation combined with abnormal voice quality decreases intelligibility. An intelligibility test has been devised to quantitate this feature, so fundamental to effective communication. The subjects read a number of phonetically balanced short words which are recorded on tape and played back to a panel of judges who are preferably not associated with speech pathology. The judges write down their concept of each word, and the scores reflect the percentage of words recognized.

Some basic principles of research design are observed in all attempts to standardize perceptual judgments. The recordings must be taken under identical conditions, if possible with high-fidelity equipment in a soundproof room. The control group and the cleft palate group must be matched as closely as possible to eliminate variables. For example, comparison of the speech of cleft palate children from mixed sociological or ethnic backgrounds with that of adult medical students would obviously be illogical. Recordings of subjects and controls must be taped randomly so that the judges have no indication of the group to which the speaker belongs. Finally, the ratings must be subjected to statistical analysis, the test's validity depending on the coefficient of correlation between the judges.

While the intelligibility test reveals over-all speech proficiency, the characteristics of defectiveness must be more specifically defined.

Faults in articulation are best defined by a carefully structured item test in which the patient reads a series of words containing all the possible articulatory sounds. His performance is checked on a standard form by a trained speech pathologist, and areas of weakness are delineated by category. Among variations of the Templin-Darley 176-item test in general use, the Iowa Pressure Articulation Test is perhaps the most valuable for patients with cleft palate. It stresses features of articulation requiring maximum impounding of breath pressure and thus affords some measurement of velopharyngeal competence. When articulation is assessed by a structured test employing such a check-list system, many variables inherent in perceptual evaluation are minimized. In several studies, careful statistical analyses have demonstrated close correlation among the judges through this method.

Voice quality has in general been evaluated according to the degree of hypernasality recognized in continuous speech samples, although as mentioned above this may be oversimplifying a complex problem. Scaling has been based on relatively gross categories such as "normal voice quality," "mildly nasal," and "severely nasal"; or on an equal-interval scale which numerically rates the degree of defectiveness. The most reliable method would appear to be "direct magnitude estimation"; a reference point is established for a given stimulus, and all examples are related to it. With well-selected sample recordings of various degrees of defectiveness, and careful prior indoctrination of the listener-judges, a panel of either trained or untrained observers can perform reliably under rigid statistical control. As Moll has pointed out, perceptual tests offer the most logical and direct means of assessing defective speech. When performed in a carefully controlled research atmosphere, they can be statistically valid. This is not necessarily the case in the more variable clinical setting, however. In fact, one observer has stated that management decisions should never be made solely on the basis of subjective evaluation.

PRESSURE AND FLOW STUDIES

Velopharyngeal incompetence is at the core of cleft palate speech. Abnormalities of both articulation and voice quality inevitably result from nasal escape of air and constant coupling of the naso- and oropharynx, since the palatal complex cannot function as an effective valve to exclude the nasal cavity from the resonating system.

Even in the earliest days of cleft palate surgery, physicians used such relatively crude diagnostic tests as blowing out a match or inflating a rubber balloon; they also held a mirror just below the nares during speech, which would cloud in the presence of nasally emitted air.

Wardill (1926), the first who attempted to quantitate the valve's incompetence, inserted collapsible balloons into the nasopharynx to measure the volume of escaping air. Buncke (1959) adapted a manometric system to measure oral and nasal breath pressure, and Chase (1960) modified it by introducing a constant air leak into the closed system to prevent the tongue's blocking the incompetent valve. The most detailed studies of valve incompetence have been made at the Speech Center of the University of Iowa. When the oral breath pressure is measured first with the nostrils open and then blocked, the ratio in normal individuals is 1:1. The Iowa group (1959) showed that the oral breath-pressure ratio varies directly with velopharyngeal competence and correlates closely with proficiency in articulating high-pressure consonants—fricatives, plosives, and affricates. This finding has been confirmed by others studying cleft palate speech in a number of dimensions. Greene's report of 263 patients with surgically repaired cleft palate, however, revealed no relation between breath-pressure studies and speech proficiency.

The manometric methods not only preclude the measurement of physiological events during connected speech but also introduce a highly artificial variable, obstruction, into the research design. These two drawbacks can be averted by use of a flow meter which directly measures oral and nasal air flow during speech. Quigley (1963) developed such an instrument which utilizes the cooling effect of an air current upon an electrically warmed sensing element. Although still in an experimental stage and requiring more complicated data-reduction methods than the manometer, this instrument is very promising, since it can measure nasal volume flow rates and thus directly quantitate nasal air emission during speech.

The cross-sectional area of the open palatopharyngeal port during speech has been precisely measured by Warren (1964). With differential pressure transducers placed in the patient's mouth and nose, he measured flow rates in a manner similar to Quigley's, making use of a simple aerodynamic formula:

$$\text{Orifice area} = \frac{\text{Rate of airflow through orifice}}{\sqrt[2]{2\left(\dfrac{\text{Orifice differential pressure}}{\text{Air density}}\right)}}$$

Not surprisingly, he found that in normal speakers the cross-sectional area is greatest during voicing of the nasal consonants and the vowels immediately preceding them. The phonetic context, rather than the vowels themselves, determines the degree of velopharyngeal opening. A report of this exquisitely sensitive method with reference to the evaluation of cleft palate patients is still to come.

The above studies confirm the importance of the palatopharyngeal mechanism in speech production. In general, velopharyngeal competence directly governs how efficiently sounds can be produced that require the greatest impounding of intraoral breath pressure. The University of Iowa group, which has considerably furthered our understanding of such phenomena, has scrupulously pointed out that these are indirect measures of speech indicating potential rather than proficiency. Their greatest clinical value would appear to be in evolving criteria for performing secondary procedures. If speech following palatoplasty is poor and palatopharyngeal incompetence is evident, secondary surgery to lengthen the palate is desirable. But if there is a speech deficit despite adequate valving, surgical measures will very likely be unavailing.

RADIOLOGIC TECHNIQUES

The functional relations, in time and space, of the speech-producing mechanism have been most effectively studied by roentgenography. Detailed measurements of parts of the mechanism not directly visualized and clarification of the relation between the palato-pharyngeal complex and speech production are among the advances made possible through this discipline. Lateral films of the head using soft tissue techniques to delineate the tongue, palate, and posterior pharyngeal wall, have excellent definition, and the patient's exposure to radiation is negligible. The velum/pharyngeal wall relation during production of sustained sounds was established principally by X-rays. Careful positioning by means of a radiolucent headholder is mandatory for cephalometric studies, as even slight rotation results in significant errors of measurement. With the use of still films, the degree of velopharyngeal competence is usually best demonstrated by sustained production of the sibilant /s/, as vowel production is accompanied by varying degrees of velopharyngeal opening in normal subjects. Only limited data are available, however, from single-exposure X-ray studies. Sustained sounds are not characteristic of normal speech, and necessary immobilization of the articulatory structures precludes a true physiological measurement.

Cineroentgenography with a 35-mm. camera provides detailed information on relations of the structures involved during the production of connected speech, and hence is a more relevant adjunct to clinical study. An image intensifier provides excellent clarity, and keeps radiation exposure to the midline of the head at safe levels (5.4 r with 70 kv machine for a 2-minute film). A frame-by-frame analyzer permits the tracing of anatomical landmarks. Synchronization of the film with a tape recording of the subject's voice reveals exact correlations between speech sequences and changing anatomical relations. This procedure is time-consuming and laborious. Rapid motion of the palate during speech, including vibration against the posterior pharyngeal wall, makes it necessary to trace every third frame of a 30-frame-per-second film strip (Fig. 22-1).

The most valuable measurements for analyzing speech-mechanism movements are: (1) *A-B*, the reference line from the posterior nasal spine to the most prominent part of the tubercle of the atlas; (2) *V-H*, the maximal height above *A-B* achieved by the palate in motion; (3) *V-P*, the velopharyngeal aperture in cases of valve in-

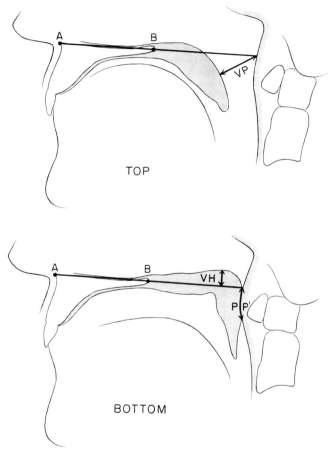

FIG. 22-1 *By means of a cineroentgenographic frame-by-frame analyzer, changing anatomical relations can be correlated with speech sequences. The most important measurements are shown in the two diagrams.*

TOP

    AB is line from anterior to posterior nasal spines extrapolated to the posterior pharynx.

    VP measures degree of velopharyngeal incompetence.

BOTTOM

    VH is maximum height that velum rises above AB.

    PP′ is extent of velar contact with posterior pharyngeal wall.

competence. Other measurements include length of the soft palate relative to the depth of the pharynx; extent of velar contact with the pharyngeal wall; thickness of the soft palate; and excursion of the pharyngeal wall itself during speech. To date, a statistical relation has been adequately established only between the velopharyngeal aperture and articulatory defectiveness. Mazaheri (1964) of the Lancaster Cleft Palate Centre is the only investigator in the field who found no such mathematical correlation, reporting varying degrees of incompetence even in the same individual.

Our clinic is interested in the palate's mobility as measured by the time required (in milliseconds) to open and close the velopharyngeal port; palatal scarring and denervation following radical retropositioning operations may be just as deleterious to speech as anatomical shortening.

A recent development in radiographic technology is recording of the image on video tape. McWilliams has recorded 5- to 10-minute samples of connected speech with far less radiation exposure than occurs with conventional fluoroscopic equipment. Sound synchronization is relatively easy, and immediate playback of the test sequence is a definite advantage. Video tapes cannot yet be played slowly or analyzed on a frame-by-frame basis, however; so either the TV image must be transferred onto film or else the assessment must be qualitative rather than quantitative.

ACOUSTIC STUDIES

Whereas measurements of pressure phenomena and anatomical relations provide indirect information about speech production, characteristics of speech itself may be directly quantitated acoustically.

The sound spectrograph (Fig. 22-2) is the most familiar instrument for speech analysis on the acoustic level. Developed by Bell Laboratories in the 1940's, it displays the power components of speech visually, plotting both frequency and intensity against time (Fig. 22-3). Cross-sectional "cuts" of the tracing permit quantitation of the relative intensity of different frequencies at a specific instant. In reproductions of spectrographic tracings, "pressure" consonants are characterized by short bursts of high-frequency energy and vowel tones by "formants"—broad sustained bands of great intensity in the lower frequencies.

Perhaps the most intensive work to date on cleft palate speech has been done at the University of Uppsala by Nylén and Bjork (1961). Synchronizing sound spectrography and cineroentgenography, they have directly related articulatory proficiency to velopharyngeal competence. With an increasing cross-sectional area of the palato-

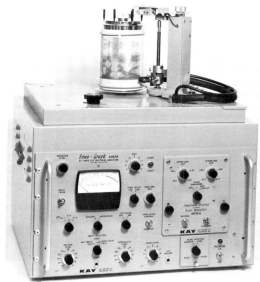

FIG. 22-2 *Sound spectrograph which analyzes speech at the acoustic level.*

pharyngeal port, the intensity of high-frequency bursts is attenuated. The Swedish studies relating voice quality to formant-band width and intensity were less productive. The wide variability in this respect in normal individuals militates against standardization of the spectrographic response to voice quality defectiveness—a finding confirmed by other investigators.

Although this technique has only recently been applied in cleft palate research, objective comparison of defective speakers will undoubtedly be achieved ultimately by means of the sound spectrograph. Only with standardized procedures, more information, and computer

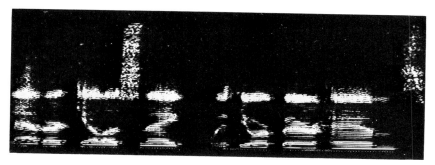

FIG. 22-3 *The power components of speech are displayed visually by spectrography, frequency and intensity being plotted against time.* (*Courtesy of Haskins Laboratory, New York City.*)

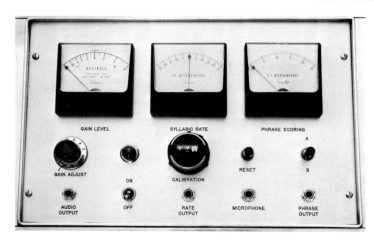

FIG. 22-4   *The Voice Systems Meter developed by the IBM Corporation has been a useful tool in objective speech analysis. This instrument defines phase relations in the speech pressure wave which imply coupling or uncoupling of the naso- and oropharynx.*

techniques of data retrieval will the problems of individual variation be overcome. The range of normality must be defined before defects can be classified.

Our own modest studies of cleft palate speech on the acoustic level have been aided by an instrument developed by the IBM Corpo-

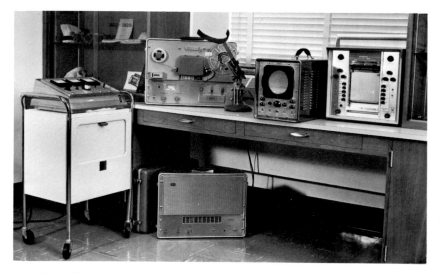

FIG. 22-5   *Voice Systems Meter, Ampex tape recorder, and oscilloscope have been used by us for objective analysis of speech.*

ration (Fig. 22-4). It "recognizes" a vocabulary of spoken words, and we have adapted the concept to calibrate certain speech features. By studying phase relations in the speech pressure wave rather than by frequency filtration techniques we have been able to define quantities of nasal resonance in a test phrase, and hence to infer coupling of the naso- and oropharynx.

In our opinion, the voice quality defect in cleft palate speech involves considerably more than excessive nasal resonance, and either perceptual or acoustic assessments of "nasality" are valueless in objectively classifying the degree of impairment. The concept of a range of voice quality appears more pertinent; normal speakers can discriminate between the desirable brilliance of normal nasal resonance and the full oral tones produced when the nasopharynx is excluded from the resonating system by a competent velopharyngeal valve. In our series, cleft palate speakers with more severe impairment could not make this discrimination; their speech was flat and monotonous, characterized instrumentally by a narrow range of voice quality.

A review of the modalities for assessment of speech following cleft palate repair reveals that limited information is gained by any single approach. Studies in depth relying on various techniques, such as those of Bzoch (1964), Nylén and Bjork, and the speech centers at Lancaster and Iowa City, give a far more accurate and comprehensive picture of the "speech profile." The heterogeneity of the cleft palate population is an important factor, since treatment of the anatomical defect is complicated by numerous geographical, educational, social, economic, and psychological variables. Finally, the perceptual nature of speech reception makes it imperative that all objective measurements include listener judgments. These, in turn, must be standardized to whatever extent is possible to facilitate consistent and reliable assessments that are free from observer bias, for comparison with physiological or acoustic measurements.

CHAPTER 23

Social
Service

MARGARET ROUILLION

In the practice of medicine today, increasing consideration is being given to the patient not only as an individual but also as a participating member of his family and his community. The social worker in a medical setting works with patients and their families when personal or environmental difficulties either predispose toward illness or interfere with maximum results from medical care. Interrelated environmental and personal factors are the basis for social evaluation and diagnosis, the substance of which is shared with the doctors, nurses, and others working closely with the patient.

The social worker studies the patient's current home situation, his background, his feelings and needs, as well as the attitudes, actions, and reactions of the parents and relatives as they relate to him and his medical condition. Social data are obtained by interviewing family members or employers as well as the patient (if he is not too young) and contacting organizations such as a school, community agency, church, court, hospital, or recreational facility. From these sources the worker may glean information helpful in evaluating the patient's and his family's attitudes and feelings toward his physical condition and the medical situation, and his potential for rehabilitation. The earlier the patient comes to the social worker's attention, the more meaningful will be her contribution to his total care. Her contact with the family varies according to the nature of the problems presented.

The over-all framework within which the cleft palate team functions at St. Luke's Hospital enables the social worker to meet with families early in their association with the doctor and the hospital. The worker is responsible for completion of a questionnaire formulated when the Cleft Palate Clinic was founded and revised from time to time, to provide information for research into possible etiological factors in cleft lip and cleft palate. This gives the worker an opportunity to begin a positive working relation with the patient's mother— or some other person close to him—which helps her to determine the parents' future attitudes. It is therefore preferable for the mother to complete the questionnaire in the social worker's presence rather than at home. If the questionnaire is mailed in, the worker tries to see the mother as soon as possible. When families live some distance from the hospital, this may be difficult; most of our patients' mothers have been accessible, however.

During the first interview, the worker expresses her interest not only in the patient but also in his family and in what lies ahead for him. This is important since through family-centered casework, she is the member of the cleft palate team most likely to help the family with the myriad social and emotional problems arising from this condition. The worker appreciates that some parts of the questionnaire may touch sensitive areas, leading the mother to talk freely and meaningfully about situations, feelings, and concerns that would otherwise be difficult to elicit. Maximum time is allowed for this initial contact, to foster a relaxed and sympathetic atmosphere in which the mother can discuss stresses and strains during her pregnancy, whether her baby was planned for and wanted. These delicate areas must be approached and explored with sensitivity and understanding if the information is to be meaningful. Such information clarifies the worker's understanding of implications in the family's feelings.

To foster satisfactory cooperation with the mother and others close to the patient, the worker attempts to convey a feeling of acceptance, interest in the patient, and availability to help them plan to meet his needs. It is a severe shock for a mother to learn that her baby is not physically perfect. She first wonders why this has happened and then becomes concerned about his future development. Anxiety and confused feelings of guilt should be handled as early as possible. When the questionnaire elicits such feelings, the worker recognizes them with the mother and helps her to view their basis and significance realistically.

During initial contacts with the mother, the worker often senses areas of tension and anxiety that may respond to casework. She arranges future appointments with the mother or other relatives and works with them at their own pace and according to their degree of concern. If a relation is to be productive, it must have meaning for the patient or relatives involved. The worker gains satisfaction as knotty problems begin to resolve, attitudes change, and a new sense of responsibility develops. From time to time she becomes frustrated, too, as she can deal only with material which the patient or family bring to a situation.

In the many cases where patients are referred to a cleft palate clinic directly after birth, the social worker usually does not encounter strong parental rejection; she can deal with certain problems before they have become distorted or deeply entrenched. The sooner a patient comes to the attention of an expert cleft palate team, the better is his chance for optimum growth and development.

We will cite several cases in point.

H. P., No. 35-38-36

Helen was born with a bilateral cleft of the primary and secondary palates, and in infancy had surgery elsewhere with residual disfigurement which became more pronounced as she grew older. She was 8 years old when first seen at St. Luke's Cleft Palate Clinic. Her appearance was marred by heavy scars, facial distortion, and protruding teeth. Fortunately, her parents had given her the love and attention so necessary for security, but she met with rejection in school and in the community. Children teased her and ridiculed her by imitating her speech. She tended to avoid them; became withdrawn, lonely, quiet, and unhappy. Through the local office of the State Department of Health, Crippled Children's Division, she was referred to St. Luke's, where surgery, dental work, and speech training were carried out. During the child's medical care, the social worker had a close relation with the mother, supporting her and helping her plan for the various treatment steps. The parents, very protective of their daughter during her early years, feared that she might suffer or be emotionally hurt while in the hospital, but, with help, they gained confidence and cooperated completely in Helen's care. She perceived this change in her parents and responded to their hope for her physical improvement. During Helen's hospitalization, the worker maintained close contact with her to help her relate more positively to people outside of her family circle. She first began to relate to other children in the hospital, then to the doctors and nurses, and eventually to people in her neighborhood and at school. The following is an excerpt from her mother's letter to the worker:

"We are only too glad to comply with the doctor's request that we attend the cleft palate conference. There are not words to express the appreciation that I feel for the hospital and its cleft palate clinic. Helen is wonderful to look at. No longer do I feel pity when I look at her. Before, her lip was such a broken, scarred sight, but now, as the days go by, she improves all the time. . . . You have been so understanding, kind and gentle to Helen and myself. Just to know that if I didn't understand things I *should* know, I could call you and you were never too busy to help me."

The parents had accepted Helen from the beginning. The mother had been instructed by a hospital nurse in the feeding and care of the baby. Such early support is likely to determine the degree to which the mother can cope with the problems attending a physical deformity. Although Helen was not seen at our cleft palate clinic until she was 8, she had continuing warmth and devotion from her parents. Her mother's enterprise in securing help and support shortly after Helen's birth undoubtedly was a large factor in her cooperation during the child's later medical care. In contrast to this case, there are many mothers of babies with bilateral cleft lips and cleft palates who have received no early help and have had to manage a frightening and difficult situation on their own.

M. Q., No. 42-42-47

Maria, the sixth of seven children born to Puerto Rican parents, was 2½ years old when transferred to St. Luke's from a hospital where she had been under care for a fractured leg. She was malnourished, had bilateral microtia, and Pierre Robin syndrome (micrognathia and cleft palate). Except for brief intervals at home, she had spent most of her life in three different hospitals prior to her admission to St. Luke's. The parents, particularly the mother, repeatedly requested that Maria be placed in an institution, and had refused to take her home because they did not want her in the family. The father showed only slight interest in Maria, visiting her occasionally. In spite of her marked physical and emotional improvement over a period of 3 years at St. Luke's, with palatoplasty and bilateral construction of the auricles, the mother steadfastly refused to have any contact with her. The father, almost a stranger to his child, in turn received little or no attention from her. He passively accepted her preference for doctors, nurses, and others in the hospital.

The father, regularly employed but at a minimum salary, tried to meet his responsibilities toward his rapidly increasing family. He spoke English; it was possible to communicate with the mother only in Spanish. Sensitive, emotional, and motherly, she felt very guilty about Maria's condition and about being afraid to undertake her care. The mother's fears and anxieties, magnified by time, had become obsessional. They originated shortly after Maria's birth, when she took the baby home from the hospital without any instructions about feeding, suggestions for care, or assurance that the condition could be improved. She described the "hush-hush" atmosphere and the father's unwillingness to discuss the baby's condition. She was left completely alone, and constantly feared that the child would choke to death. Today, any talk of Maria's returning home revives her feeling of panic. The father does not want the child home because he fears that his wife will have another nervous breakdown necessitating hospitalization. After a thorough evaluation of the total family situation, it was recognized that Maria's best chance for maximum growth and development lay outside the home. As no foster home suitable for her needs could be found, she is to be placed in an institution.

Maria has developed considerably over the past 3 years and has learned to walk. Thanks to expert plastic surgery, she is beginning to talk—slowly and using a limited vocabulary. She has a hearing aid and receives regular training through the hearing and speech department. She is becoming a bright, affectionate child who needs and responds to individual attention. Because of retarded emotional development, she was transferred to the hospital's convalescent branch where there is a nursery school. The social worker was alert to the implications of overindulgence and spoiling from too much concentrated attention in the hospital and discussed these factors with the doctors and team members.

Maria's ability to cope with new situations, following her 3 years of coordinated care, is evident from the nursery school teacher's report:

"We work with Maria on an individual basis as much as possible. The head teacher tries to take her downstairs early in the morning, and although this causes much jealousy on the part of the other children if they see her go, she feels it benefits her greatly. In the classroom, Maria holds her own very well. She makes her wants known with sounds, gestures, and using her lovely eyes. She is made to use words as much as possible. She can be aggressive, i.e., hitting and pushing, but is amenable to suggestion. She loves the field trips and is quite unafraid of new situations. She absorbs new experiences like a sponge."

During Maria's hospitalization period, the worker maintained contact with the parents. Her attempts to help the mother accept a changed child—no longer a helpless, deformed baby—were unavailing, so plans proceeded for a foster home or institutional placement. If the other hospital where Maria was born had had a cleft palate team to lend help and support, the mother would not have been left alone to cope with a situation beyond her comprehension and control. It is believed that intensive emotional trauma could have been avoided and a climate created that would foster parental acceptance.

Parents can be saved much unhappiness if they are aware of resources for helping handicapped children. Through the initiative of the Children's Bureau in Washington, D.C., a program for the medical care of crippled children was included in the Social Security Act of 1935 (Title 5, Part 2). States can obtain matching Federal funds for an approved medical program for handicapped persons under 21 years of age. The states administer their own programs and have wide latitude in fitting it to their particular needs. Today, Arizona is the only state that does not have such a program which covers care of children with congenital anomalies, including cleft palate. The aim is to locate children eligible for help and supply the type of care needed.

The program provides diagnostic services, maintains a state register of crippled children, and recommends hospitals, convalescent homes, and foster homes offering skilled medical care. Medical, nursing, medical-social, and physiotherapy services are available to children not in need of hospital care. In cooperation with other agencies, arrangements can be made for educational and vocational training. Professional groups, both public and private, work together under the program to help the crippled child. Dr. Martha Eliot, former Director of the Children's Bureau, described this approach as follows:*

> From our experience with the administration of the state crippled children's programs, we have learned much about the importance of a multiprofessional approach to the patient . . . an approach which considers his individual personality and stage of growth, his handicaps or illness, his family and the community in which he lives and what kind of an adult he may become.

The Cleft Palate Clinic at St. Luke's has operated on this basis since its inception. The timetable of services for patients is reviewed periodically in regular conferences of the team. When it is desirable for patients to be there for observation, discussion, and planning, the social worker makes the arrangements. For patients living some dis-

* From a speech given at a meeting of State and Territorial Health Officers, Washington, D.C., November 1955.

tance from the hospital, transportation expenses may be paid, at her discretion, from a special fund.

The worker expends considerable effort to ensure continuity of care. The parents' initial contact with the doctor is a positive experience, for they are relieved to learn that something can be done for their child. The social worker's initial interview follows, usually in relation to the anomaly questionnaire. Her contact with the family thereafter depends on how well they are able to accept the child's condition and cooperate in treatment. She helps to handle individual family problems that come to her attention. Brief contacts include the patient's attendance at cleft palate conferences, plans for a summer camp, follow-up on medical care, completion of the questionnaire, and clinic attendance. Some families need more intensive casework to help resolve such problems as cultural adjustment, school difficulties, poor housing, interpretation of medical care, anxiety about the patient's condition, emotional difficulties, financial insecurity, vocational training and employment, family or environmental difficulties. The worker may also explain community resources such as the Visiting Nurse Service, nursery schools, the Homemaker Service, and the Legal Aid Society.

As medical social casework is family-centered, the patient's home situation is assessed—particularly as it bears on his development and well-being. Conditions that undermine family health must be dealt with because they affect his development and growth. An illustration of family-centered casework follows.

B. R., No. 44-39-83

> Bertha, 8 years old and the middle child in a family of five, was born with a left total cleft of primary and secondary palates. She was born in Puerto Rico and came to the United States at the age of 3 with her mother, brothers, and sister; the father had preceded them. Bertha's cleft lip was repaired at 6 months. The father had strenuously opposed any further operation despite her serious speech impairment. She was accepted readily by her family. Her brothers and sister, taking her physical condition as a matter of course, included her in their play and other pursuits. She seldom sought the companionship of neighborhood children, preferring the security of her family. Bertha had not been accepted at school because of her speech impairment, which was increasingly a handicap.
>
> This family of seven shared a small tenement apartment in poor condition. Although the father worked regularly, his small earnings were inadequate for the family's needs and had to be

supplemented from time to time. Since he dominated the family, it was difficult for any member to act individually. Nevertheless, the mother persuaded him to let her take Bertha to St. Luke's Cleft Palate Clinic. With help from the social worker, the father accepted the doctor's medical recommendations and gave his consent for operations (revision of upscar, closure of oronasal fistula, palatoplasty and primary pharyngeal flap), speech training, and guidance, now long overdue. This coordinated care so changed his attitude that he cooperated fully in medical planning for the child.

During Bertha's hospitalization, she was found to have primary tuberculosis. Physical examination of all family members revealed active tuberculosis in the mother and a primary condition in the other siblings. Since the worker had established a positive relation with the parents at the time of Bertha's admission, she helped arrange individual medical care. This necessitated separation of the closely knit family. The mother went to a tuberculosis hospital and the boys to a preventorium. The older girl went to a home for adolescent girls, as the father believed his work would prevent his giving her adequate supervision. The father lived in a furnished room until his family was reunited. During this difficult period, while he kept his job and visited his family in four different places, the worker continued to give him support and guidance in dealing with what seemed to him a bewildering situation.

As Bertha continued to receive care at St. Luke's and its convalescent home in the country, she became more outgoing, friendly, and independent. Her need for speech motivation was appreciated by those around her. At school, her relations with other children improved steadily. After a year, the mother was discharged. Both parents strongly desired to have the entire family reunited. Better living quarters were finally secured in a city housing project. The worker continued to assist the family with current problems: readjustment to a new neighborhood, behavior difficulties of the older daughter, furnishing the new home, planning Bertha's schooling, and better employment for the father.

The father, always dominant in his family, was sustained throughout the period of breaking up his home and providing a new one when the members' health permitted. Many different emotional problems in this family required casework service. The worker's cooperation with her counterparts in the various institutions made it easier for her to assume full casework responsibility for the reunited family. When the family could cope with their own problems, the worker's role was limited to helping the patient when needed.

The social worker must consider the needs and feelings of each patient with a cleft palate in helping him toward full utilization of available educational facilities. His road is a difficult one at best, and those around him must be understanding and patient. When they recognize and encourage his strivings toward improved speech, acceptable performance, and relating to others, his efforts continue and he gains in self-confidence. When this situation is not obtained, difficulties and problems inevitably arise.

F. M., No. 44-44-32

Florence first came to St. Luke's at the age of 17, with a disfigured face and a severe speech impairment. Previous operations had done little to improve her appearance. In her extremely unstable home she was made to feel unattractive and unwanted. She was sent to a school that proved somewhat helpful in offering a degree of warmth, understanding, and security, but on returning home she was still faced with serious difficulties in relationships and adjustments. Long-term casework was indicated in view of many frustrations in her previous life experiences. The worker therefore focused on helping Florence secure employment which would satisfy her longing to prove she could be productive, earn, and feel worthwhile. She held several jobs for short periods only. Her clinic attendance was irregular. She cooperated well only in relation to immediate environmental difficulties. The worker therefore emphasized the need for continuity of medical care and was available to help as needed. This patient would have progressed much more quickly and smoothly if she had been cared for at a cleft palate clinic at an early age when it is much easier to establish productive cooperation with the team members.

The worker has found that mothers who are managing adequately often turn to the social worker for help on a specific problem which may be interrupting or interfering with the patient's adjustment and growth.

The following are examples of such brief contacts. The mother of a 9-year-old girl with a cleft palate had long felt that the child's schoolteacher was "abusive" but had hesitated to confront her. The school problem steadily worsened until she finally asked the worker to intercede. The worker explained ways of interpreting to the teacher the child's physical and emotional needs arising from the deformity.

The mother then talked with the teacher, who recognized that her impatience and undue demands had restricted the child's performance and caused anxiety and withdrawal. The mother was encouraged to return to discuss the girl's progress from time to time.

In another instance, the young wife of a serviceman, who was moving to the west coast, called to enquire about further medical care for their baby with multiple anomalies. Both parents wanted to have everything possible done for the child. The worker directed them to the medical social consultant of the Crippled Children's program in the new area, explaining that the child would be referred for expert care and that the expenses could be handled through the state program for crippled children. When the couple had become settled, the mother wrote a warm and affectionate letter to the worker saying that their child was receiving excellent care, and that they had a healthy new baby—"a blessing."

In another case, a mother sought help because she felt that her only child, with a cleft palate, should have the companionship of other children. She wanted to enroll the little girl in a nursery school and take a job to defray the expense. After consulting with the doctor and the speech therapist, the worker helped the mother with this plan.

Continuity of care for cleft palate patients encompasses not only medical and dental treatment and speech training but also their adjustments to the daily demands of living—an area in which the social worker's services are mainly required. In the case of a baby or young child, the worker's relation is mainly with the mother, helping with her immediate feelings and reactions to the baby's defect and with future planning. When the child is of school age, the worker's relations may be numerous: with the parents and/or close relatives, with the child, and with community resources, such as school, camp, recreational facilities, and specialized agencies. When the patient is an adult, the worker primarily helps him to meet his own needs and cope with his own problems of adjustment. Families or community agencies become involved only as their services are needed to assist the patient in self-help. Throughout all contacts with each patient, the worker emphasizes the importance and value of periodic clinic visits, as well as cooperating with the doctors by attending conferences to evaluate his progress and to review the timing of various treatment phases. Home visits are made for follow-up purposes as well as for planned casework services. School visits are sometimes needed in relation to the child's adjustment. The worker confers with the doctor and other members of the team in specific situations. She attends the regular cleft palate conferences and presents pertinent social data when indicated. She is available in emergencies and accessible to patients or relatives who feel they cannot wait for the next regular appointment to discuss certain problems. The worker cooperates with community agencies on behalf of patients and helps them make the best use of services such as vocational counseling and employment facilities. She may have periodic or prolonged contact with the patient and his family, depending on the individual situation.

In summary, the social worker in the St. Luke's Cleft Palate Clinic attempts to help the patient and his family cope with the myriad social and emotional problems which arise from his condition. She gives guidance and emotional support, where indicated, to enable the patient to make the best adjustment to his medical care and daily living. She establishes early a relation with the mother and makes clear that she is available to help with problems hindering the child's adjustments at home, at school, or in the community.

As our cleft palate team is concerned with the patient's over-all development, members from the different disciplines work closely toward the goal of habilitation. The social worker keeps abreast of the patient's personal and environmental adjustments and reports relevant material at the cleft palate conferences or to individual team members. She renders many brief services to ease tensions or resolve minor problems, and handles the more difficult and deeply rooted problems through intensive casework over a longer period of time.

Questionnaire No. _____

THE ST. LUKE'S HOSPITAL ANOMALY QUESTIONNAIRE

INVESTIGATION OF POSSIBLE CAUSATIVE FACTORS
PRODUCING HUMAN MALDEVELOPMENT

CLEFT PALATE CENTER*

St. Luke's Hospital Center
in the City of New York

Patient's Deformity: _____

Patient's Name: _____

Date of Birth: _____ Sex: _____

Address: _____

Telephone: _____

Hospital Number: _____

Father's Name: _____

Mother's Name: _____

Father's Race: _____

Mother's Race: _____

Questionnaire Completed by: _____

Date Questionnaire Completed: _____

FAMILY

Q. Are you single? _____

    Are you married? _____

    Are you separated? _____

    Are you divorced? _____

    Is your husband the father of this child? _____

    Is the father of this child a cousin or a relation to you? _____

    If so, what relation is he to you? _____

GEOGRAPHICAL NATIVITY

Q. In what country were you born? _____

    In what country were your parents born? _____

    In what country was the father of this child born? _____

    In what country were the parents of the father of this child born? _____

RELIGION

Q. What is your religion?_____

    What is the religion of your parents?_____

    What is the religion of the father of this child? _____

    What is the religion of the parents of the father of this child? _____

PARENTAL AGE

Q. How old are you? _____

    How old is the father of this child? _____

    How old were you when this child was born? _____

    How old was the father of this child when it was born? _____

* Approved for care of patients with cleft palate by Department of Health, City of New York: 1957–1965

Original Questionnaire:	June 1, 1957
First Revision:	October 1, 1958
Second Revision:	January 1, 1962
Third Revision:	January 1, 1966

HISTORY OF MORTALITY AND PERIODS OF RELATIVE INFERTILITY

Q. In what year were you married? _____

How many children have you? _____

Have you had any miscarriages or unsuccessful pregnancies? _____

Have any of your children been born dead? _____

Have any of your children died after they were born? _____

If so, what did they die of? _____

How long was your pregnancy with this baby? _____

How much did your baby weigh at birth? _____

List the names of all of your children and the years they were born.

Name	Year	Name of Father
_____	_____	_____
_____	_____	_____
_____	_____	_____
_____	_____	_____

List all the miscarriages you have had and the year they occurred.

Miscarriage	Year
_____	_____
_____	_____
_____	_____

FAMILY PLANNING

Q. Do you want this child? _____

Did you want the child when you first discovered you were pregnant? _____

Does the father of this child want this child? _____

Did you use any birth control methods before you became pregnant? _____

What did you use? _____

INTRAUTERINE TRAUMA

Q. After you became pregnant did you try to get rid of this baby? _____

What did you do? _____

If you took pills or medicine, how much did you take? _____

In what months of pregnancy did you do this? _____

HEREDITARY HISTORY

Q. Did anyone in your family have the same condition as your baby? _____

Who? _____

Has anyone in your family or in the family of the father of this child had any of the following?

	What relation to you?
Hare lip	_____
Too many fingers	_____
Too many toes	_____
Club feet	_____
Cleft palate (hole in the roof of the mouth)	_____
Mental retardation	_____
Fingers that are stuck together (web fingers)	_____
Toes that are stuck together (web toes)	_____
Deformed ears	_____
Bumps or holes in front of the ears	_____

Heart murmur _____
Heart deformity _____
Birth marks on the face—what color _____
Tumors or growths of any kind _____
Undescended testicles _____
Any other deformity _____

HEALTH OF THE PARENT AT THE TIME OF CONCEPTION

Q. Were you well at the time you became pregnant? _____

Was the father of the child well at the time you became pregnant? _____

If you or the father were not well, what was the matter? _____
_____

Were you sick just before you knew you were pregnant? _____

How many months before you became pregnant did you get sick? _____

Describe how you felt. _____
_____

What kind of medicine did you take? _____

How long were you sick? _____

VOMITING

Q. Did you have any vomiting during your pregnancy? _____

What months of pregnancy did you vomit? _____

What meals made you sick? _____

Did you lose any weight the 1st 3 months? _____   If so, how much? _____

Did the doctor give you pills to stop vomiting? _____

What was the name of the pills? _____

WORK

Q. Did you work while you were pregnant? _____

What kind of work were you doing? _____

What months of pregnancy did you work? _____
_____

Was it light or heavy work? _____

ANEMIA

Q. Have you ever had anemia? _____ low blood _____, weak blood _____

Did you have it when you were pregnant with this baby? _____

Did the doctor give you pills for it? _____

What was the name of the pills? _____

What months of pregnancy did you take the medicine? _____

BLEEDING

Q. Did you have any bleeding (vaginal) during this pregnancy? _____

Did you have any spotting (vaginal) during this pregnancy? _____

Did you bleed in month 1—2—3? _____   Which month? _____

Did you have to be a patient in the hospital because of the bleeding? _____

How much bleeding did you have? (pads per day) _____

Were you given any medicine for the bleeding? _____

What? _____

CONTRACTIONS

Q. Did you feel any contractions in your first three months of pregnancy? _____
_____

Pressure pains or cramps? _____

What month did you feel them? _____

HYPOXIA

Q. Did you ride in a boat and get seasick in the first three months you were pregnant?
_____
Did you live in the mountains the first three months you were pregnant?_____
Which mountains? _____
Did you fly in an airplane the first three months you were pregnant? _____
What airlines did you fly with? _____
Where were you flying to? _____
Were you airsick? _____
Did you go to the dentist in the first four months of pregnancy? _____
Did he give you novacaine, something to put you to sleep or numb the gum? _____
What did he give you?_____
Did you have any X-rays of your teeth at this time?_____ How many?_____
Did you have any operations while you were pregnant with this baby?_____
If so, what was the operation?_____
Did you have the operation in the first three months your were pregnant?_____
Did you feel dizzy in the beginning of your pregnancy? _____
Did you faint in month 1—2—3? _____

IRRADIATION

Q. Did you have an X-ray of your chest taken while you were pregnant? _____
What month of pregnancy? _____
Did you have an X-ray of your stomach taken while you were pregnant? _____
What month of pregnancy? _____
Did you have any other X-rays while you were pregnant with this baby? _____
_____
What were the X-rays of? _____
What month of pregnancy were they taken? _____

INFECTIONS AND DISEASES

Q. Did you have a cold in the first three months of pregnancy? _____
Did you take any pills for the cold? _____
What pills did you take? _____
Did you have a fever with this cold? _____
_____
When you were pregnant were you ever exposed to the German measles? _____
Did you ever have them in the first three months of pregnancy?_____
Did you ever have any of these illnesses in the first three months of pregnancy
with this child? _____
Whooping cough _____
Regular measles _____
Mumps   _____
Smallpox   _____
Encephalitis   _____
Chicken pox   _____
Flu   _____
Do you have diabetes (sugar in the blood)? _____
Do you take anything for it? _____
How long have you had it? _____
Have you ever had any thyroid condition? _____
Was your thyroid over-active or under-active?_____
Do you take medicine for it?_____ Did you take medicine for it when you were
pregnant with this baby? _____
Do you know whether your blood is Rh Negative or Rh Positive? _____
Did you have high blood pressure when you were pregnant? _____

What month of pregnancy? _____

Have you ever had rheumatic fever? _____

What operations have you had and when? _____

Did you have worms or parasites in the first three months of pregnancy? _____

Did you have diarrhea when you were pregnant? _____

How long did you have it? _____ What months of pregnancy? _____

Did you have any rectal bleeding in month 1—2—3? _____

How much did you bleed? _____

Did you get many headaches in early pregnancy? _____

What did you take for them? _____

INJECTIONS

Q. During the first three months of pregnancy were you given any injections of:

    Gamma globulin _____

    Cortisone   _____

    ACTH   _____

    Did you receive any flu shots in the first three months of pregnancy? _____

    _____

    Did you receive any polio shots in the first three months of pregnancy? _____

    _____

    Did you have any smallpox vaccinations in the first three months of pregnancy?_____

    _____

    Did you have any Asian flu shots in the first three months of pregnancy? _____

    _____

DIET

Q. Did you eat meat, vegetables and potatoes regularly when you were pregnant?_____

    _____

    How many months were you pregnant? _____

    How much weight did you gain when you were pregnant? _____

    Did you lose any weight while you were pregnant? _____

    If so, how much? _____

    Does your religion cause you to eat any special foods or fast for any long period

    of time? _____

ALCOHOL

Q. Do you drink anything alcoholic? _____

    Does your husband? _____ Or the father of this child? _____

    How many drinks a day do you have? _____

    How many drinks a day does the father of this child have? _____

VITAMINS

Q. When did you start taking vitamins during your pregnancy?_____

    What kind do you take? _____

    Did you take the vitamins regularly or only occasionally?_____

    Did you ever take more than you were supposed to during your pregnancy?_____

    _____

ALLERGIES

Q. Do you have an allergy? _____ to what?_____

    Penicillin   _____

    Hay fever   _____

    Tomatoes   _____

    Sea food   _____

    Soap   _____

    Dogs, cats, bees _____

    Were you allergic during your pregnancy? _____

    Did you take any medicine for it?_____ If so, what?_____

Did you have an allergy reaction when you were pregnant? _____

During what month? _____

Describe how you felt _____

Were you sick just before you got pregnant? _____

Describe the illness _____

EMOTIONAL STRESS

Q. Were you upset or nervous during your pregnancy? _____

If so, what was the matter? _____

When during your pregnancy did this occur?_____

Do you consider yourself to be a nervous person or a calm person? _____

If you were unhappy, nervous, or tense during your pregnancy, were you_____

Slightly upset?_____ Very upset?_____ Extremely upset?_____

Do you have headaches when you are upset? _____

Does your stomach hurt when you are upset? _____

Do you get a rash or diarrhea when you are upset? _____

PSYCHIATRIC

Q. Have you ever been to see a psychiatrist? _____

Did you see one while you were pregnant? _____

For what reason were you seeing the psychiatrist? _____

Have you ever had a nervous breakdown or have you ever been put in the hospital

for your nerves?_____ What year_____

MISCELLANEOUS

Q. What does the father of this child do for a living? _____

How long has he worked there? _____

What is his job? _____ What does he have to do?_____

Do you smoke? _____

Did you smoke when you were pregnant? _____

How many cigarettes a day? _____

Were you exposed to fresh paint in the first three months of pregnancy? _____

What was being painted?_____ How long were you exposed?_____

Did you use dye on your hair in the first three months you were pregnant?_____

What was the dye you used? _____

Did you take any pills or medicines to bring on your period just before you realized

you were pregnant? _____

If so, what was the name of the pills? _____

At what month did you take them? _____

Did you take any sleeping pills in the first three months of pregnancy?_____

If so, what was the name of the pills? _____

Did you take any pills for your nerves when you were pregnant?_____

What month did you take them? _____ What is the name of them?_____

Did you ever have syphilis?_____ When?_____

Were you treated for it? _____

Did you ever have gonorrhea during your pregnancy?_____ When?_____

Were you treated for this?_____

Did you have any infections in the uterus? _____ At what month?_____

Did you have a kidney infection while you were pregnant? _____

Did you have a kidney X-ray (IVP)?_____ What month of your pregnancy? _____

PLEASE ADD ANY OTHER INFORMATION YOU MIGHT THINK WOULD BE USEFUL.

CHAPTER 24

Etiological
Factors

MARGIE DE FOREST HAIGHT

It is in the interest of any cleft palate clinic to look into possible causes of congenital lip and palate anomalies in the human population. Whereas surgical and dental techniques of repair have been refined in the last 15 years to the point where satisfactory results can be achieved, the actual causes of congenital malformations remain relatively mysterious. Careful evaluation of environmental influences in the early months of pregnancy may reveal common factors in the production of anomalies. This information could be used for the education of all concerned and especially for the care of the pregnant patient. With widespread knowledge of the causative factors, the incidence of anomalies should be lowered.

The St. Luke's Cleft Palate Clinic is making a continuing study based on prepartum history of mothers of children with such defects, and is using as controls an equal number of patients in the eighth or ninth month of pregnancy from the prenatal clinic of the Woman's Hospital Division of St. Luke's. The information is obtained by means of a questionnaire composed of 26 primary and 236 secondary questions; the questionnaire has been revised three times since the clinic started in 1956. The questions cover virtually all factors known to produce malformations in experimental animals or in man, plus several that are believed to do so. Although the best leads regarding environmental etiological factors come from the science of teratology, we cannot, and indeed must not, extrapolate data from the laboratory to clinical practice. In fact, the investigator must be careful to dispel from the minds of the mothers interrogated the impression that these questions are based on proved cause-and-effect relations, lest the doors to malpractice litigation be flung wide open.

The research associate and the social worker are responsible for interviewing a parent (usually the mother) or other close relative of the child with cleft lip or palate and for interviewing the control group. Both groups answer the same questionnaire. The hospital records of the control group are examined postpartum for the presence of any anomalies in the child and for medical information not revealed in either the questionnaire or the interview.

Many problems have been encountered in the course of the study. Owing to the ethnic makeup of the hospital neighborhood, the control group is composed largely of Puerto Rican and Negro women ward patients. Women in the test group (mothers of patients with facial clefts) have more diverse social, economic, and ethnic backgrounds, since the families were referred from the entire state of New York. The principal objection to the test-group data is that the women were interviewed after the birth of a malformed child, which quite naturally influenced their answers by inserting a memory bias. The control-group women, interviewed in the last trimester of pregnancy, were optimistically confident of delivering a normal healthy baby.

Language was a barrier in many cases. When possible, an interpreter was called in, but it has been found that disruption of communication between the mother and the interviewer may result in misunderstanding and distortion. Many of the children brought to our clinic were reared by relatives who had no knowledge of the mother's prenatal history. Furthermore, when the patient with an anomaly was an older child or adolescent at the time of admission, the mother could not recall details of her pregnancy. Some of the mothers in the control group had visited either a private doctor or another institution so that pertinent information on the early months of pregnancy was not available.

The quantity and range of information obtained in this study depended largely on the interviewer's interest and skill. Her's is a difficult task, requiring quick, sound observation. For example, it is useful to evaluate the mother at first sight. Is she nervous, sullen, loquacious, ill at ease? Her attitude may govern the manner in which the interviewer should direct questions. To establish good rapport with the mother she should create a climate of confidence and trust, maintaining a respectful manner yet appearing friendly and natural. Each mother requires a different approach.

Unless all questions are clearly understood, the interview is valueless. If the mother is confused, the question should be simplified until it is clear. Often it is advantageous to depart from the usual order of questions, especially when the mother is nervous or is mentally retarded. The nervous mother first should be asked friendly impersonal questions to encourage relaxation. A retarded mother's answers are often vague and her story changes frequently. Here, repetition and additional clarifying questions are needed. Sometimes it is wise not to press for an immediate reply to a troublesome question, but rather to proceed with others and return to it later. In such situations the interviewer must be patient and take additional time.

Because of the numerous possibilities for error in this study, stringent criteria were applied in determining the significance of answers. Only teratogenic factors occurring in the first trimester of pregnancy were noted. Other factors which required precise definition to be considered significant were infertility lasting over 4 years, conception at age 40 or older, severe anemia, vaginal bleeding of any amount, vomiting more than one meal a day, smoking 40 or more cigarettes a day, or drinking more than 1 pint of alcoholic liquor a day. The quantitation of emotional stress we found to be virtually impossible, although we made the attempt. The stressful episode had to have occurred in the first trimester, and it had to be a well-documented psychological trauma such as desertion by the father, who ofttimes was not the husband; knowledge of malignancy in the husband; separation from the husband; aversions to the husband; sudden unemployment of the husband; psychiatric treatment of the mother; rejection of the baby; a stormy eviction by the landlord.

The psychological impact of economic deprivation and discrimination, real or imagined, is hard to assess. However, in the end the mother must be judged as an individual, not as a type. All people are to some degree sensitive, insecure, and afraid of the unknown; some are weaker and more easily affected physically by their emotional state than others. In all instances their vulnerability must be assessed if their emotional stress is to be evaluated. Although the assignment of psychological stress as an etiological factor rests on insecure grounds, we should point out that in a study published in *Surgical Forum* in 1962 we reported that in C-57 black mice which had been subjected three times daily to psychological trauma by electric shocking (by spark-gap gun), no anomalous offspring were born, but there was a rather high rate of resorption (21 out of 88, or a 22.5 per cent resorption, as opposed to 7 per cent in the control group). We postulate that resorption, along with small litters, is a lesser manifestation of a teratogenic effect.

Among the 100 children with cleft lip and/or palate, whose mothers formed our test group, 25 had associated anomalies, and 11 of these had three or more anomalies. The total number of anomalies was 48; the number of different anomalies was 20. The most common associated anomalies were club feet, mental retardation, micrognathia with Pierre Robin syndrome, and congenital heart disease (Table

TABLE 24-1. ANOMALIES ASSOCIATED WITH CLEFT LIP OR PALATE

Club feet	6
Mental retardation	6
Micrognathia	5
Congenital heart disease	5
Microcephalia	3
Deformed ears	3
Hyperplasia of facial bones	3
"Deformities" of eyes	3
Coloboma	2
Hypertelorism	1
Ptosis	1
Craniosynostosis	2
Umbilical hernia	1
Syndactylia	1
Agenesis of teeth	1
Tracheoesophageal fistula	1
Spina bifida	1
Polydactylia	1
Dislocation of hip	1
Duplication of kidney	1
Total	**48**

24-1). Microcephalia occurred in three children with median cleft of the lip (arrhinencephalia syndrome). Table 24-2 list the anomalies present in the offspring of the control mothers.

An hereditary factor, as evidenced by the questionnaire, was present in 15 of the children of the test-group mothers (Table 24-3) compared with 3 of the children of the control mothers. Cytogenetic studies of karyotypes performed in 7 of the 15 test-group children whose malformations had an hereditary basis have revealed malformations in either the second or third pair of autosomal diploids, usually shortening of the arms as measured from the centromere.

TABLE 24-2. ANOMALIES IN OFFSPRING OF CONTROL GROUP

Hydrocele	4
Umbilical hernia	3
Hemangioma	3
Undescended testes	2
Congenital dislocation of hip	1
Tibial torsion	1
Accessory nipple	1
Congenital heart disease	1
Skin tag	1
Total	**17**

TABLE 24-3. POSSIBLE CAUSATIVE FACTORS IN PATIENTS
WITH CLEFT LIP AND/OR PALATE

Factors	CL (17)	CL/CP (50)	CP (33)
Heredity	5	8	2
Prematurity	1	4	4
Emotional stress	5	17	11
Anemia	1	5	7
Threatened abortion	1	1	1
Age			
Female	1	2	3
Male	0	1	2
Allergic reaction	2	3	0
Virus	1	5	3
Other		4	

Nine of the children of the test-group mothers had been born prematurely, compared with three children of the control mothers.

In virtually no case did the history of the pregnancy provide positive data concerning the relation of environment to the malformation. However, both groups of mothers went to their obstetricians late—very few, if any, sought help during the first trimester, and, as a result, virtually none were taking supplemental vitamins during this all-important period of organogenesis.

Through this particular research project one fact was made clear. Much can be done to lower the incidence of birth defects by stressing the importance of early prenatal care to all women. At the present time information for expectant mothers is not available until the time the mother presents herself to the prenatal clinic. Unfortunately most women do not attend the prenatal clinic until the first trimester of pregnancy is over, when most of the potential damage to the fetus has occurred. Ignorance and old wives' tales lead to foolish and often damaging mistakes.

Is it not possible to establish a public education program stressing the importance of early prenatal care, such as has been developed through the mass media for the early detection of cancer, of muscular dystrophy, etc.? Such a program could cut the incidence of malformations. For example, when a German measles epidemic broke out recently, a statement was televised requesting all pregnant women to see their doctors or go to the hospital if they had been exposed to rubella. Such a program could reduce the incidence of malformation due to German measles.

A wide range of research continues in the field of congenital anomalies. Generally speaking, chromosomal defects, viral infections, uterine failures, and a variety of other environmental factors are implicated in birth deformities; yet there remains much to be learned in the exciting field of genetics and biochemistry. A careful and skeptical study of prenatal care is necessary to shed more light upon deleterious conditions and products of this modern age which may be harmful to the fetus.

BIBLIOGRAPHY

ABBE, R. New plastic operation for the relief of deformity due to double harelip. *Med. Rec. 53:*477, 1898.

ADAIR, F. L. Fetal malformations in multiple pregnancy. *Amer. J. Obstet. Gynec. 20:*539, 1930.

ADAMS, W. M., and ADAMS, L. N. The misuse of the prolabium in the repair of bilateral cleft lip. *Plast. Reconstr. Surg. 12:*225, 1953.

ADISMAN, K. Cleft palate—an interdisciplinary problem. M.S. thesis, New York University College of Dentistry, 1960.

ADRIANI, J., and GRIGGS, T. S. An improved endotracheal tube for pediatric use. *Anesthesiology 15:*466, 1954.

ALCOCK, T. Case of congenital division of the palate in which union of the divided parts was effected. *Trans. Ass. Apoth. 1:*377, 1823.

ANDERSON, S. M. Pediatric anesthesia, Vol. 2. In Evans, F. T., and Gray, C. *General Anesthesia.* London: Butterworth, 1959, p. 159.

ANNANDALE, T. On the closure of congenital fissures in the hard and soft palate. *Edinburgh Med. J. 10:*621, 1865.

ASTOUL, R., and BLANCHART, A. Sabre et tratemiento de las fissuras palatinos, y sus resultados foneticas. *Rev. Chir. Esp. 26:*277, 1947.

AYRE, P. The T piece technic. *Brit. J. Anaesth. 28:*520, 1956.

BAECKDAHL, M., and NORDIN, K. E. Replacement of the maxillary bone defect in cleft palate, a new procedure. *Acta Chir. Scand. 122:*131, 1961.

BAILEY, P., and CUSHING, H. *A Classification of the Tumors of the Glioma Group on a Histological Basis with a Correlated Study of Prognosis.* Philadelphia: Lippincott, 1926.

BARR, M. L., and CARR, D. H. Sex chromatin, sex chromosomes and sex anomalies. *Canad. Med. Ass. J. 83:*979, 1960.

BARSKY, A. J. Pierre Franco, father of cleft lip surgery: His life and times. *Brit. J. Plast. Surg. 17:*335, 1964.

BARSKY, A. J., KAHN, S., and SIMON, B. E. Early and late management of the protruding premaxilla. *Plast. Reconstr. Surg. 29:*58, 1962.

BAUER, T. B., TRUSLER, H. M., and TONDRA, J. M. Changing concepts in the management of bilateral cleft lip deformities. *Plast. Reconstr. Surg. 24:321*, 1959.

BAXTER, H. A new method of elongating short palates. *Canad. Med. Ass. J. 46:322*, 1942.

BAXTER, H., and CARDOSA, M. A method of minimizing contracture following cleft palate operations. *Plast. Reconstr. Surg. 2:214*, 1947.

BERKELEY, W. T. The cleft lip nose. *Plast. Reconstr. Surg. 23:567*, 1959.

BERNARD, C., and HUETTE, C. *Precis Iconographique de Medicine Operatoire et d'Anatomie Chirurgicale. Paris: Mequignon-Marvis Fils, 1846.*

BERRY, J. On sixty-seven cases of congenital cleft palate treated by operation with special reference to the after results. *Brit. Med. J. 2:853*, 1905.

BERRY, J. Discussion on the treatment of cleft palate by operation. *Proc. Soc. Exp. Biol. Med. 10:127*, 1926.

BERRY, J., and LEGG, T. P. *Harelip and Cleft Palate.* Philadelphia: Blakiston, 1912.

BILL, A. H., MOORE, A. W., and COE, H. E. The time of choice for repair of cleft palate in relation to the type of surgical repair and its effect on the bony growth of the face. *Plast. Reconstr. Surg. 18:469*, 1956.

BILLROTH, T. Ueber Uranoplastik. *Wien. Klin. Wschr. 2:241*, 1889.

BJORK, L. Velopharyngeal function in connected speech. *Acta Radiol. Suppl.* 202, 1961.

BLAIR, V. P., and BROWN, J. B. Mirault operation for single harelip. *Surg. Gynec. Obstet. 51:81*, 1930.

BLAKELY, R. W. The complementary use of speech prostheses and pharyngeal flaps in palatal insufficiency. *Cleft Palate J. 1:194*, 1964.

BOTREY, R. Tratamiento quirurgico de la insuficiencia velo-palatine. *Rev. Coen Med. Barcel. 33:433*, 1907.

BOUCHER, C. O. *Current Clinical Dental Terminology.* St. Louis: Mosby, 1963.

BRADFORD, L. J., BROOKS, A. R., and SHELTON, R., JR. Clinical judgement of hypernasality in cleft palate children. *Cleft Palate J. 1:329*, 1964.

BRAUER, R. O. A consideration of the LeMesurier technique of single harelip repair with a new concept as to its use in incomplete and secondary harelip repairs. *Plast. Reconstr. Surg. 11:275*, 1953.

BRAUER, R. O. A comparison of the Tennison and LeMesurier lip repairs. *Plast. Reconstr. Surg. 23:249*, 1959.

BRAUER, R. O., CRONIN, T. D., and REAVES, E. L. Early maxillary orthopedics, orthodontia and alveolar bone grafting in complete clefts of the palate. *Plast. Reconstr. Surg. 29:625*, 1962.

BREINE, U., and JOHANSON, B. Tibia as donor area of bone graft in infants, influence on the longitudinal growth. *Acta Chir. Scand. 131:230*, 1966.

BRENT, R. L. The effect of irradiation on the mammalian fetus. *Clin. Obstet. Gynec. 3:928*, 1960.

BRENT, R. L., FRANKLIN, J. B., and BOLDEN, B. T. Modification of irradiation effects on rat embryos by uterine vascular clamping. *Radiat. Res. 18:* 58, 1963.

BROADBENT, B. H. A new X-ray technique and its application to orthodontia. *Angle Orthodont. 1:*35, 1951.

BROADBENT, T. R. In *Treatment of Patients with Clefts of Lip, Alveolus and Palate.* 2nd Hamburg Internat. Symp. Stuttgart: Thieme, 1966.

BROADBENT, T. R., and SWINYARD, C. A. The dynamic pharyngeal flap. *Plast. Reconstr. Surg. 23:*301, 1959.

BROPHY, T. W. Surgical treatment of palatal defects. *Trans. World Columbian Dent. Cong.* (1893) *2:*532, 1894.

BROPHY, T. W. A new operation for cleft palate. *Med. Rec. 50:*532, 1896.

BROPHY, T. W. Early operation for closure of cleft palate. *Ann. Otol. 6:*39, 1897.

BROPHY, T. W. *Oral Surgery.* Philadelphia: Blakiston, 1915.

BROPHY, T. W. *Cleft Lip and Palate.* Philadelphia: Blakiston, 1923.

BROWN, J. B. Elongation of partially cleft palate. *Surg. Gynec. Obstet. 63:* 768, 1936.

BROWN, J. B., and MCDOWELL, F. Secondary repair of cleft lips and their nasal deformities. *Ann. Surg. 114:*101, 1941.

BUEHRING, J. Beitrag zum organischer wiederersatz der defecte des harten gaumens vermittelst knochensubstanz. *Deutsch. Klin.* 472, 1850.

BUNNELL, S. Cleft palate repair—The cause of failure in infants and its prevention. *Surg. Gynec. Obstet. 45:*530, 1927.

BURDICK, C. G. Harelip and cleft palate. *Ann. Surg. 92:*35, 1930.

BURIAN, F. On the disturbances of growth of the upper jaw in operated cleft-lips and palates. In *Trans. Internat. Soc. Plast. Surg., 1st Cong.* Baltimore: Williams & Wilkins, 1957, p. 224.

BURSTON, W. R. The early orthodontic treatment of cleft palate conditions. *Dent. Pract. 9:*41, 1958.

BURSTON, W. R. The presurgical orthopedic correction of the maxillary deformity in clefts of the primary and secondary palate. In *Trans. Internat. Soc. Plast. Surg., 2nd Cong.* Edinburgh: Livingstone, 1960, p. 28.

BUSZARD, F. A. A case of successful operation for fissure of the palate in an infant six months old. *Brit. Med. J. 1:*350, 1868.

BYRNE, M. L., SHELTON, R. L., JR., and DIEDRICH, W. M. Articulatory skill, physical management and classification of children with cleft palate. *J. Speech Hearing Res. 26:*326, 1961.

BZOCH, K. R. Clinical studies of the efficacy of speech appliances as compared to pharyngeal flap surgery. *Cleft Palate J. 1:*275, 1964.

BZOCH, K. R. The effects of a specific pharyngeal flap operation upon phonation, articulation and resonance characteristics of the speech of 40 cleft palate persons. *J. Speech Hearing Dis. 29:*111, 1964.

CALDWELL, J., and LETTERMAN, G. Vertical osteotomy in the mandibular rami for correction of prognathism. *J. Oral Surg. 12:*185, 1954.

CALNAN, J. Submucous cleft palate. *Brit. J. Plast. Surg. 6:*264, 1954.

CALNAN, J. The error of Gustav Passavant. *Plast. Reconstr. Surg. 13:*275, 1954.

CANNON, B., and FISHER, D. Plastic surgery: Harelip and cleft palate. *New Eng. J. Med. 245:*179, 1951.

CHASE, R. A. An objective evaluation of palato-pharyngeal competence. *Plast. Reconstr. Surg. 26:*23, 1960.

CHORIN, M. Account of a case of double harelip, accompanied with fissure of the palate; with remarks. *J. Chir. 1:*97, 1791.

CLIFFORD, R. M., and POOL, R. The analysis of the anatomy and geometry of the unilateral cleft lip. *Plast. Reconstr. Surg. 24:*311, 1959.

CLOQUET, J. New operation for cleft palate. *N.Y. Dent. Recorder 8:*209, 1854.

COCCARO, P. J. A serial cephalometric study of the growth of the soft palate in cleft palate children. M.S. Thesis, University of Rochester, Rochester, N.Y., 1960.

COHLAN, S. Q. Excessive intake of vitamin A as a cause of congenital anomalies in the rat. *Science 117:*535, 1953.

COLLES, M. H. Use of chloroform. *Dublin Quart. J. Med. Sci. 44:*345, 1867.

CONWAY, H. One stage push-back operation for congenital insufficiency of the palate. *Surgery 22:*341, 1947.

CONWAY, H. Combined use of push-back and pharyngeal flap procedure in complicated cases of cleft palate. *Plast. Reconstr. Surg. 7:*214, 1951.

CONWAY, H., BROMBERG, B., HOEHN, R. J., and HUGO, N. E. Causes of mortality in patients with cleft lip and cleft palate. *Plast. Reconstr. Surg. 37:*51, 1966.

CONWAY, H., and STARK, R. B. Inferiorly based pharyngeal flap in the speech rehabilitation of complicated cleft palate cases. In *Trans. Internat. Soc. Plast. Surg., 1st Cong.* Baltimore: Williams & Wilkins, 1957.

CONWAY, H., and WAGNER, K. S. Incidence of clefts in New York City. *Cleft Palate J. 3:*284, 1966.

COOPER, H. H., LONG, R. E., COOPER, J. A., MAZAHERI, M., and MILLARD, R. T. Psychological orthodontic and prosthetic approaches in rehabilitation of the cleft palate patient. *Dent. Clin. N. Amer.* July, p. 381, 1960.

COUNIHAN, D. T. Articulation skills of adolescents and adults with cleft palates. *J. Speech Hearing Res. 25:*181, 1960.

COUPE, T. B., and SUBTELNY, J. D. Deficiency or displacement of tissue. *Plast. Reconstr. Surg. 26:*600, 1960.

CRIKELAIR, G. F., BOM, A. F., LUBAN, J., and MOSS, M. Early orthodontic movement of cleft maxillary segments prior to cleft lip repair. *Plast. Reconstr. Surg. 30:*426, 1962.

CRONIN, T. D. Surgery of the double cleft lip and protruding premaxilla. *Plast. Reconstr. Surg. 19:*389, 1957.

CRONIN, T. D. Method of preventing raw area on nasal surface of soft palate in push-back surgery. *Plast. Reconstr. Surg. 29:*40, 1962.

CURTIN, J. W. A surgeon's evaluation of the cleft palate team. *Plast. Reconstr. Surg. 29:*289, 1962.

CURTIS, T. A., and CHIERICI, G. Prosthetics as a diagnostic and in pharyngeal flap surgery. *Cleft Palate J. 1:*95, 1964.

CUSACK, J., and CRAMPTON, P. A case of cleft palate successfully operated on by Dr. James Cusack, and two cases, on which the operation was successfully performed by Sir Philip Crampton. *Dublin J. Med. Sci.* p. 321, 1843.

CUTHBERT, J. Transposed flaps in cleft palate repair. *Brit. J. Plast. Surg.* *4:*185, 1951.

DANFORTH, C. H., and CENTER, C. Nitrogen mustard as a teratogenic agent in the mouse. *Proc. Soc. Exp. Biol. Med. 86:*705, 1954.

DAVENPORT, H. T. Management of respiratory obstruction following removal of a tracheostomy tube. *Canad. Med. Ass. J. 91:*1074, 1964.

DAVIES-COLLEY, N. C. On a method of closing cleft of the hard palate by operation. *Brit. Med. J. 2:*950, 1890.

DAVIES, R. M., and DANKS, S. Anaesthetic care in cleft lip and palate surgery; Review of 500 cases. *Anaesthesia 8:*275, 1953.

DAVIS, J. S., and RITCHIE, H. P. Classification of congenital clefts of the lip and palate. *J.A.M.A. 70:*1323, 1922.

DAVIS, W. B. Methods preferred in cleft lip and cleft palate repair. *J. Int. Coll. Surg. 3:*116, 1940.

DE HAAN, C. R. J. Marion Sim's first scientific publication, operation for double congenital harelip. *Bull. Woman's Hosp. 1:*54, 1959.

DEMING, M. V., and OECH, S. R. Steroid and antihistaminic therapy for post-intubation subglottic edema in infants and children. *Anesthesiology 22:*933, 1961.

DERICHSWEILER, H. Some observations on the early treatment of harelip and cleft palate cases. In *Trans. European Orthodont. Soc.,* 1958.

DICKSON, D. R. An acoustic study of nasality. *J. Speech Hearing Res. 5:*103, 1962.

DIEFFENBACH, J. F. Ueber das Gaumensegel des Menschen und der Saeugethiere. *Litt. Ann. Ges. Heilk. 4:*298, 1826.

DIEFFENBACH, J. F. Beitraege zur Gaumennath. *Litt. Ann. Ges. Heilk. 10:* 322, 1828.

DINGMAN, R. O. Surgical correction of developmental deformities of the mandible. *Plast. Reconstr. Surg. 3:*124, 1948.

DORRANCE, G. M. Lengthening the soft palate in cleft palate operations. *Ann. Surg. 82:*208, 1925.

DORRANCE, G. M. The repair of cleft palate; Concerning the palatine insertion of the superior constrictor muscle of the pharynx and its significance in cleft palate; With remarks on the "push-back" operation. *Ann. Surg. 95:*641, 1932.

DORRANCE, G. M. *The Operative Story of Cleft Palate.* Philadelphia: Saunders, 1933.

DORRANCE, G. M., and BRANSFIELD, J. M. The push-back operation for repair of cleft palate. *Plast. Reconstr. Surg. 1:*145, 1946.

DUNN, F. S. Observations on the pharyngeal flap operation for the improvement of speech in cleft palate patients. *Plast. Reconstr. Surg. 7:*530, 1951.

DUNN, F. S. Management of cleft palate cases involving the hard palate so as not to interfere with the growth of the maxilla. *Plast. Reconstr. Surg. 9:*108, 1952.

EBEL, DR. Beitraege zur gaumennath. *Chir. Augenh. 6:*79, 1824.

ECKENHOFF, J. E. Same anatomic considerations of the infant larynx influencing endotracheal anesthesia. *Anesthesiology 12:*401, 1951.

ECKSTEIN, H.   Ueber subkutane und submukoese hartparaffin-prothesen. *Deutsch. Med. Wschr. 28:*573, 1902.

EDGERTON, M. T.   Surgical lengthening of the cleft palate by dissection of the neurovascular bundle. *Plast. Reconstr. Surg. 29:*551, 1962.

ERNST, F.   Zur Frage der gaumenplastik. *Centrabl. Chir. 52:*464, 1925.

FENNELL, G.   Management of tracheostomy in infants. *Lancet 2:*808, 1962.

FERGUSSON, W.   Observations on cleft palate and on staphylorrhaphy. *Med. Times Gazette 2:*256, 1844.

Five Decades of Action for Children. U.S. Dept. of Health, Education and Welfare, Children's Bureau Publication No. 358, 1962.

FLETCHER, S. G., SHELTON, R. L., JR., SMITH, C. L., and BOSMA, J. F.   Radiography in speech pathology. *J. Speech Hearing Dis. 25:*135, 1960.

FOGH-ANDERSON, P.   *Inheritance of Harelip and Cleft Palate.* Copenhagen: Nyt. Nordisk Forlag-Arnold Busch, 1942.

FOGH-ANDERSON, P.   In *Treatment of Patients with Clefts of Lip, Alveolus and Palate.* 2nd Hamburg Internat. Symp. Stuttgart: Thieme, 1966.

FORBES, W. S.   On a new operation for certain cases of cleft palate and bifid uvula. *Trans. Coll. Phys.* (Philadelphia) *1:*70, 1875.

FORSHALL, I., OSBORNE, R. P., and BURSTON, W. R.   Observations on the early orthopaedic treatment of cleft lip and palate conditions. In Hotz, R. (ed.) *Early Treatment of Cleft Lip and Palate.* Berne: Huber, 1964, p. 68.

FRANCIS, W. W.   Repair of cleft palate by Philibert Roux in 1819, A translation of John Stephenson's "De Velosyntheses." *J. Hist. Med. 18:*209, 1963.

FRANCO, P.   Bec de lièvre. In Nicaise, E. (ed.) *Chirurgie Composée en 1561.* Paris: Alcan, 1895, p. 313.

FRASER, F. C.   Causes of congenital malformations in human beings. *J. Chron. Dis. 10:*97, 1939.

FRASER, F. C.   Analysis of prenatal histories of babies with cleft lip with or without cleft palate. Presented at 2nd Ann. Meet. Teratology Soc., Gainesville, Fla., Mar. 16–17, 1962.

FREUND, H.   Gaumensplatenoperation nach Schoenborn-Rosenthal. *Centrabl. Chir. 54:*3206, 1927.

GAINES, F. P.   Frequency and effect of hearing losses in cleft palate cases. *J. Speech Dis. 5:*141–149, 1940.

GANZER, H.   Wolfsrachenplastik mit Ausnutzung des Gesamtem Schleimhautmaterials zur Vermeidung des Verkuerzung des Gaumensegels. *Berl. Klin. Wschr. 57:*619, 1920.

VON GAZA, W.   Ueber Freie Fettgewebstransplantation in den retropharyngeal Raum bei Gaumenspalte. *Arch. Klin. Chir. 142:*590, 1926.

GEORGIADE, N., PICKRELL, K., and QUINN, G.   Varying concepts in bone grafting of alveolar palatal defects. *Cleft Palate J. 1:*43, 1964.

GEORGIADE, N., and QUINN, G.   Newer concepts in surgical correction of mandibular prognathism. *Plast. Reconstr. Surg. 27:*185, 1961.

GERSUNY, R.   Ueber eine Subcutane Prothese. *Ztschr. Heilk. 21:*199, 1900.

GILBERT, C., and GILLMAN, J.   The morphogenesis of trypan blue induced defects of the eye. *S. Afr. J. Med. Sci. 19:*147, 1934.

GILLIES, H., and EVANS, A. J. Experience of tube pedicle flap in cleft palate. In *Trans. Internat. Soc. Plast. Surg., 1st Cong.* Baltimore: Williams & Wilkins, 1957, p. 208.

GILLIES, H., and FRY, W. A new principle in the surgical treatment of congenital cleft palate and its mechanical counterpart. *Brit. Med. J. 1:* 335, 1921.

GILLIES, H., and HARRISON, S. H. Operative correction by osteotomy of recessed malar maxillary compound fracture in a case of oxcephaly. *Brit. J. Plast. Surg. 3:*123, 1950.

GILLIES, H., and MILLARD, D. R. *The Principles and Art of Plastic Surgery.* Boston: Little, Brown, 1957, Vol. II, p. 324.

GIRARD (of Berne). Sur L'Uranostaphylorraphie. *Ass. Franc. Chir. Proc. Verb.* p. 410, 1901.

GLOVER, D. M. A long range evaluation of cleft palate repair. *Plast. Reconstr. Surg. 27:*19, 1961.

GNUDI, M. T., and WEBSTER, J. P. *The Life and Times of Gaspare Tagliacozzi.* New York: Reichner, 1950, p. 486.

GRABER, T. M. Craniofacial morphology in cleft palate and cleft lip deformities. *Surg. Gynec. Obstet. 88:*359, 1949.

GRABER, T. M. Congenital cleft palate deformity. *J. Amer. Dent. Ass. 48:* 375, 1954.

GRABER, T. M., BZOCH, K. R., and AOBA, T. A functional study of the palatal and pharyngeal structures. *Angle Orthodont. 29:*30, 1959.

GRACE, L. Frequency of occurrence of cleft palates and harelips. *J. Dent. Res. 22:*495, 1943.

VON GRAEFE, C. F. Kurze Nachrichten und Auszuge. *J. Pract. Arznek. Wundarzk. 44:*116, 1817.

VON GRAEFE, C. F. Die Gaumennath, ein Neuentdecktes Mittel gegan Angeborene Fehler der Sprache. *J. Chir. Augenh. Partl. 1:*556, 1820.

VON GRAEFE, C. F. Die Gaumennath. *J. Chir. Augenh. 10:*371, 1827.

GRAHAM, G. R. Circulatory and respiratory physiology in infancy and childhood. *Brit. J. Anesth. 32:*97, 1960.

GRAYSON, M., POWERS, A. M., and LEVI, J. Mother-child relationship in rehabilitation of the physically handicapped. *Soc. Casework 32:*261, 1951.

GREENE, M. C. L. Speech analysis of 262 cleft palate cases. *J. Speech Hearing Dis. 25:*43, 1960.

GREGG, N. MCA. Congenital cataract following German measles in the mother. *Trans. Ophthal. Soc. Aust. 3:*35, 1941.

GRISWOLD, M. L., and SAGE, W. F. Extraoral traction in the cleft lip. *Plast. Recontr. Surg. 37:*416, 1966.

GROSS, K. M. Respiratory patterns: Mechanism of congenital malformation. In *2nd Conf. N.Y. Ass. for Aid of Crippled Children,* 1954.

GRUNEWALD, P. Mechanisms of abnormal development. *Arch. Path. 44:*398, 495, 648, 1947.

GUERRERO-SANTOS, J., VAZQUEZ PALLARES, VERA, A. S., MACHAIN, P. O., and CASTANEDA, A. Tongue flap in reconstruction of the lip. In *Trans. Internat. Confed. Plast. Surg., 3rd Cong.* Amsterdam: Excerpta Medica, 1964.

GURLT, E. J. *Geschichte der Chirurgie und ihrer Ausubung.* Berlin: Hirschwald, 1898, p. 646.

HAGEDORN. Uber eine modification der hasenschartenoperation. *Central. Chir. 11:*756, 1884.

HAGERTY, R. F. Unilateral cleft lip repair. *Surg. Gynec. Obstet. 106:*119, 1958.

HAGERTY, R. F. Cartilage pharyngoplasty in cleft palate patients. *Surg. Gynec. Obstet. 112:*350, 1961.

HAGERTY, R. F., and HILL, M. J. Pharyngeal wall and palate movements in postoperative cleft palates and normal palates. *J. Speech Hearing Dis. 3:*59, 1960.

HALE, F. The relation of vitamin A to anophthalmos in pigs. *Amer. J. Ophthal. 18:*1087, 1935.

HALLE. Gaumennaht und Gaumenplastik. *Ztschr. Hals-Nasen-Ohrenh. 12:* 377, 1925.

HANHART, E. Zur Vererbung der Lippen-Kiefer Gaumenspalten (Hasenscharten u. Wolfsprachen) beim Menschen. *Arch. Julius Klaus-Stift. 21:*333, 1946.

HANSON, M. L. A study of velopharyngeal competence in children with repaired cleft palates. *Cleft Palate J. 1:*217, 1964.

HARKINS, C. S. *Principles of Cleft Palate Prosthesis.* Philadelphia: Temple University, 1960.

HARKINS, C. S., BERLIN, A., HARDING, R. L., LONGACRE, J. J., and SNODGRASSE, R. M. A classification of cleft lip and cleft palate. *Plast. Reconstr. Surg. 29:*31, 1962.

HARRISON, R. G. Experiments in transplanting limbs and their bearing upon the problems of the development of nerves. *J. Exp. Zool. 4:*239, 1907.

HEISTER, L. *A General System of Surgery.* London: Innys, 1739.

HILL, M. J., and HAGERTY, R. F. Speech following pharyngoplasty in postoperative cleft palate patients. *J. Speech Hearing Res. 5:*179, 1962.

HOLDER, T. M. Problems peculiar to infants. In Gibbon, J. H. (ed.) *Surgery of the Chest.* Philadelphia: Saunders, 1962, Ch. 7.

HOLDSWORTH, W. G. *Cleft Lip and Palate,* 2nd ed. New York: Grune & Stratton, 1957.

HOLLAND, W. W., and JOUNG, I. M. Neonatal blood pressure in relation to maturity, mode of delivery and condition at birth. *Brit. Med. J. 2:*1331, 1956.

HOLLWEG, E. Beitrag zur Behandlung von Gaumenspalten. Inaug. Diss., Tuebingen, 1912.

HONIG, C. A. *On Pharyngoplasty.* Utrecht: Bosen, 1963.

HORTON, C. E., CRAWFORD, H. H., and ADAMSON, J. E. John Peter Mattauer—America's first plastic surgeon. *Plast. Reconstr. Surg. 27:*268, 1961.

HORTON, C. E., CRAWFORD, H. H., ADAMSON, J. E., BUXTON, S., COOPER, R., and KANTER, J. The prevention of maxillary collapse in congenital lip and palate cases. *Cleft Palate J. 1:*25, 1964.

HYNES, W. Pharyngoplasty by muscle transplantation. *Brit. J. Plast. Surg. 3:*128, 1950.

HYSLOP, V. B., and WYNN, S. K. Bone flap technique in cleft palate surgery. *Plast. Reconstr. Surg. 9:*97, 1952.

INGALLS, T. H., and PHILBROOK, F. R. Monstrosities induced by hypoxia. *New Eng. J. Med. 259:*558, 1958.

INKSTER, J. S. The T piece technic in anesthesia. *Brit. J. Anaesth. 28:*512, 1956.

It's Your Children's Bureau. U.S. Dept. of Health, Education and Welfare, Children's Bureau Publication No. 357, 1962.

IVY, R. H. Modern concept of cleft lip and cleft palate management. *Plast. Reconstr. Surg. 9:*121, 1952.

IVY, R. H. Influence of race on the incidence of certain congenital anomalies, notably cleft lip and palate. *Plast. Reconstr. Surg. 30:*581, 1962.

JAVERT, C. T. *Spontaneous and Habitual Abortion.* New York: Blakiston, 1957.

JOHANSON, B., and OHLSSON, A. Bone grafting and dental orthopaedics in primary and secondary cases of cleft lip and palate. *Acta Chir. Scand. 122:*112, 1961.

JOLLEYS, A. A review of the results of operations on cleft palate with reference to maxillary growth and speech functions. *Brit. J. Plast. Surg. 7:*229, 1954.

JORDAN, E. P. Articulation test measures and listener ratings of articulation defectiveness. *J. Speech Hearing Dis. 3:*303, 1960.

KALTER, H. Factors influencing the frequency of cortisone-induced cleft palate in mice. *J. Exp. Zool. 134:*449, 1957.

KALTER, H. The multiple causation of congenital malformation. Presented at Teratology Conference, New York, N.Y., Apr. 9, 1960.

KARNOFSKY, D. A. Assay of chemotherapeutic agents on the developing chick embryo. *Cancer Res. Supp. 3:*83, 1955.

KATZ, R. L., MATTEO, R. S., and PAPPER, E. M. The injection of epinephrine during general anesthesia with halogenated hydrocarbons and cyclopropane in man. 2. Halothane. *Anesthesiology 23:*597, 1962.

KERNAHAN, D. A., and STARK, R. B. A new classification for cleft lip and cleft palate. *Plast. Reconstr. Surg. 22:*435, 1958.

KIEHN, C. L., DES PREZ, J. B., TUCKER, A., and MALONE, M. Experiences with muscle transplants to incomplete soft palates. *Plast. Reconstr. Surg. 35:*123, 1965.

KILDUFF, C. J., WYANT, G. M., and DALE, R. H. Anaesthesia for repair of cleft lip and palate in infants using moderate hypothermia. *Canad. Anesth. Soc. J. 3:*102, 1956.

KILNER, T. P. Cleft lip and palate repair technique. *St. Thomas Hosp. Rep. 2:*127, 1937.

KILNER, T. P. Quoted by Edgerton, M. T. Surgical lengthening of the cleft palate by dissection of the neurovascular bundle. *Plast. Reconstr. Surg. 29:*551, 1962.

KINNIS, G. D. Emotional adjustments of the mothers to the child with a cleft palate. *Med. Soc. Work 3:*67, 1954.

KOTTGEN, U., and BOLT, W. Krieslauf. In Brock, J. (ed.) *Biologische Daten Fur Den Kinderarzt,* 2nd ed., Vol. 2. Berlin-Gottigen-Heidelberg: Springer, 1954.

KRIMER, W. Einige Bemerkungen zu Graefe's Gaumennath. *J. Chir. Augenh. 10:*619, 1824.

KROGMAN, W. M.   The problem of the cleft palate face. *Plast. Reconstr. Surg.* *14:*370, 1954.

KUESTER, E.   Ueber die Beseitigung der Functionsstoerungen des weichen Gaumens. *Berl. Klin. Wschr. 10:*172, 1882.

LABORIT, H., and HUGUENARD, P.   L'hibernation artificielle par moyens pharmacodynamiques et physiques en chirurgie. *J. Chir. 67:*631, 1951.

LANE, W. A.   Cleft palate. *Clin. J. 5:*65, 1897.

VON LANGENBECK, B.   Operation der Angeboremen Totalen Spaltune des Harten Gaumens nach einer Neuer Methode. *Deutsch. Klin. 8:*231, 1861.

VON LANGENBECK, B.   Wetere Erfahrungen in Gebiete der Uranoplastik Mittelst Abloesung des Mucoesperiostalen Gaumenueberzuges. *Arch. Klin. Shir. 5:*1, 1864.

LANGMAN, J.   Appearance of antigens during the development of the lens. *J. Embryol. Exp. Morph. 7:*264, 1959.

LEIBOWITZ, J. O.   Amatus lusitanus and the obturator in cleft palate. *J. Hist. Med. 13:*492, 1958.

LEIGH, M. D., and BELTON, M. K.   *Pediatric Anesthesiology.* New York: Macmillan, 1960.

LEIGH, M. D., MCCOY, D. D., BELTON, M. K., and LEWIS, G. B., JR.   Bradycardia following intravenous administration of succinylcholine chloride to infant and children. *Anesthesiology 18:*698, 1957.

LEMESURIER, A. B.   A method of cutting and suturing the lip in the treatment of complete unilateral clefts. *Plast. Reconstr. Surg. 4:*1, 1949.

LEMESURIER, A. B.   The treatment of complete unilateral harelips. *Surg. Gynec. Obstet. 95:*17, 1952.

LIMBERG, A.   Neve Wege in der Radikale Uranoplastik; Osteotomia interlaminaris; Resectio Marginis Foraminis palati; Plaettchennaht; Fissura ossea occults. *Zentralbl. Chir. 54:*1745, 1927.

LINDSAY, V. K., LEMESURIER, A. B., and FARMER, A. M.   A study of the speech results in a large series of cleft palate patients. *Plast. Reconstr. Surg. 29:*273, 1962.

LIS, E. F., PRUZANSKY, S., KOEPP-BAKER, H., and KOBES, H. R.   Cleft lip and cleft palate: Perspectives in management. *Pediat. Clin. N. Amer. 3:*995, 1956.

LISTON, R.   Congenital deficiencies and deformities. In *Practical Surgery.* London: Churchill, 1846.

LONGENECKER, C. G., RYAN, R. F., and VINCENT, R.   The incidence of cleft lip and cleft palate in Charity Hospital. *Plast. Reconstr. Surg. 35:*548, 1965.

LU-CH'IEN, S., and TAO-HSIEH, C.   Electroacupuncture anesthesia in oral surgery: A preliminary report. *Chinese Med. J. 80:*97, 1960.

LYNCH, J. B., LEWIS, W. R., and BLOCKER, T. G.   Maxillary bone grafts in cleft palate patients. *Plast. Reconstr. Surg. 37:*91, 1966.

MAC COLLUM, D. W., and RICHARDSON, S. O.   Management of the patient with cleft lip and cleft palate. *Pediatrics 20:*573, 1958.

MAC COLLUM, D. W., RICHARDSON, S. O., and SWANSON, L. T.   Habitation of cleft palate patient. *New Eng. J. Med. 254:*531, 1956.

MAC MAHON, B., and MC KEOWN, T. The incidence of harelip and cleft palate related to birth rank and maternal age. *Amer. J. Hum. Genet. 5:*176, 1953.

MARCKS, K. M., TREVASKIS, A. E., and DACOSTA, N. Further observations in cleft lip repair. *Plast. Reconstr. Surg. 12:*392, 1953.

MARCKS, K. M., TREVASKIS, A. E., and PAYNE, M. J. Bilateral cleft lip repair. *Plast. Reconstr. Surg. 19:*401, 1957.

MASON, F. *On Harelip and Cleft Palate.* London: Churchill, 1877.

MASTERS, F. W., BINGHAM, H. G., and ROBINSON, D. W. The prevention and treatment of hearing loss in the cleft palate child. *Plast. Reconstr. Surg. 25:*503, 1960.

MATTHEWS, D. The premaxilla in bilateral clefts of the lip and palate. *Brit. J. Plast. Surg. 5:*77, 1952.

MATTHEWS, D., and GROSSMANN, W. A. A combined orthodontic and surgical approach to the problem of the collapsed maxilla in cases of cleft palate. In *Trans. 3rd Internat. Cong. Plast. Surg.* Amsterdam: Excerpta Medica, 1964, p. 239.

MAZAHERI, M., MILLARD, R. T., and ERICKSON, D. M. Cineradiographic comparison of normal to non-cleft subjects with velopharyngeal inadequacy. *Cleft Palate J. 1:*199, 1964.

MC DONALD, I. H. Infant physiology and anesthesia. *Brit. J. Anesth. 32:*22, 1960.

MC NEIL, C. K *Oral and Facial Deformity.* London: Pitman, 1954.

MC NEIL, C. K. Congenital oral deformities. *Brit. Dent. J. 101:*191, 1956.

MC WILLIAMS, B. J., and BRADLEY, A. P. A rating scale for evaluation of video-tape recorded X-ray studies. *Cleft Palate J. 1:*88, 1964.

MC WILLIAMS, B. J., and GIRDANY, B. The use of Televex in cleft palate research. *Cleft Palate J. 1:*398, 1964.

MEARS, J. E. Clefts of the hard and soft palates. *Southern Med. Rec. 24:*59, 1894.

MEISSNER, A. Nouvelle methode d'allongement du voile palais et de retrecissement du pharyng. *Revue de Stomatolagie 35:*405, 1933.

METTAUER, J. P. On staphylorrhaphy. *Amer. J. Med. Sci. 21:*309, 1837.

MILLARD, D. R., JR. Radical rotation in single harelip. *Amer. J. Surg. 95:*318, 1958.

MILLARD, D. R., JR. Adaptation of the rotation-advancement principle in bilateral cleft lip. In *Trans. Internat. Soc. Plast. Surg., 2nd Cong.* Edinburg: Livingstone, 1960, p. 50.

MILLARD, D. R., JR. Complete unilateral clefts of the lip. *Plast. Reconstr. Surg. 25:*595, 1960.

MILLER, M. H. Hearing losses in cleft palate cases. *Laryngoscope 66:*1492, 1956.

MILLER, M. H. Hearing problems associated with cleft palate. *Ann. Otol. 68:*90, 1959.

MILLER, M. H., and POLISAR, I. A. *Audiological Evaluation of the Pediatric Patient.* Springfield, Ill.: Thomas, 1964.

MIRAULT, G. Lettre sur l'operation du bec-de-lièvre. *J. Chir. Malgaigne.* Sept. 1844, p. 237.

MOLL, K. L. Cineflourographic techniques in speech research. *J. Speech Hearing Res. 3:*227, 1960.

MOLL, K. L. Velopharyngeal closure on vowels. *J. Speech Hearing Res. 5:*30, 1962.

MOLL, K. L. Cineradiography in research and clinical studies of the velopharyngeal mechanism. *Cleft Palate J. 1:*391, 1964.

MOLL, K. L. Objective measures of nasality—A letter to the editor. *Cleft Palate J. 1:*371, 1964.

MOLL, K. L., HUFFMAN, W. L., LIERLE, D. M., and SMITH, J. K. Factors related to the success of pharyngeal flap procedures. *Plast. Reconstr. Surg. 32:*581, 1963.

MONNIER, J. P. Zur Technik der Gaumenspaltenoperation. *Schweiz. Med. Wschr. 59:*595, 1929.

MONTIN. Bec-de-lievre avec écartement des os du palais. *Bull. Gén. Thérap. 2:*231, 1836.

MOORE, F. T. A new operation to cure nasopharyngeal incompetence. *Brit. J. Surg. 47:*424, 1960.

MORAN, R. E. The pharyngeal flap operation as a speech aid. *Plast. Reconstr. Surg. 7:*202, 1951.

MORESTIN, H. Operation complementaire de l'uranostaphylorraphie, amelioration phonetique considerable obtenue par l'allongement de pilier posterieurs. *Bull. Mem. Soc. Chir. 36:*621, 1910.

MORGAN, T. H., BRIDGES, C. B., and STURTEVANT, A. H. The genetics of Drosophila. *Bibl. Genet. 2:*1, 1924.

MORRIS, H. C., and SMITH, J. K. A multiple approach for evaluating velopharyngeal competence. *J. Speech Hearing Dis. 27:*218, 1962.

MORRIS, H. C., SPRIESTERSBACH, D. C., and DARLEY, F. L. An articulation test for assessing competence of velopharyngeal closure. *J. Speech Hearing Res. 4:*48, 1961.

MOSCARELLA, A. A., and STARK, R. B. Anemia, cortisone, and maternal stress as teratogenic factors in mice. *Surg. Forum 111:*469, 1962.

MOSKOWICZ, L. Zur Technik der Uranoplastik. *Arch. Klin. Chir. 83:*572, 1907.

MUIR, I. F. K. Repair of the cleft alveolus. *Brit. J. Plast. Surg. 19:*30, 1966.

NORDIN, K., and JOHANSON, B. Freie Knockentransplantation bei Defekten im Alveolarkamm nach Kieferorthopaedischer Einstellung der Maxilla bei Lippen-Kiefer-Gaumenspalten. *Fortschr. Kiefer Ges. Chir. 1:*168, 1955.

NYLEN, B. O. Cleft palate and speech. *Acta Radiol. supp.* 203, 1961.

OLDFIELD, M. C. Modern trends in harelip and cleft palate surgery with a review of 500 cases. *Brit. J. Surg. 37:*178, 1949.

OLIN, W. H. *Cleft Lip and Palate Rehabilitation.* Springfield, Ill.: Thomas, 1950, Ch. 11.

OLIVER, P., RICHARDSON, J. R., CLUBB, R. W., and FLAKE, C. G. Tracheotomy in children. *New Eng. J. Med. 267:*631, 1962.

OMBREDANNE, L. Technique de l'urano-staphylorrhaphie. *J. Chir. 8:*1, 1912.

OWEN, E. *Cleft Palate and Harelip.* London: Kerner, 1904.

PADGETT, E. C. The repair of cleft palate cases after unsuccessful operations with reference to cases with an extensive loss of palatal tissue. *Arch. Surg. 20:*453, 1930.

PADGETT, E. C. Repair of cleft palate primarily unsuccessfully operated upon. *Surg. Gynec. Obstet. 4:*63, 1936.

PADGETT, E. C., and STEPHENSON, K. L. *Plastic and Reconstructive Surgery,* 1st ed. Springfield, Ill.: Thomas, 1948.

PARÉ, A. *The Works of That Famous Chirugeon Ambroise Paré.* Translated by Thomas Johnson. London: Clark, 1678.

PARÉ, A. *Oeuvres Complètes* (ed. by J. Malgaigne). Paris: Beillière, 1840, Vol. 2, p. 607.

PASSAVANT, G. Zweiter Artikel Ueber die Operation der Angeborenen Spalten des Harten Gaumens und er Damit Complicirten. *Arch. Heilk. 3:*305, 1862.

PASSAVANT, G. Ueber die operation der Angeborenen Spalten des Harten Gaumens und der Damit Complicirten Habenscharten. *Arch. Heilk. 3:*193, 1892.

PECK, C. H. The operative treatment of cleft palate with report of eight cases. *Ann. Surg. 43:*5, 1906.

PEER, L., HAGERTY, R., HOFFMEISTER, F. D., COLLITO, M. B., and MANLEY, R. S. An evaluation of the Warren Davis osteoplastic technique in cleft palate repair. *Plast. Reconstr. Surg. 14:*1, 1954.

PEER, L. A., WALKER, J. C., and MEIJER, R. The Dieffenbach bone-flap method of cleft palate repair. *Plast. Reconstr. Surg. 34:*472, 1954.

PEET, E. The Oxford technique of cleft palate repair. *Plast. Reconstr. Surg. 28:*282, 1961.

PEŠKOVÁ, H., and FÁRA, M. Lengthening of the columella in bilateral cleft. *Acta Chir. Plast. 2:*18, 1960.

PEYTON, W. T. Dimension and growth of the palate in infants with gross maldevelopment of the upper lip and palate. *Amer. J. Dis. Child 47:*1265, 1934.

PFEIFER, G. Classification of Northwest German Jaw Clinic. In *Treatment of Patients with Clefts of Lip, Alveolus and Palate.* 2nd Hamburg Internat. Symp. Stuttgart: Thieme, 1966.

PFEIFFER, G., and SCHUCHARDT, K. Growth of the nose, upper jaw and teeth after primary osteoplastic completion of the cleft alveolar ridge in patients with cleft lip and palate. In *Trans. 3rd Internat. Cong. Plast. Surg.* Amsterdam: Excerpta Medica, 1964, p. 282.

PHAIR, G. M. The Wisconsin Cleft Palate Program. *J. Speech Dis. 12:*410, 1947.

PICKERELL, H. P. On a new method of treating cleft palate. *New Zeal. Med. J. 11:*125, 1912.

PICKERELL, K., MASTERS, F., GEORGIADE, N., and HORTON, C. Restoration of lip contour using fascia, tendon, and dermal grafts. *Plast. Reconstr. Surg. 14:*126, 1954.

POHLMANN, G. A dissertation on the embryology of the face. Leipzig, 1910.

PORTERFIELD, H. W., TRABUE, J. C., TERRY, J. L., and STIMPERT, R. D. Hypernasality in noncleft palate patients. *Plast. Reconstr. Surg. 37:*216, 1966.

POTTER, R. K., KOPP, G. A., and GREEN, H. C.   *Visible Speech.* Princeton, N.J.: Van Norstrand, 1947.

POWERS, G. R.   Cinefluorographic investigations of articulatory movements of selected individuals with cleft palates. *J. Speech Hearing Dis. 5*:59, 1962.

PRATHER, E. M.   Scaling defectiveness of articulation by direct magnitude-estimation. *J. Speech Hearing Dis. 3*:380, 1960.

PRECECHTEL, A.   Contributions to operative correction of short palate. *Otol. Slavica 4*:23, 1932.

PRINCE, D.   *Plastic and Orthopedic Surgery.* Philadelphia: Lindsay & Blakiston, 1876.

PRUZANSKY, S.   Description, classification and analysis of unoperated clefts of the lip and palate. *Amer. J. Orthodont. 39*:590, 1953.

PRUZANSKY, S.   Factors determining arch form in clefts of the lip and palate. *Amer. J. Orthodont. 41*:827, 1955.

PRUZANSKY, S.   *Congenital Anomalies of the Face and Associated Structures.* Springfield, Ill.: Thomas, 1961.

PRUZANSKY, S.   Pre-surgical orthopedics and bone grafting for infants with cleft lip and palate: A dissent. *Cleft Palate J. 1*:164, 1964.

QUIGLEY, L. F., JR., SHIERE, F. R., WEBSTER, R. C., and COBB, C. M.   Measuring palato-pharyngeal competence with the nasal anemometer. *Cleft Palate J. 1*:304, 1964.

QUIGLEY, L. F., JR., WEBSTER, R. C., COFFEY, R. J., KELLEHER, R. E., and GRANT, H. P.   Velocity and volume measurements of nasal and oral airflow in normal and cleft palate speech, utilizing a warm-wire flowmeter and a two-channel recorder. *J. Dent. Res. 42*:1520, 1963.

RANDALL, P.   A triangular flap operation for the primary repair of unilateral clefts of the lip. *Plast. Reconstr. Surg. 23*:331, 1959.

RANDALL, P.   Surgery and speech. *Surgery 56*:910, 1964.

RANK, K. B., and THOMSON, J. A.   Cleft lip and palate in Tasmania. *Med. J. Aust.* 1961.

REIDY, J. P.   370 personal cases of cleft lip and palate. *Ann. Roy. Coll. Surg. 23*:341, 1958.

REIDY, J. P.   Pharyngoplasty in speech. *Brit. J. Plast. Surg. 17*:389, 1964.

RETHIE, A.   Operative Rachenverengerung zur Behebung der Rhinolalia Aperta. *Monatschr. Ohrenh. 66*:842, 1932.

RICHARDSON, W. R.   Thoracic emergencies in the newborn infant. *Amer. J. Surg. 105*:524, 1963.

RITCHIE, H. P.   Congenital clefts of the face and jaws. In Lewis, D. (ed.) *Practice of Surgery.* Hagerstown, Md.: Prior, 1955, Vol. 5, Chap. 9.

ROBERTS, J. B.   Congenital clefts of the face. *Ann. Surg. 67*:110, 1918.

ROBERTSON, E. L. S.   Racial incidence of cleft lip and palate in Trinidad. In *Trans. 3rd Internat. Cong. Plast. Surg.* Amsterdam: Excerpta Medica, 1954, p. 300.

ROBINSON, D. W., BYRNE, M., and MCLELLAND, W. D.   Speech evaluation of the posterior pharyngeal flap. *Plast. Reconstr. Surg. 15*:114, 1955.

ROGERS, B. C.   Harelip repair in colonial America, a review of 18th Century and earlier surgical techniques. *Plast. Reconstr. Surg. 34*:142, 1964.

ROSENTHAL, W. Zur Frage der Gaumenplastik. *Zentralbl. Chir. 51*:1621, 1924.

ROSSELLI, S. Divisione palatina e sua aura chirurgico alu. *Cong. Internaz. Stomatal 36*:391, 1935.

ROTH, R. E., SAUNDERS, D. E., STARK, R. B., and DE HAAN, C. R. Operative blood loss in common plastic surgical procedures. *Plast. Reconstr. Surg. 31*:399–406, 1963.

ROUX, P. J. Observation sur une division congenitale du voile du palais et de la luette guérie au moyen d'une opération analogue a celle du bec-de-lièvre, pratiquée par M. Roux. *J. Universal Sci. Med. 15*:356, 1819.

ROUX, P. J. Memoire sur la staphylorrhaphie ou la suture du voile du palais. *Arch. Gén. Med. 7*:516, 1825.

SALANITRE, E., and RACKOW, H. H. Changing trends in anesthetic management of the child with cleft lip-palate malformation. *Anesthesiology 23*:610, 1962.

SARNAT, B., and ENGEL, M. B. A serial study of mandibular growth after removal of the condyle in the Macaca Rheusus monkey. *Plast. Reconstr. Surg. 7*:364, 1951.

SARNAT, B., and GANS, B. J. Growth of bones: Methods of assessing and clinical importance. *Plast. Reconstr. Surg. 9*:140, 1952.

SATALOFF, J., and FRASER, M. Hearing loss in children with cleft palates. *Arch. Otolaryng. 55*:61, 1952.

SCHMID, E. Kongressbericht der Suedwest-Deutschen Zahn-und Kieferaerztl. Fortbildung Frankfurt 1949, *Deutsch. Zahnaerztl. Zeitschrift 11*:624, 1950.

SCHMID, E. Die Annaherung der Kieferstuempfe bei Lippen-Kiefer-Gaumenspalten, Ihre-Schaedlichen Folgen und Vermeidung. *Fortschr. Kiefer Ges. Chir. 1*:37, 1955.

SCHMID, E. Die Osteoplastik bei Lippen-Kiefer-Gaumenspalten. *Arch. Klin. Chir. 295*:868, 1965.

SCHMID, E. The use of ear cartilage grafts and composite grafts in repairs of the upper lip with special reference to formation of the philtrum. In *Trans. 3rd Internat. Cong. Plast. Surg.*, Amsterdam: Excerpta Medica, 1964.

SCHOENBORN. Ueber eine Neue Methode der Staphylorraphie, Verhandl. *Deutsch. Gesellsch. Chir. 4*:235, 1875.

SCHRUDDE, J., and STELLMACH, R. K. Funktionelle Orthopedische Gesichtspunkte bei der osteoplastik der defecte des Kiefefbogens bei Lippen-Kiefer-Gaumenspalten. *Fortschr. Kieferothop. 20*:372, 1959.

SCHUCHARDT, K. Die Entwicklung der Lippen-Kiefer-Gaumenspalten. *Arch. Klin. Chir. 295*:850, 1960.

SCHUCHARDT, K. *Treatment of Patients with Clefts of Lip, Alveolus and Palate.* 2nd Hamburg Internat. Symp. Stuttgart: Thieme, 1966.

SCHULTZ, L. T. A cephalometric evaluation of 100 patients who have had cleft palate repair. *Cleft Palate Bull. 18*:174, 1955.

SERCER, Z. Beitrag zur Technik der Operativen Therapie der Rhinolalia Aperta. *Rev. Chir. Structive* July, 1935, p. 5.

Services for Children. U.S. Dept. of Health, Education and Welfare Publication, 1963.

Services for Children with Cleft Lip and Cleft Palate. Amer. Pub. Health Ass. Comm. on Child Health, 1955.

SEZGIN, M. Z., and STARR, R. B. The incidence of congenital defects. *Plast. Reconstr. Surg. 27:*259, 1961.

SHATKIN, S., and STARK, D. B. Cleft lip and palate moulages. *Plast. Reconstr. Surg. 36:*225, 1965.

SHERMAN, D., SPRIESTERBACH, D. C., and MOLL, J. D. Glottal stops in the speech of children with cleft palates. *J. Speech Hearing Dis. 24:*37, 1959.

SLAUGHTER, W. B., and BRODIE, A. G. Facial clefts and their surgical management in view of recent research. *Plast. Reconstr. Surg. 4:*311, 1949.

SLAUGHTER, W. B., and PRUZANSKY, S. Velar closure in cleft palate surgery. *Plast. Reconst. Surg. 13:*341, 1954.

SMITH, C. The bifurcation of trachea in young infancy; A statistical study. Paper delivered at Internat. Anesth. Res. Soc. Bel Harbor, Fla., March, 1962.

SMITH, C., ROWE, R. D., and VLAD, P. Sedation of children for cardiac catatherization with ataractic mixture. *Canad. Anaesth. Soc. J. 5:*35, 1958.

SMITH, H. L. *A System of Operative Surgery.* Philadelphia: Lippincott, Grumbo, 1852.

SMITH, H. L. Cleft palate. *Boston Med. Surg. J. 132:*478, 1895.

SMITH, J. K., HUFFMAN, M. C., LIERLE, D. M., and MOLL, K. L. Results of pharyngeal flap surgery in patients with velopharyngeal incompetence. *Plast. Reconstr. Surg. 32:*493, 1963.

SMITH, R. E. *Anesthesia for Infants and Children.* St. Louis: Mosby, 1963, 2nd ed.

SMITH, T. On the use of chloroform in the cure of cleft palate. *Lancet 2:* 226, 1869.

SNELL, G. D., and PICKEN, D. I. Abnormal development in the mouth caused by chromosome imbalance. *J. Genet. 31:*213, 1935.

SOIVIO, A. In *Treatment of Patients with Clefts of Lip, Alveolus and Palate.* 2nd Hamburg Internat. Symp., 1964.

SPARROW, S. S. Effect of filming rate and frame selection in cineradiographic velopharyngeal analysis. A.A. Thesis, 1964.

SPEMANN, H. *Embryonic development and induction.* New Haven: Yale Univ. Press, 1938.

SPRAGUE, E. W. Management of cleft lip and palate cases. *Surg. Clin. N. Amer. 6:*1481, 1926.

SPRIESTERBACH, D. C., MOLL, K. L., and MORRIS, H. C. Heterogenicity of the cleft palate population and research designs. *Cleft Palate J. 1:*210, 1964.

SPRIESTERBACH, D. C., MOSS, K. L., and MORRIS, H. C. Subject classification and articulation of speakers with cleft palate. *J. Speech Hearing Res. 362:*1961.

SPRIESTERBACH, D. C., and POWERS, G. R. Articulation skills, velopharyngeal closure and oral breath pressure of children with cleft palates. *J. Speech Hearing Res.* 2:318, 1959.

STANLEY-BROWN, E. G. *Pediatric Surgery for Nurses.* Philadelphia: Saunders, 1961, Ch. 5.

STARK, R. B. The pathogenesis of harelip and cleft palate. *Plast. Reconstr. Surg.* 13:20, 1954.

STARK, R. B. The pathographic expansion principle as applied to the advancement flap. *Plast. Reconstr. Surg.* 15:222, 1955.

STARK, R. B. Embryology, pathogenesis and classification of cleft lip and cleft palate. In Pruzansky, S. (ed.) *Congenital Anomalies of the Face and Associated Structures.* Springfield, Ill.: Thomas, 1961.

STARK, R. B. *Plastic Surgery.* New York: Hoeber, 1962.

STARK, R. B. Congenital anomalies. *Rev. Surg.* 22:305, 1965.

STARK, R. B. The historic basis for contemporary cleft palate surgery. In *Symposium on Orofacial Abnormalities.* Wilmington, Del.: Alfred I Du Pont Institute, April 24, 1965, p. 13.

STARK, R. B., DEFOREST, M., HARRIS, E., and VOLLENWEIDER, H. Investigation of possible causative factors producing human maldevelopment. *Plast. Reconstr. Surg.* 30:543, 1962.

STARK, R. B., and DEHAAN, C. R. The addition of a pharyngeal flap to primary palatoplasty. *Plast. Reconstr. Surg.* 26:378, 1960.

STARK, R. B., DEHAAN, C. R., and WASHIO, H. Forked flap columellar advance. *Cleft Palate J.* 1:116, 1964.

STARK, R. B., DEHAAN, C. R., WEATHERLEY-WHITE, R. C. A., and WASHIO, H. Pharyngeal flap in the primary treatment of cleft palate. In *Trans. 3rd Internat. Cong. Plast. Surg.* Amsterdam: Excerpta Medica, 1964, p. 324.

STARK, R. B., and EHRMANN, N. A. The development of the center of the face with particular reference to surgical correction of bilateral cleft lip. *Plast. Reconstr. Surg.* 21:177, 1953.

STEFFENSEN, W. H. A method for repair of the unilateral cleft lip. *Plast. Reconstr. Surg.* 4:144, 1949.

STEFFENSEN, W. H. Further experience with the rectangular flap operation for cleft lip repair. *Plast. Reconstr. Surg.* 11:49, 1953.

STEVENS, A. H. Staphylorraphe or palate suture, successfully performed by A. H. Stevens, Prof. of Surgery in the College of Physicians and Surgeons, New York. *N. Amer. Med. Surg. J.* 3:233, 1827.

STOBWASSER, C. Die Hasenscharten in der Göttingen Chirurgische Klinik von October 1875 bis Juli 1882. *Deutsch. Zeilschrift Chir.* 19:11, 1883–1884.

STOCKARD, C. R. Human types and growth reactions. *Amer. J. Anat.* 31:261, 1923.

STRAITH, R. E., TEASLE, J. L., and MOORE, L. T. Local anesthesia in the newborn. *Plast. Reconstr. Surg.* 16:125, 1955.

SUBTELNY, J. D. Width of the naso-pharynx and related anatomical structures in normal and unoperated cleft palate children. *Amer. J. Orthodont.* 41:889, 1955.

SUBTELNY, J. D.   Physico-acoustic considerations in the radiographic study of speech. *Cleft Palate J. 1:*402, 1964.

SUBTELNY, J. D., and KOEPP-BAKER, H.   Palatal function and cleft palate speech. *J. Speech Hearing Dis. 26:*213, 1961.

SULLIVAN, D. E.   Bilateral pharyngoplasty as an aid to velopharyngeal closure. *Plast. Reconstr. Surg. 27:*31, 1961.

SWANSON, L. T.   A cephalometric evaluation of 100 patients who have had cleft palate repair. *Cleft Palate Bull. 18:*174, 1955.

TENNISON, C. M.   The repair of the unilateral cleft lip by the stencil method. *Plast. Reconstr. Surg. 9:*115, 1952.

TJIO, J. M., and LEVAN, A.   The chromosome number of man. Hereditas (Lund) *42:*1, 1956.

TÖNDURY, G.   Über die Genese der Lippen-, Kiefer-, Gaumenspalten. *Fortschr. Kiefer Gesichtschir. 1:*1, 1955.

TOOLAN, H. W.   Experimental production of mongoloid hamsters. *Science 131:*1446, 1960.

TRASLER, D. G., and FRASER, F. C.   Factors underlying strain, reciprocal cross, in maternal weight differences in embryo susceptibility to cortisone induced cleft palate in mice. *Proc. 10th Internat. Cong. Genoa 2:*296, 1958.

TRETSVEN, V. E.   Incidence of cleft lips and palate in Montana Indians. *J. Speech Hearing Dis. 28:*52, 1963.

TRUSLER, H. M., BAUER, T. B., and TONDRA, J. M.   The cleft lip palate problem. *Plast. Reconstr. Surg. 16:*174, 1955.

TSCHMARKE, G.   Zur Operativen Behandlung der angeborenen Gaumenspalte. *Arch. Klin. Chir. 144:*697, 1927.

VAN DEMARK, D. R.   Misarticulations and listener judgements of the speech of individuals with cleft palates. *Cleft Palate J. 1:*232, 1965.

VAUGHAN, N. S.   The importance of the premaxilla and the philtrum in bilateral cleft lip. *Plast. Reconstr. Surg. 1:*240, 1946.

VEAU, V.   *Division Palatine*. Paris: Masson, 1931.

VEAU, V.   *Ztschr. Anat. Entwich. 108:*459, 1938.

VEAU, V.   *Bec de Lievre*. Paris: Masson, 1938, p. 323.

VEAU, V., and RUPPE, C.   Technique de l'urano-staphyorrhaphie. *J. Chir. 20:* 113, 1922.

VECCHI, V., and FRANZ, A.   In Calderini (ed.) *Rassegna Storica dell'Anesthesiologia*. Bologna, 1957, p. 105.

VELPEAU, A. L. M.   *New Elements of Operative Surgery* (Translated by P. S. Townsend). New York: Samuel S. & William Wood, 1847.

VILAR-SANCHO, B.   A proposed new international classification of congenital cleft lip and cleft palate. *Plast. Reconstr. Surg. 30:*263, 1962.

WALDRON, C. W.   Management of unilateral cleft of the palate. *Plast. Reconstr. Surg. 5:*522, 1950.

WALKER, J. C., COLLITO, M. B., MANCUSI-UNGARO, A., and MEIJER, R.   Physiologic considerations in cleft lip closure: The C-W technique. Plast. Reconstr. Surg. *37:*552, 1966.

WARDILL, W. E. M.   Discussion on the treatment of cleft palate by operation. *Proc. Roy. Soc. Med. 5:*178, 1926–1927.

WARDILL, W. E. M. Cleft palate. *Brit. J. Surg. 16 :*127, 1928.

WARDILL, W. E. M. Cleft palate. *Brit. J. Surg. 21 :*347, 1933.

WARDILL, W. E. M. Techniques of operation for cleft palate. *Brit. J. Surg. 25 :*117, 1937.

WARKANY, J., and KALTER, H. Maternal impressions and congenital malformations. *Plast. Reconstr. Surg. 30 :*628, 1962.

WARKANY, J., and NELSON, R. C. Appearance of skeletal abnormalities in the offspring of rats reared on a deficient diet. *Science 92 :*383, 1940.

WARREN, D. W., and DUBOIS, A. B. A pressure flow technique for measuring velopharyngeal orifice area during connected speech. *Cleft Palate J. 1 :*52, 1964.

WARREN, J. C. On an operation for the cure of natural fissure of the soft palate. *New Eng. Quart. J. Med. Surg. 1 :*1, 1928.

WARREN, J. M. Operations for fissures of the soft and hard palate (palatoplastie). *New Eng. Quart. J. Med. Surg. 1 :*538, 1843.

WEATHERLEY-WHITE, R. C. A., DERSCH, W. C., and ANDERSON, R. H. Objective measurement of nasality in cleft palate patients—A preliminary report. *Cleft Palate J. 1 :*120, 1964.

WEATHERLEY-WHITE, R. C. A., STARK, R. B., and DE HAAN, C. R. The objective measurement of nasality in cleft palate patients—Correlation with listener judgments. *Plast. Reconstr. Surg. 35 :*588, 1965.

WEATHERLEY-WHITE, R. C. A., STARK, R. B., and DE HAAN, C. R. Acoustic analysis of speech: Validation studies. *Cleft Palate J. 3 :*291, 1966.

WEBSTER, J. P. Crescentic peri-alar cheek excision for upper lip flap advancement with a short history of upper lip repair. *Plast. Reconstr. Surg. 16 :*434, 1955.

WEBSTER, R. C. Cleft palate, part I. *Oral Surg., Oral Med., & Oral Path. 1 :*3, 1948.

WEBSTER, R. C. Cleft palate, part II, treatment. *Oral Surg., Oral Med., & Oral Path. 1 :*4, 1948.

WEBSTER, R. C., COFFREY, R. J., RUSSELL, J. A., and QUIGLEY, L. C. Methods of surgical correction of velopharynteal sphincter incompetency using palatal and posterior pharyngeal tissues. A proposed system of classification. *Plast. Reconstr. Surg. 18 :*474, 1956.

WEINSTEIN, M. L., and ADAMS, E. L. Further observations on use of rectal sodium pentothal. *Anesth. Analg. 20 :*229, 1941.

WHETNALL, E., and FRY, D. B. *The Deaf Child.* Springfield, Ill.: Thomas, 1964.

WHITEHEAD, W. R. Remarks on a case of extensive cleft of the hard and soft palate, closed at a single operation. *Amer. J. Med. Sci. 62 :*114, 1871.

WISHNIK, S. M. To restore the child with a cleft palate. *Child,* Apr. 1951, p. 141.

WOLSTENHOLME, G. E. M., and O'CONNOR, C. M. Ciba foundation symposium on congenital malformations. Boston: Little, Brown, 1960.

ZICKENFOOSE, M. S. Feeding problems of children with cleft palate. *Child. 4 :*225, 1957.

INDEX

AREA OF SPEECH PATHOLOGY-AUDIOLOGY
DEPARTMENT OF SPEECH AND DRAMATIC ART
UNIVERSITY OF MISSOURI-COLUMBIA
COLUMBIA, MISSOURI 65201